13 For Patients of Moderate Means
A Social History of the Voluntary Public General Hospital in Canada, 1890–1950
David Gagan and Rosemary Gagan

14 Into the House of Old
A History of Residential Care in British Columbia
Megan J. Davies

15 St Mary's
The History of a London Teaching Hospital
E.A. Heaman

16 Women, Health, and Nation
Canada and the United States since 1945
Edited by Georgina Feldberg, Molly Ladd-Taylor, Alison Li, and Kathryn McPherson

17 The Labrador Memoir of Dr Henry Paddon, 1912–1938
Edited by Ronald Rompkey

18 J.B. Collip and the Development of Medical Research in Canada
Extracts and Enterprise
Alison Li

19 The Ontario Cancer Institute
Successes and Reverses at Sherbourne Street
E.A. McCulloch

20 Island Doctor
John Mackieson and Medicine in Nineteenth-Century Prince Edward Island
David A.E. Shephard

21 The Struggle to Serve
A History of the Moncton Hospital, 1895 to 1953
W.G. Godfrey

22 An Element of Hope
Radium and the Response to Cancer in Canada, 1900–1940
Charles Hayter

23 Labour in the Laboratory
Medical Laboratory Workers in the Maritimes, 1900–1950
Peter L. Twohig

24 Rockefeller Foundation Funding and Medical Education in Toronto, Montreal, and Halifax
Marianne P. Fedunkiw

25 Push!
The Struggle for Midwifery in Ontario
Ivy Lynn Bourgeault

26 Mental Health and Canadian Society
Historical Perspectives
Edited by James Moran and David Wright

27 SARS in Context
Memory, History, and Policy
Edited by Jacalyn Duffin and Arthur Sweetman

28 Lyndhurst
Canada's First Rehabilitation Centre for People with Spinal Cord Injuries, 1945–1998
Geoffrey Reaume

29 J. Wendell Macleod
Saskatchewan's "Red Dean"
Louis Horlick

30 Who Killed the Queen?
The Story of a Community Hospital and How to Fix Public Health Care
Holly Dressel

31 Healing the World's Children
Interdisciplinary Perspectives on Health in the Twentieth Century
Edited by Cynthia Comacchio, Janet Golden, and George Weisz

32 A Canadian Surgeon in the Army of the Potomac
Francis M. Wafer
Edited by Cheryl A. Wells

33 A Sadly Troubled History
The Meanings of Suicide in the Modern Age
John Weaver

34 SARS Unmasked
Risk Communication of Pandemics and Influenza in Canada
Michael G. Tyshenko with assistance from Cathy Patterson

35 Tuberculosis Then and Now
Perspectives on the History of an Infectious Disease
Edited by Flurin Condrau and Michael Worboys

36 Caregiving on the Periphery
Historical Perspectives on Nursing and Midwifery in Canada
Edited by Myra Rutherdale

37 Infection of the Innocents
Wet Nurses, Infants, and Syphilis in France, 1780–1900
Joan Sherwood

38 The Fluorspar Mines of Newfoundland
Their History and the Epidemic of Radiation Lung Cancer
John Martin

39 Small Matters
Canadian Children in Sickness and Health, 1900–1940
Mona Gleason

40 Sorrows of a Century
Interpreting Suicide in New Zealand, 1900–2000
John C. Weaver

Sorrows of a Century

Interpreting Suicide in New Zealand, 1900–2000

JOHN C. WEAVER

McGill-Queen's University Press
Montreal & Kingston • London • Ithaca

Bridget Williams Books
Wellington, New Zealand

Sorrows of a Century is published in Canada by McGill-Queen's University Press (for the world excluding New Zealand) and in New Zealand by Bridget Williams Books Limited.

ISBN 978-0-7735-4275-4 (cloth)
ISBN 978-0-7735-8995-7 (ePDF)
ISBN 978-0-7735-8996-4 (ePUB)

Legal deposit first quarter 2014
Bibliothèque nationale du Québec

Printed in Canada on acid-free paper that is 100% ancient forest free (100% post-consumer recycled), processed chlorine free

Published simultaneously in New Zealand by Bridget Williams Books Ltd, PO Box 12474, Wellington 6144, New Zealand. www.bwb.co.nz
ISBN 9781927277232; ISTC A022013000006284

This book has been published with the help of a grant from the Canadian Federation for the Humanities and Social Sciences, through the Awards to Scholarly Publications Program, using funds provided by the Social Sciences and Humanities Research Council of Canada.

McGill-Queen's University Press acknowledges the support of the Canada Council for the Arts for our publishing program. We also acknowledge the financial support of the Government of Canada through the Canada Book Fund for our publishing activities.

Bridget Williams Books would like to acknowledge the generous support of the Box Trust for Mental Health, and the ongoing support of the BWB Publishing Trust and the G & N Trust.

Library and Archives Canada Cataloguing in Publication

Weaver, John C., author
Sorrows of a century : interpreting suicide in New Zealand, 1900-2000 / John C. Weaver.

(McGill-Queen's/Associated Medical Services studies in the history of medicine, health, and society ; 40)
Includes bibliographical references and index.
Issued in print and electronic formats.
ISBN 978-0-7735-4275-4 (bound). –
ISBN 978-0-7735-8995-7 (ePDF). – ISBN 978-0-7735-8996-4 (ePUB)

1. Suicide – New Zealand – History – 20th century. 2. Suicide – Social aspects – New Zealand – History – 20th century. 3. Suicide – Economic aspects – New Zealand – History – 20th century. I. Title. II. Series: McGill-Queen's/Associated Medical Services s studies in the history of medicine, health, and society ; 40

HV6548.N49W43 2013 362.280993'0904 C2013-906748-5
C2013-906749-3

National Library of New Zealand Cataloguing-in-Publication Data

Weaver, John C.

Sorrows of a century : interpreting suicide in New Zealand, 1900-

2000 / John C Weaver.

ISBN 978-1-927277-23-2

Suicide – New Zealand – History – 20th century. I. Title.

362.2809930904 – dc 23

Typeset by Jay Tee Graphics Ltd. in 10.5/13 Sabon

Contents

Tables, Graphs, and Figures

TABLES

GRAPHS

FIGURES

Acknowledgments

This book relies on witnesses' depositions and related evidence held in New Zealand inquest files. On two occasions Coronial Services transferred blocks of ever more recent files to Archives New Zealand. Each time that an accession occurred, I advanced the cutoff date for this study, until it was feasible to conclude in 2000. The prospect of covering a century was an opportunity too important to ignore; however, that ambition strained the budget by adding roughly four thousand files to my initial estimate. The ten years of travel needed to assemble notes and data sets required assistance from three sources. Initial core funding came from the Social Sciences and Humanities Research Council of Canada. I am grateful for this essential assistance. McMaster University, through the offices of the Provost and the Vice-President of Research, contributed too. McMaster supported a research leave for six months in 2010 when I computed data and wrote several chapters. Vital support came from Adam Weaver, who hosted my stays in Wellington during thirty months spread from June 2003 to June 2013. Adam's intellectual and moral support was also significant; his reactions to my conjectures and accounts of unhappy narratives were measured and serious. Affected both by the post-war experiences of an uncle, Albert Tamorria, who fought in the Solomon Islands, and by the Vietnam War's impact on her childhood Maryland community, Joan Weaver kept the trauma of veterans prominent in our discussions over this project.

This book evolved as circumstances fell into place. Adam's appointment to Victoria University was a fortuitous circumstance. Other helpful developments followed. An early good turn of fortune occurred when Richard Hill, director of the Treaty of Waitangi Research Unit of the Stout Research Centre for New Zealand Studies at Victorian University, recommended Dr Doug Munro as a research assistant. An experienced scholar and tenacious researcher, Doug found time amidst other projects to read files, code information, prepare notes, offer points of interpretation, and bring New Zealand publications to my attention. Our encounters with heartbreaking misfortunes and disturbing violence required mutual support. Several categories of destructive conduct reinforced a shared and rising abhorrence of male violence. We formed a conviction too about the social and psychological importance of decent employment. From Doug and his wife Teloma, I started to learn about the people of the Pacific Islands. As well, through Doug I met remarkable individuals, including the late Donald Munro, bass-baritone and "New Zealand icon." At the archives Doug introduced me to a stream of visiting researchers. As the book review editor for the *Journal of Pacific History*, it seemed that he knew "everyone." Lunches at the Single File Café and Friday pub evenings at the Hotel Bristol occasionally resembled purposeful history seminars. Thankfully this was not always the case. Conversations slipped into discussions about films, current politics, rural life, rugby, and more.

Doug's gregariousness led to a second opportunity that ultimately proved essential for refining the ideas in this book. Curious about current proceedings in the coroner's court, Doug contacted Wellington Coroner Garry Evans and attended a court session. Subsequently, I joined Doug in meetings with Garry. Exchanges with Garry and Chief Coroner Neil McLean clarified the principles of evidence used in New Zealand inquests. Furthermore, it was Garry's dedication to quests for truth by open discussion that helped clear several obstacles to our access to specific items. The inquest files are accessible to *bona fide* researchers, but some material – for example, recriminatory suicide notes – had prudently been placed in sealed envelopes. Garry insisted that we should apply for access to these notes because he maintained that they held important evidence beyond summaries or selected quotations in police occurrence reports. He was correct. Garry's own inquest findings and supporting explanations show an astute mind and compassionate sensibility. It is hard to imagine families finding comfort through inquest proceedings, yet Garry's well-chosen words addressed to the court convey a heartfelt sense of loss, respect for individuals, and the objective of saving lives. In recent years, New Zealand's coroners have developed a model independent service concerned with learning from misfortune, exposing negligence, and advancing public discussion.

A third essential development was intrinsic to this book's analysis of suicide. It was important to have ages for individuals since life stages affected the specific motives or explanations for self-destruction; however, inquest forms did not routinely require a statement on age or date of birth. Alison Ainsworth at the office of the Registrar of Births, Deaths, and Marriages arranged for missing ages to be supplied from official data sets that summarized death certificates. Without this information the book would have lost depth and credibility. Staff members at Archives New Zealand provided exemplary service. Doug and I placed considerable demands on retrieval and conservation services. Heidi Kuglin, Graham Langton, Vernon Wybrow, and Uili Fecteau aided this project from the beginning; in more recent times, I also benefited from the attention of Jenifer Lash, Norm Goug, Donal Raethel, Jonathan Newport, and Andrew Wright. Jocelyn Chalmers, seconded to Archives from the Turnbull Library in the National Library during the latter's renovation, was helpful and has assisted with my plans for future New Zealand research in the Turnbull Library collections. The coroners' inquests constitute an archival treasure of international significance, but more collections await the attention of historians keen to craft new understandings of the past that are anchored in fact. The records are plentiful and the search engine "Archway" is a fine tool for scholars and genealogists alike. Staff members at Archives New Zealand have attempted to secure sensible access rules when dealing with government departments. Thus, I was able to probe the politics of a youth suicide panic in the late 1980s and early 1990s, and to develop a fuller account of shifting medical practices during the twentieth century than would have been possible otherwise. Jennie Ensor assisted with securing permission to reproduce illustrative material for Queen Mary Hospital at Hanmer Springs and Bruce Shephard did likewise for material held at the Porirua Hospital Museum. Editorial cartoonists Frank Greenall and Tom Scott each permitted me to use a pointed graphic statement from their lively works that chronicle public affairs. I am indebted to New Zealand artist Richard Killeen for permission to use his painting "Three Coloured Blocks" on the cover of the MQUP edition. I also thank Laurence Aberhart for use of the photograph on the cover of the Bridget Williams Books edition.

The generosity and flexibility of individuals whom I met in New Zealand's public service and public life made this study feasible. I am profoundly indebted to them. Many assisted because they had an awareness of suicide as a well-publicized issue in New Zealand and hoped that this project would offer guidance. My skeptical stance with respect to prevention, founded on a belief in the power of shifting historical contingencies, prevents me from endorsing specific policies or making any firm recommendations. The past suggests that the future forms of distress are unpredictable. Nevertheless, I hope that the well-documented observations and lines of argument offered on the following pages will not disappoint those who championed this project in expectation of solutions. It is my belief that suicide studies have become complacent and tautological, chugging in circles along the rails of set methods and presumptions. That contentious claim does not mean that all contributions to the extensive literature lack wisdom, but rather that few investigations have explored large numbers of actual cases of suicide and many publications make exaggerated claims for findings based on indirect observations. Alleged breakthroughs in understanding struck me as lacking substantial direct evidence. I accept responsibility for these critical outlooks and for the comparably tart conclusions dispersed throughout the book.

Preliminary drafts of chapters were presented as lectures at the Stout Centre on the topics of shell shock during World War I and youth suicides in the 1980s and 1990s. On both occasions, the interest shown was encouraging. Suggestions by Jean-Christopher Somers led to a re-evaluation of my approach to youth suicide. At the University of Waikato, Cathy Colborne and Giselle Byrnes arranged a seminar; the discussion assisted my efforts to understand the 1980s and 1990s in New Zealand. In Canada, I had the benefit of discussions at a seminar at the University of Western Ontario. McMaster colleagues commented following several departmental talks. David Wright, now at McGill University, generously shared his extensive knowledge on the history of psychiatry. Articulate and energetic, David inspires. Following a lecture at the University of Manitoba, a congenial psychiatrist remarked that he accepted much of what I described in relation to trends in his field. He surely expressed a controversial opinion. Questions posed at Manitoba caused me to consider ethnicity with care. This subject was raised again by one of the anonymous reviewers of the manuscript. Commentary by another reviewer resulted in more work on illness and self-euthanasia. I am thankful for these constructive suggestions. The publications of New Zealand's social, economic, and medical historians have been invaluable. I am particularly indebted to the work of James Belich, Barbara Brookes, Tom Brookings, Cathy Colborne, Bronwyn Dalley, Jim McAloon, and Warwick Brunton.

Don Akenson and Phil Cercone at McGill-Queen's University Press believed in the urgency of a book that dealt with suicide, domestic violence, self-euthanasia, and psychiatry's shifting tendencies. They have given me much needed encouragement in this and previous endeavours. The diverse auspices of illustrations and the substantial use of graphs and tables required attention to production details. To help me along, Ryan Van Huijstee provided advice and direction. Innumerable improvements in style and many timely questions were the products of Grace Seybold's careful reading of the manuscript. Ruth Pincoe prepared an excellent index. As on other occasions I am grateful to have had access to the talented individuals who comprise the Canadian academic publishing field.

I am indebted to Wellington friends who tolerated my reflections on life and history. In these respects I acknowledge the cordiality of Don Loveridge, Matt Trundle, Arthur Pomeroy, Richard Hill, Brigitte Bonisch-Brednich, Julie Warren, Colin Jeffcott, Meren Luehrs, Gareth Roderick, Juliet Scoble, and members of an informal bush tramping group from Rutherford House at Victoria University.

Preface

A timely access to personal information can advance knowledge and understanding in the humanities and the social sciences. From time to time, academics lay claim to providing information of value on public issues; we can and we should. Where bureaucratic obstruction and the imposition of fees impede investigation, rational debate is curbed.

Without extensive and forthright testimony on life's many troubles, even the most skilful investigations remain forever hemmed in and must operate indirectly by theoretical conjecture, manipulation of mute aggregate data, probes of selected cases that may be unrepresentative, and questionnaires and interviews that by their brevity or limited number cannot canvass deeply many people's experiences. In an age of privacy, timely access is rare. The defence of privacy is well understood, for it is under pressure from state agencies and commercial bodies alike. The well-resourced and powerful can collect and analyze while independent and potentially critical parties face obstacles. Privacy can be balanced by freedom of information. Such a balance was maintained during research for this book.

Timely access was the position taken by New Zealand Coronial Services, an agency that may now be unique among common-law jurisdictions on account of its spirit of judicial independence, belief in disclosure, and history of records preservation. However, I hope that what I encountered is not exceptional, and that this book will provoke quests for comparable records and the application of access regulations in ways that facilitate a wave of new research on social questions. Privacy was maintained by my voluntary decision to change names; there was no requirement that I do so. Public records were used throughout the study and no citations have been altered. Other researchers can retrace my steps.

My access to case files and an associated frankness in reporting words and conduct will surely irritate and exasperate some, as will my critiques of much suicide research, my recurrent attention to individual reasoning rather than mental illness, a discussion of medically assisted suicide, and scepticism about short-term suicide prevention measures. My intentions are to bring to light abundant evidence, to use that evidence to open a host of debates, and ultimately to advance inquiry into society, the economy, and the individual.

SORROWS OF A CENTURY

Introduction

Our attachment to life depends on our interest in it.

William Hazlitt

Our first task is peace; our second task is to see that nobody be hungry; and the third task is fairly full employment. The fourth task is, of course, education.

Karl Popper

Rarely can an ambition to know how people thought about their lives be achieved. Self-reflections by individuals are rare. In these circumstances, coroners' inquests into suicides provide a matchless means for a reconstruction of existential feelings. In New Zealand, there are approximately twenty-five thousand suicide inquest files for the twentieth century. With unusual care, they relate tales of discontent, misery, and independence. Their scope and detail are remarkable because in New Zealand, coroners have long been involved in investigations at an early stage and they may question witnesses at an open hearing. Their process has been described as "inquisitional" rather than passive.[1] To complete social history from the bottom up, other writers by different means will find ways to recount pleasures and joys. Histories of sports and entertainment have laid that foundation.[2] Inquests certainly pull the evidence to the bleak side, but that may capture essential dimensions of life because, as a coroner remarked about suicide in 2000, "it is so common that there are few extended families who have not at some time been in your position [a grieving family] and that is a very sad thing."[3]

Beyond their intrinsic importance, inquests produce keyholes to the past that expose more than might be imagined. Witnesses' explanations for fatal decisions portray eras through idioms of speech, and descriptions of settings and circumstances. These revelations and more contribute to a sense of location and what life was like there and then, at a time and place inaccessible to us now. People's reflections on the motives for self-destruction even touch the life-affirming values of the times. The inquests reveal individuals' encounters with love through love lost, work through work lost, aspirations through opportunities lost, health through illness, and ideas of sanity through mental illness. The instinctive drive for play, the basis for the recreations that bring pleasures and joy, surfaces in depositions. Admittedly, the activities so revealed are mainly gambling, drinking, and sexual pursuit of someone other than a spouse. Trouble ensued. But life is filled with risky encounters.

There is no exaggerating the wealth of information. All material in every inquest file for the twentieth century was accessible. The entire country is covered. We developed our own data set from the bottom up, case by case. We reviewed accidental deaths to see if any were suicides. Some surely were and they entered our study; we compiled a data set independent of coroners' findings and are confident that few violent deaths known to authorities escaped our attention. There may have been deaths in remote areas that went unreported, but most disappearances were of interest to someone, and even remains discovered years after a death prompted an inquest.[4]

Coroners worked with the police and medical practitioners to collect information and thus assembled statements, medical reports, and physical evidence. However, they occasionally steered clear of a suicide finding while still accepting evidence that to any neutral observer inclined decisively toward a finding of suicide. We encountered findings like this one: "the deceased died by a gun shot self-inflicted." Such a statement was drafted to leave open the possibility of an accident. "The deceased died by drowning. How he came to be in the water is unknown." That statement too avoided upsetting family members.[5] In these instances and many more that involved poisons, medication, or coal gas, the evidence of a motive or several motives plus an indication of intention were often plain enough to allow us to make a judgement, independent of coroners' findings, as to whether a death was an accident or a suicide. To assemble the data set, we went beyond the guidance of indices or abstract ledgers to locate suicide case files. Although guides to the files prepared by clerks exist and helped with the selection of many clear-cut instances of suicide, the data set was the product of thorough independent searches and careful assessments extending over seven years of research.

The research methods are described in an appendix; however, it is essential to state now that in the last fifteen to twenty years of the twentieth century, the case files contained not only the witnesses' depositions, but where applicable they held medical reports, psychiatric assessments, and arrest records, in addition to obligatory autopsy reports. There were thousands of suicide notes, an occasional diary, a few audio and video tapes, and several student "friendship books."[6] Information abounds for the 1980s and 1990s; by then police investigations and inquests had become exceedingly thorough. In all years, the files disclose the strains of daily living and the physical and mental states of men and women of diverse ages, cultures, and walks of life as they encountered disappointments. They also capture changes in such matters as hazardous vices, the sources of shame, work credentials, sexual freedom, attitudes about self-euthanasia, and trends in youth culture including nihilism. We discuss these phenomena as they relate to individuals' lives; we assess the meaning and quality of life as individuals contemplated their past and future in relation to their own times. Crucially, we stress that cultural and economic changes are central to understanding self-destruction, and that the background pressures and anxieties adversely affecting individuals altered over the decades. Amidst changing cultural circumstances, people thought about their pains, their illnesses, and an afterlife. Changes on the economic and cultural fronts, products of the human factor in history, undermine theories about suicide. The changes were often sudden. For economic conditions, that may be well understood and easily accepted, but cultural change could also transpire suddenly, as it did with respect to youth culture in the 1980s. The wider lesson is that there can be no static characterizations of suicidal persons.

World and national historical events inflicted considerable misery on ordinary people in the twentieth century. New Zealand shared in global crises, but also global palliatives. Medical information in the case files, and that includes mental health assessments, shows that despite geographic isolation, New Zealand was immersed intellectually in the "Western world." The shared history means that the sources of torment unearthed here are close to those that operated in many other jurisdictions. In fact, medical records in the case files denote conflicting academic perceptions of people's mental states.

There are limits to comparisons and parallels. New Zealand was and is a land of plenty, a condition that makes it exceptionally fortunate. Simultaneous with the elements of global integration and relative prosperity, the country's unique cultural makeup also surfaces in these records. New Zealand is multicultural in its own dynamic way. Commonalities with other places across the globe still remain striking. The patterns of suicide motives, the evidence of medical treatment, and ideas about life after death may not be perfectly universal, but for much of Europe, North America, and Australia, there were and are tremendous similarities. In one respect, New Zealand's experience with suicide may even have been ahead of other economically advanced countries, because the country's financial crises in the 1980s and internationally watched neo-liberal policy responses adversely affected the immediate employment prospects of young people and contributed to a soaring youth suicide rate. Comparable periods of adjustment and pessimism in other countries possibly have had a similar impact, although without the rigorous practices of coroners and the survival of case files, the investigative methods developed in this book cannot be duplicated everywhere.

The century's hard times are well-known. In addition to witnessing the impact of wars, epidemics, and economic crises on men and women, we encountered mundane events that dragged down individuals of all ages, from all classes, and at all periods. The insomnia of critical self-reflection or the impulsiveness of anger always had background origins, and more times than not, witnesses indicated what in their estimation had gone wrong. We want to emphasize the word *estimation* in the previous sentence, because it is impossible to know for sure what motivated people. That problem will always obstruct suicide studies. However, witnesses at inquests were usually close to the deceased and there is a ring of authenticity in their remembrances of last words or descriptions of conduct. Some men and women who populate the following pages could not endure their self-assessment, their physical pain, or their mental suffering. Some did not reflect long on their condition but acted impetuously; others hesitated and planned. Their troubles frequently went beyond the century's big events and they occasionally surpassed our imagination.

Suicide serves as a point of access to a socio-medical history of the human condition. The exceptional scope of the New Zealand records – a resource of world heritage standing – makes the current undertaking feasible. General practitioners, psychiatrists, clinical psychologists, and social workers have encountered suicide in their professional routines; sociologists, psychiatrists, and psychologists have attempted theoretical or rationalized understandings. The study of suicide has also engaged a few historians who believed that a society's management of suicides could disclose distinct cultural periods in "national" history.[7] Other historians have noted what suicides reveal about the pressures of everyday life.[8] We pursued this objective of social historians by collecting information on over eleven thousand individuals from the overall set of approximately twenty-five thousand suicide inquest files. Several sections of *Sorrows of a Century* incorporate New Zealand cases recounted in a prior companion book, *A Sadly Troubled History: The Meanings of Suicide in the Modern Age*.[9] To cover men and substance abuse for the entire century, it was necessary in chapter two to revisit alcoholism and *delirium tremens*, going over incidents that occurred before 1950. Likewise, the discussion of war trauma in chapter five includes an account of cases from World War I drawn from the earlier book.

The files are abundant, but the secondary literature on suicide is simply immense. Many publications were reviewed and discussed in *A Sadly Troubled History*. Some of that material plus more recent publications are worked into *Sorrows of a Century*, but secondary literature is largely relegated to endnotes. Flesh and blood, voice and thought, should be privileged and left unobstructed as far as possible. The diversity of human thought on display has also contributed to a sidelining of a considerable body of so-called theory, or what Karl Popper and his intellectual heirs might call pseudo-science. While insights have been gleaned from the work of sociologists and psychologists, and no doubt subliminally absorbed into our own thinking, any suggestion that knowledge about suicide can be encapsulated in a theory seems hubristic. Insights, yes; theory never.

To challenge an aspiration of "suicidology" is to tempt a reasonable reply from "suicidologists." They would be justified in asking the following questions. On what basis can history secure legitimacy in an area densely populated with specialists working in extensive intellectual traditions? What validates interlopers who barge in through openings from the past? Howard Kushner confronted these matters in *Self-Destruction in the Promised Land* by lamenting the splintering of suicide studies into the rival fields of sociology and psychology. He advocated a synthesis. Historians could participate prominently in working toward a synthesis due to their familiarity with sifting and sorting evidence, as well as their lack of a vested interest in seeing suicide as a topic fundamental to their discipline, which is the case for sociology and somewhat for clinical or medical psychology. Specialization had impeded breakthroughs since 1900, Kushner claimed; however, "specialists have provided us with the insights essential for the construction of a synthesis."[10] While this book shares his willingness to look for clues in several disciplines, there is much yet to be said to recommend a historical undertaking. In her study of mental illness and suicide in Japan, Junko Kitanaka reaches a conclusion similar to Kushner's, although she felt it necessary to re-insert emphatically the study of society because the medicalization of suicide had gone far since the publication of *Self-Destruction in the Promised Land.*[11] For Kitanaka, the diversity of human nature decreed that we take "a more nuanced view of mental illness – one that remains simultaneously biological, psychological, and thoroughly *social.*"[12] Her emphasis on social factors is shared in this book.

Trust in history, as an essential path to understanding society, for a study of suicide comes down to three considerations: the scope and quality of the case-based evidence, a commitment to recreate events with humility rather than certainty, and a knowledge of circumstances at specific times and places. The first of these three considerations provides the best justification for a license to write with confidence on the topic.

What makes the inquests so valuable? An absolute requirement for a full inquest into a suspected suicide was demanded in New Zealand and only relaxed in 2006; other common-law countries minimized coronial activity earlier, typically before 1950. On account of the possibility that an inquest could be reopened, the Ministry of Justice collected and retained all inquest files centrally. Miraculously, files for the twentieth century have survived. With exceedingly rare exceptions they seem complete.[13] In the vast majority of instances, witnesses' depositions, suicide notes, medical reports, and autopsies enabled us to find one motive and often more for a suicide. Motives alone are insufficient to explain the act. Plenty of people endure comparable crushing difficulties to the ones brought out at an inquest; in fact, that very proposition encourages us to believe that what we are describing are common challenges, losses, and disappointments. The particular troubles of the century that we describe enveloped many more people, and that likelihood increases their value to social and medical history. However, that claim prompts a question that will be asked on several occasions in this book. If troubles were common, why were most people in pain able to endure while others could not and opted for suicide?

A mere accumulation of observations cannot answer this question. Analysis requires informed conjectures about the reasoning behind a decision to act. To comprehend suicide calls for a two-step approach and an imaginative piecing together of shards of testimony. First, there are the crises that cause despair. Second, there are the internal reasoning processes needed to surmount a primal instinct to survive; we can attempt to reconstruct people's reasoning processes from witnesses' accounts, deathbed statements, and suicide notes. Motives that make up the first step can be addressed by quantitative analysis and accompanying extracts from statements, but an investigation of the reasoning that constitutes the second step must rely wholly on our patching together themes from statements, alas without statistical references to frequency. Some documents relate in detail how individuals reasoned their way to suicide as a solution; some show that people relied on ideas about life after death to get them past a threshold. However, numerous suicides came as the concluding deed in an impulsive outburst. Individuals raced out the door in a fit of passion. Many files are rich in details about the thought processes while others are silent on the subject; that circumstance makes it impossible to attempt to find a frequency pattern in the reasoning processes. Even if it were technically possible to lump reasoning into categories, our preference would be to stress the individuality of thought.

As the previous sentence suggests, this book takes positions that may offend critical readers from outside the discipline of history, readers who aspire to distill events into models and theories. We privilege world, national, local, and household events in understanding how individuals thought about themselves, and about family members, friends, employers, and even eternal life. Suicide is partly situational and history is devoted to situations in time. This claim challenges the idea of a motionless world implicit in psychologists' attempts to comprehend suicide though quests for the timeless personality traits of people at risk. Furthermore, testimony frequently describes situations that highlight material conditions. In contrast to tangibles, psychologists consider perceptions. Here there is need for the synthesis that Kushner recommended. Consider shame. People felt shame due to a transgression that put them at odds with associates, but they also perceived that they let themselves down and could not live with self-reproach.[14] There is a dual or interactive quality to the emotion: there is an external reality and an internal processing. The same consideration of interaction applies to the perception of being a burden.

In *Why People Die by Suicide*, Thomas Joiner wrote that one condition necessary for "the desire for death" was "perceived burdensomeness."[15] This proposition means that suicidal people are described as having perceived that they were a burden; it can be extended to the notion that they perceived that their lives had been ruined, or perceived that they were failures. The case files show that individuals who perceived damaging things about themselves were often not wide of the mark in self-judgement. If it is acknowledged that many suicidal individuals needed support in some form, then by extension they were a burden to someone. Perception presented alone is not revealing; it projects verisimilitude but is an unbounded word. It can embrace many things that seem reasonable, but alone it presents only incomplete situations. It is wisest to look at the situation and the human interactions, and then note how perception entered the picture. From case files, situations were reconstructed and categorized.

In plenty of cases, the so-called perceptions captured realities, not chimeras. People really could be a burden and insensitive people told them so. Some individuals experienced financial failure through their own actions. They had ruined their prospects, and creditors or partners erupted with displeasure. Even when perceptions were patently fantastic and at odds with "reality," the basis for a misconception or erroneous perception has to be considered in relation to family circumstances, cultural values, the legal system, the character of work, and labour's rewards. Each of these elements was subject to change over time. Something had initiated the perception and coloured it in heart-rending shades via historically contingent values. Some older men and women perceived that they were dying from cancer, but they had received no such diagnosis; however, they knew loved ones who had suffered from cancer. There were popular fears about unsuccessful invasive treatments. Individuals perceived things through layers of circumstances that included the great events of the century, the nature of labour, family lore, and tensions within a household.

There is another controversial position. A suicide is a premature death. Sympathy and compassion are understandable; after all, the lives under consideration ended before their time. That constitutes tragedy. Studies in psychology and sociology have wrapped suicide with colourless language that avoids saying anything that is not nice about the deceased.[16] Many case files support the victim hypothesis, although testimony also discloses violent cruel figures, deserving of help, surely, but also meriting statements on the hard truth about what they had done to others in the lead-up to their deaths. Suicides take place amidst situations covering a wide range of human conduct and not everyone is pleasant.

To highlight patterns and analysis, the dates and locales of events are mentioned sparingly. The chapters are thematic rather than chronological. The year in which a particular death occurred can be discerned from the endnotes, since each case number consists of a sequence number within a year. An individual's personal information is seldom presented unless it adds to the point being argued. One of this book's leading contentions is that chronology is important when it comes to understanding suicides. Therefore, time in the form of eras is discussed in chapter one, where we wrestle with the problem of defining the periods of the twentieth century and listing their leading traits.

Time in people's lives is also an essential consideration, so this initial chapter also introduces the life-course with its phases. In "*This Rash Act*," Victor Bailey commented on the challenge of defining phases in the Victorian era and on the significance of these phases in any analysis of suicide.[17] Defining the phases is a compounded problem when dealing with the entire twentieth century, because improved health care and greater longevity require an occasional adjustment to the ages that comprise phases such as the prime of life or old age. Chapter one includes a discussion of the strategy for defining phases in the life-course. Once past the two conceptualizations of time, this initial chapter moves on to identify a number of continuities and changes in long-term trends. The principal factors tracked across the century include motive for suicide by the phase in the life-course, occupation, gender, ethnicity, and method. In later chapters more attention is given to situations; the variables introduced in chapter one are reconsidered through the words of the witnesses and the individuals who committed suicide. In these later chapters, there is a risk of allowing well-documented cases to guide analysis; however, the words of the deceased and witnesses are the best means to integrate the economic and cultural transformations that caused despair or precipitated rage. Graphs and tables hem in the bias of selection that would come from building on the more extraordinary and insightful statements.

The second chapter considers gender in detail. It shows how some men considered women as their property, how with perverse reasoning they threatened to end lives, including their own, to retain that "property." Naturally, this chapter reports on domestic violence and sexual abuse. Chapter three surveys the importance of work for men, and the consequences of major shocks to employment and financial well-being in the post-war recession of the early 1920s, and the Great Depression of the 1930s. It identifies the significance of a prolonged era of prosperity that extended from roughly 1950 into the 1970s. That especially prosperous time forms the essential backdrop for understanding the high rate of suicide for young people that occurred in subsequent crisis years.

Chapter four considers illnesses and injuries as motives for suicide. Under the heading of trauma it looks at the impact of the two world wars on the lives of service personnel and civilians. Unquestionably, war had extensive consequences captured in the biographical profiles of men and women who committed suicide, but at times it was difficult to sort out the war influences from other, more commonplace, motives. On account of the tendency of many mental health professionals to assert that most suicides are products of mental disorders, chapter five focuses on mental illnesses. This chapter suggests that the emphasis placed on this one item has diverted attention from background stresses. Life can be hard. The emphasis that psychiatrists and psychologists placed on mental illness as a leading factor in suicides is challenged. However, not all of our arguments and findings align with critics of psychiatry and psychology. Much of chapter five points to depression as a mental illness with a long history; it was not a recent invention of drug companies. Whether it has been over-diagnosed is another question altogether; the inquest information shows the great difficulty that lay people as well as medical professionals had when determining whether depression in specific instances was an illness or great sadness caused by a tragedy.

Chapter six recounts how an assortment of factors helped to make suicide, especially youth suicide, a public issue in the late twentieth century. There were intense inter- and intra-professional disputes as well as political manoeuvring to exploit the crisis. In chapter seven, we set aside the guesswork explanations of contemporaries who ended up accenting mental illness. Instead, we explain the rise in youth suicides through information found in the case files. Now more thorough than in prior years, the inquests indicate a convergence of unemployment, difficulties at school, family troubles, and broken relationships. In this chapter, we offer our most emphatic corrective to explanations that focus on mental health, but we retain mental health as a substantial concern. It just was not paramount. Moreover, it was not always the illness alone which brought people down, but the failings of a health care system in the throes of a major transformation. Because most of the events in this chapter occurred during an abruptly imposed regime of austerity, its findings should be of concern to social service and medical agencies, and the interested public, in countries practicing comparable belt-tightening.

Chapter eight looks at life histories, last words, and suicide notes to explain how individuals came to think that death was not final, not painful, and that the suffering of those left behind was not compelling enough to deter action. An argument running throughout the book maintains that there is an interaction among such leading motives as economic stress, marital discord, physical debilities, and mental illness. As a result, there is 'cross-stitching' among the thematic chapters. In chapter eight, points from previous chapters are mentioned and lines of reasoning from subsequent sections alluded to.

The abundant personal details and occasional criticisms of medical practices and failures in the medical system will upset guardians of privacy and members of medical and kindred professions. It is difficult for us to endorse the idea that the trust of patients will be enhanced by covering up errors or pretending that there are no uncertainties among therapeutic philosophies in psychiatry nor imperfections in the practice of clinical psychology. Privacy interpreted as the closure of information (as opposed to the protection of a patient's identity) is unjustified in a society committed to public welfare. We found instances where psychiatric patients, family members, and dissenting doctors were sceptical of treatments and all had good cause for their questioning attitude.

The fact that we could carry this study forward into recent times will incite concern among guardians of privacy. Always when explaining this research, we are asked about confidentiality. There are oft-proclaimed reasons for closing records of an intimate nature for fifty to a hundred years. These justifications include respect for a patient's privacy; some claim too that there is a need for physicians to have the trust of their patients. A deceased person, however, is no longer a patient, and trust must be earned. There are arguments in favour of access. The discussion of mental health issues is in the public interest and secrecy may be self-serving. These counter-positions legitimize access to these exceptional records. Furthermore, the proceedings of New Zealand's coroners' court are open.

We have taken the precaution of making the names of individuals anonymous in all years except in rare instances where names were disclosed in newspapers. Even then we disguised names if we thought that family members at the time were reticent about public reports or that disclosure would harm the living. All files in this study were publicly accessible, although some contain restricted information in sealed envelopes to which we were granted access.

1

Long-Term Perspectives: Chronology, Gender, Life-Course, Ethnicity, and Method

Initially life and death must be portrayed in bold strokes without the colour of detail, because of the unprecedented, almost unmanageable, time span. Particulars flesh out all subsequent chapters. On the pages of this chapter, we array statistics to identify patterns among the lives of thousands who took their own lives. Broad trends prepare the way for the intimate observations that populate the remainder of the book. To work with events spread across a century requires organization and prejudgement about what is important. A decade-by-decade or year-by-year analysis would fragment discussion, therefore we recast the twentieth century into "types of years" based on suicide rates, shifting arrays of motives, and historical trends.

The scope of this study imposed an additional challenge; the improving state of health across the century and particularly after 1950 meant that the ages which constituted phases in the life-course changed. The prime of life extended over more of an individual's years in 2000 than in 1900. To investigate rigorously people's troubles over the life-course, it was necessary to recalibrate several life-course phases. The adjustments to time periods and to life's phases sharpen findings, but tinkering places demands on readers. Moreover, adjustments cannot deal with premature aging. In 1930, men nicknamed "old Jim" and "old Bill" were sixty; labour and drink had aged them.[1] To a small degree, age is relative to circumstances.

Complexities in the data set are exposed in this chapter, but so too are advantages that originate from a long-term study based on case files. Due to them, it was possible to work with numerous variables confident that each was linked through an individual.

Researchers who have attempted to connect suicide rates to an assortment of variables such as age, marital status, unemployment, literacy, religion, wars, disasters, isolation, and so forth frequently have depended on statistical inferences among separate data sets. In these studies, the variables lack organic relationships. With case-file data we do not have to engage in statistical gymnastics and contortions to see if, for example, high unemployment affected suicide rates. Witnesses' depositions and a police investigation indicated individuals' employment status and motives; we can directly observe how unemployment, work conditions, or financial troubles contributed to an individual's despondency.

COUNTING AND SORTING LIFE'S TROUBLES

The number of cases per year that we established is usually more reliable than the official count, and thus our suicide rates are more accurate too. Official reports originated from a count of death certificates that coroners had to submit to the Registrar General of Births, Deaths, and Marriages within three days of an inquest's conclusion. The cause of death written on a certificate embodied a coroner's finding. A few findings presented 'courtesy verdicts' that stated a dubious finding of accidental death or left the cause of death open on the grounds that there were several explanations. During the first half of the century, these suspicious findings often involved death by drowning and occasionally by gunshot.[2] Some accidental and open findings were glaringly misleading; to a reasonable witness the deaths could only have been suicides.[3]

In strict accordance with the law, coroners accepted the possibility of an accidental death if there was no firm evidence for a finding of suicide and nothing to rule out an accident.[4] From time to time family members offered alternate explanations as to why, in their estimation, a death might have been accidental. "My sister was always top heavy," declared a witness in 1954, "and I have known her to fall on her face." Allegedly she went for a walk and fell face-first into the sea.[5] In the second half of the century, family doctors could sow doubt around drug overdoses.[6] "To my knowledge," stated one practitioner in 1960, "there is accepted medical opinion that these drugs can cause mental confusion which may lead a patient to take more tablets than they intended to take. Other authorities disagree."[7] In 2000, family members successfully insisted that a young man had mistakenly taken too much medication despite the emphatic statement of a pathologist that the level of drugs in the blood "was due to a deliberate self-action rather than through therapeutic misadventure."[8] Contrary to a general practitioner's report in 2000 that an elderly man with Paget's disease had admitted to taking a whole bottle of Halcion "deliberately," the coroner attributed death to medical causes.[9] In these instances and many more, we rejected the coroner's finding and coded for a suicide.

Priests were biased witnesses. Father John Fowler testified that "because deceased was a good and devout Catholic I do not think he would consciously take his own life."[10] Some suicides of devout Catholics were treated gingerly by coroners in an effort to find a way around a suicide finding.[11] The presence of a solicitor who insisted on absolute proof of deliberate self-destruction could influence a coroner.[12] Often a mental illness that left a coroner wondering if an individual was capable of appreciating the quality of his or her action provided the grounds for an open verdict. By and large, at the end of the century we accepted the high standard of evidence required by New Zealand coroners; however, there were cases where we believed that the preponderance of evidence for a suicide was substantial and yet a coroner chose to ignore it.[13] Since inquests could be sensational and findings controversial, coroners in cities were well-known, subjected to criticism, caricatured, and occasionally front-page news (Figures 1.1 to 1.4). More so than in other common-law jurisdictions, New Zealand coroners have been public figures and exposed to controversy and scrutiny. If the attention and openness of process could still not preclude courtesy findings, then we seriously wonder about the value of aggregate data collected in other jurisdictions and based on coroners' inquests or even less scrupulous procedures. There should be a moratorium on suicide research reliant on such weak information.

There was a short-term problem with the files. During World War II, the mandatory practice of sending them promptly at the conclusion of the inquest to the Department of Justice in Wellington broke down. Some files were submitted years later, and a few possibly not at all. Instances of delayed transfers and misplaced files, though rare, were encountered during research.[14] The resulting deviation from a pattern of more suicides in the case files than in published reports was short-term (Graph 1.1).[15] By the end of the twentieth century, the difference between the number of suicides that we determined

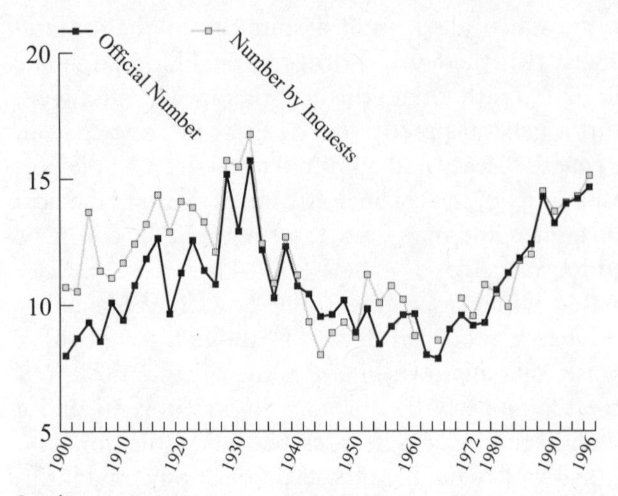

Graph 1.1
Suicide rates (men and women combined) based on official count and assessment based on Reading Inquest files, 1900–2000

from a close reading of case files and the number based on coroners' findings narrowed (Table 1.1).

Until late in the century, official reports under-counted actual suicides. Even in the late 1970s, the published count was unreliable due to an unofficial but well-understood practice of coroners avoiding a suicide finding. Family sensitivity and religious qualms continued, but there is also firm evidence of coroners avoiding suicide findings in order to allow the next of kin to benefit from the country's Accident Compensation Commission (ACC). The multi-purpose commission functioned as an accident- and life-insurer.[16] No benefits could be provided when there was a finding of suicide. "Our problem is this," wrote the commission's solicitor to the Department of Justice's Chief Advisor, Legal Section. "The Accident Compensation Commission Act provides that (with certain exceptions) no compensation is payable where death was due to suicide and that it shall be presumed, in absence to the contrary, that a death is not due to suicide. As you pointed out in a recent telephone discussion in most cases a Coroner will stop short of a clear-cut 'suicide' finding and simply record that a death was by drowning, shooting (or whatever) and will then, in appropriate cases, [list it] as 'self inflicted.'"[17] The commission's solicitor was informing the department that the phrasing of the ACC Act meant that when coroners used a courtesy finding,

Table 1.1
Likely undercounting of suicides due to coroners' courtesy verdicts

Decade	*% of cases in data set that were suicides by coroner's official finding*	*% of cases in data set that were deemed suicides by researchers on basis of a preponderance of evidence*
1900s	83.0	17.0
1910s	85.1	15.0
1920s	90.1	9.9
1930s	90.0	10.0
1940s	89.6	10.4
1950s	86.1	13.9
1960s	93.3	6.7
1970s	91.2	8.8
1980s	94.2	5.8
1990s	96.5	3.5
2000	97.4	2.6

Table 1.2
Six types of years that organize the century

	Years	*Characteristics*
National development	1900–18; 1924–26	National suicide rate of 12 to 13 per 100,000; men with work and alcohol problems
The Great Depression	1928–38	National suicide rate of 15 to 16; men with work and finance troubles
War recovery years	1920–24; 1946–48	Troubles for repatriated men include war trauma
The Long Prosperity ("Golden Weather")	1940–44; 1950–74	Suicide rate plummets to 9 to 10. For men, work and finance troubles ease
The era of economic crises	1976–98	Rate rises to 10 to 14; youth rate is unprecedented
Recovery begins	2000	Youth rate starts to drop

the commission was obliged to pay compensation. The commission might do so in any event, but it wanted to have available the option to deny compensation. Coroners by the 1980s demonstrated more professionalism and generally less concern for local sensitivities.

Suicide rates can be regarded as a barometer for the times, and as such they helped define six types of years that assist with coordinating the discussion (Table 1.2). The conventional chronology of wars and political change retains importance and from time to time enters analysis. However, trends in the suicide rates suggest time markers based on national moods of optimism, satisfaction, or despair. The conception of six types of years involved more than fluctuations in the suicide rates; we considered alterations among the leading motives. Additionally, we reflected on the tenor of witnesses' statements and suicide notes, and we formed impressions of periods. From the language of witnesses' statements, we detected changes in the mood of national life. The reach of these moods varied with phases in the life-course. Good economic times with an optimistic mood were not happy times for everyone; a number of older people with chronic illnesses, for example, experienced physical suffering, and some experienced the loss of a loved one. To take another example, in the years before the welfare state, serious economic crises affected older working people with family responsibilities, whereas unemployment crises were mitigated by the welfare state. However, while welfare was a boon to older individuals, economic crises left young people deeply pessimistic about their future.

Before delving into moods, people's ages, and suicide motives, we need to describe the six types of years. The periods had unequal lengths, and the war recovery periods were separated by roughly twenty-five years; the period of national development was also split. It included 1900 to 1914 as well as 1924 to 1926. These years of national development saw good prices for the wool clip, the emergence and consolidation of the dairy and frozen meat industries, and surges of business confidence. Recessions in 1907–08 and 1912–13 and the uneven spread of prosperity complicate the picture, but on the whole the economy showed growth.[18] A serious post-war depression interrupted expansion and undermined business confidence. For that reason, the post-war years are gathered into a separate category. During national development, suicide rates stood at around twelve to fourteen suicides per hundred thousand people. The Great Depression stands out as a distinct period; suicide rates reached sixteen to seventeen per hundred thousand. There was a mitigating circumstance late in the Great Depression. The First Labour Government, elected in 1935 and re-elected in 1938, introduced welfare measures, price support mechanisms for agriculture, and import controls. Economic recovery was not immediate, but the burst of action promoted an intangible sense of better times ahead. Optimism and pessimism cannot be quantified for historical periods; however, the suicide files are replete with evidence that despair and hope reverberated through a spirit of the times.

World War II brought full employment; with the exception of a short post-war adjustment, this fair-weather condition lasted a quarter of a century. The state-directed economy was advanced by conservative National Party Governments through public works and the expansion of state-owned enterprises.[19] A remarkable period of optimism bolstered by national self-congratulations witnessed singularly low suicide rates of eight to ten per hundred thousand. In the early 1970s came the opening phases of a protracted period of economic crises. Exports of food and wool to the United Kingdom had fallen and the country had to import petroleum at higher prices. Borrowing abroad forestalled a crisis, but by the late 1970s the country began to haemorrhage capital. The response was a sudden radical trimming of the state.

The state-managed economy that had all but guaranteed full employment depended on increasingly inefficient domestic industries, public works, and export revenue from agricultural staples. Income from the latter crumbled. A new economic order that shed some state enterprises and price support mechanisms was introduced by the Fourth Labour Government (1984–89). A subsequent National Party Government initially made deeper cuts to government spending. In the early 1980s, shortly before the election of the Fourth Labour Government, unemployment had become very serious. Young people were hit hard; for the first time in several generations, no jobs at state enterprises awaited school leavers. A palpable gloom descended on young people. During the last two decades of the century, the overall suicide rate increased to the levels found at the century's start. One staggering fact about suicides separated the beginning and the end of the century. The mean age dipped from the high forties to the high thirties.

The eras we identify mainly consist of contiguous years; however, the war and recovery years call for special treatment. At the conclusions of both world wars, the country faced imminent challenges. The government and voluntary organizations had the task of reintegrating into civilian life tens of thousands of men. Families had to adjust when men came home, and so did the men themselves. Suicide must be understood in relation to changing times. On account of the unusual types of problems that burdened people affected by the wars, their consequences for self-destruction are singled out for attention in a section of chapter four on ailments and injuries. The particular crises affecting young people in the 1980s and 1990s are so distinct and interconnected among themselves that they require a separate chapter. This exception aside, life's troubles, the sources of sorrow and rage, are organized by themes rather than periods. To round out the century, we examined the suicide inquests held in 2000. By this year, a strong economic recovery had begun. It would last until 2008.

For each of the six types of years, we computed the percentage of suicides accounted for by the leading motives (Table 1.3). The use of the word "motive" will be controversial throughout the book. It is normally defined as a reason for action, but we have applied it in a wider sense. Specifically, when we have designated a mental illness as a motive, it may truly have been a motive in the sense of a reason for the action. Some individuals aware of their conditions chose to end their suffering. In many cases, however, mental illness describes the mental state that affected judgement. To an unknown degree, our decision to categorize some instances of suicide as motivated by mental illness inflates that category, unless one assumes that most suicides are irrational, non-intentional, and *ipso facto* products of mental illness. We oppose that latter position and argue that frequently suicide was an intentional solution. Mental illness is a problem-laden concept. As a motive it is an expedient that opens the way for extended discussion in chapter five.

Coroners were not required to indicate a motive for suicide, although most provided explanations to support their findings of death by suicide. The frequency of these explanations was spotty. They were rare in the early decades and nearly universal in the closing decades. If no motive was supplied, the overwhelming majority of files contained evidence which we could assess to arrive at a motive or motives. Even in rustic situations, coroners called in witnesses and took depositions. In the railway town of Taumaranui in 1906, the public was offended by post-mortems conducted on railway tracks. Despite this "insult to civilization," the coroner held a thorough inquiry that included a doctor's testimony about the deceased's physical injuries and "depression."[20]

Motives organized by the types of years elucidate important changes in economic and social life during the century. There are patterns among the suicide motives that signal social and cultural transformation in three thematic areas: work and stress, relationships and sex, and medicine and health. First, there were currents in work-related stress. Even in the first era, that of national development, substantial

Table 1.3
Percentage of suicides of men and women by leading motives in the six types of years

	Alcohol or Drugs	*Work or Finance*	*Marital or Romantic*	*Mental Illnesses*	*Physical Ailments*
National development	16.7	15.2	6.3	19.9	20.3
The Great Depression	6.9	17.4	9.0	23.3	22.7
War recovery years	5.8	11.6	8.0	29.0	26.5
The Long Prosperity	10.4	12.4	7.5	23.9	20.9
The era of economic crises	6.9	9.6	19.4	33.9	13.0
Recovery begins	10.5	8.9	25.0	23.6	11.5

work-related and financial problems blighted lives and brought some individuals to the brink of self-destruction. Surprisingly, at the end of the twentieth century, during years of high unemployment and youth despair, work-based and financial problems had only a slight direct role in fatal despondency. Why had work-related troubles surfaced in an era of national development, but diminished in an era of hard times? Work in the era of national development was insecure and predominantly physical; however, with the election of the First Labour Government, the introduction of welfare mitigated abject financial desperation, or at least primed feelings of hope. To explain the pattern of motives for the late twentieth century, we have to include sex, the second important area of socio-cultural transformation. Changes in values about sex and family had begun in the 1960s but really attained firm standing during the 1980s and 1990s. An escalation in marital and romantic motives for suicide points to the importance of this development, a development that coincided with the onset of the era of economic crises.

The third prominent transformation involved medicine and health. Multiple medical developments affected the proportions of suicide motives. On the surface, mental illnesses or mental disorders seem to have grown in importance while physical ailments declined as motives, notably so in the last decades of the century. We must be careful when discussing mental illnesses as motives, however, because it is probable that they were under-diagnosed and under-reported for much of the century, while later in the century doctors were more inclined to dwell on mental illness rather than note the life-circumstance stresses that could have precipitated mental depression. Undoubtedly, mental illness was consistently important as a motive, although reports of it at inquests were subject to complex outlooks that changed over time. Case files show that from at least the 1900s forward, doctors and family members remarked on forms of depression that debilitated far more distressingly than transient sadness. Nevertheless, it is likely that witnesses spoke about mental illnesses with less candour early in the century and with greater forthrightness later.

The economic crises of the 1980s and 1990s added stress and precipitated breakdowns. At the same time, the greater willingness to speak of mental illness at century's end elevated the number of times that suicides were attributed to a mental illness. In earlier decades, witnesses would have highlighted the background stress of unemployment, physical ailments, or marital unhappiness. Mental illness entered popular discourse with greater frequency and honesty in the 1980s and 1990s, but that also favoured a misleading focus on the mental state rather than on factors that brought on the all-too-evident mental distress. Medical professionals in the 1980s and 1990s incorporated suicide prevention into their activities. That cultural change contributed to a trend in assigning more cases to a medical motive. To sum up, improved work conditions and social security changed lives for the better; a sexual revolution changed relationships and family arrangements, but with costs as well as benefits. Economic disappointments, related stress, and publicity about mental health increased the proportion of mental-illness attributions.

The foregoing currents are suppositions based on trends covering a century. A more detailed account of eras and motives exposes more about life's troubles. During the years of national development, alcohol abuse, work and finance problems, mental illnesses, and physical illnesses were prominent primary motives, each accounting for fifteen to twenty percent of male suicides. Marital or romantic problems comprised a relatively minor array of serious troubles at this time. Underlying the limited presence of this latter group of motives is the fact that during these years, the percentage of married men among suicides was 33.1 percent. By comparison, it was 44.2 percent during the period of the long prosperity. Men who took their own lives early in the century were predominantly single; alcohol abuse as a motive attained its greatest prominence early in the century. Testimony from the case files adds weight to an impression of an insecure labour force with a substantial number of single men in short-term or seasonal work. Many shifted often to stay employed. Some laboured on construction sites in cities and were subject to building cycles. Labourers experienced insecurity even in a period of economic growth. They were numerous and vulnerable; national prosperity was unevenly shared. Farmers, farm labourers, unspecified labourers, and men without a stated occupation accounted for nearly half of male suicides (46.4 percent) during the years of national development. Hardship flourished amidst plenty.

There was gruelling unsteady work. Accessible entertainment and companionship consisted of drinking at pubs. Witnesses' accounts of alcohol abuse and terrible withdrawal symptoms were never more abundant than during these years, particularly before World War I. Family life for some labouring men was deferred for many years. Physical ailments constituted a substantial assortment of dreadful burdens. Moreover, particular diseases not only wrecked the body but inspired fear at their merest mention as a possible diagnosis. Cancer, tuberculosis, and venereal diseases frightened men and women. Outdoor physical labour wore men down by their mid-forties; injuries left older men at a disadvantage when pursuing manual work. During the years of national development, roughly a third of males who committed suicide had rural occupations (30.6 percent).

As one would expect, in the Great Depression work and finance troubles appeared as a prominent motive cluster; neither before nor after this period did work and finance problems of male suicides reach the Great Depression level of twenty percent of motives. In later eras, both physical and mental illnesses surpassed the work or finance cluster of motives seen in the Great Depression. During this era, the leading occupations of men who took their own lives remained much the same as in prior years. Farmers, farm labourers, unspecified labourers, pensioners, and men reported as simply unemployed now accounted for half of male suicides (49.8 percent). The sheer bulk of the labouring population meant that in this era of broad-based distress, white-collar employees, professionals, and businessmen were no more prominent than before the collapse. To compensate for falling prices or wages, some men worked longer and harder. This fatigue-inducing tactic precipitated or exposed injuries. The extreme economic crisis strained the mental and physiological states of men who toiled, but alcohol abuse as measured by suicide motives plummeted. Wartime prohibition measures may have had a lingering impact and contributed to a general sobering-up; declining incomes likely helped curtail consumption too. Marital problems, many connected to the strains of the economic crisis, rose when compared to the prior era of national development, but the increase was slight.

World War II initiated the long prosperity, an extended era when high commodity prices, the safety net of the new welfare state, and the promotion of New Zealand as a highly favoured destination for immigrants conspired to create an unprecedented and unsurpassed mood of optimism. The Korean War pulled the economy into even greater growth. The suicide rate plunged. Work and finance motives for suicide sank to new lows. Marital and romantic motives were marginally higher than in previous eras; more of the men who committed suicide were married than previously. During the long prosperity, the dislocation of casual labour and the harm of alcohol abuse faded as leading motives for self-destruction. Physical and mental illnesses were more prominent than in previous groups of years. The mean age for men and women who took their own lives climbed (Graph 1.2). Men in their prime found work; older men remained at risk due to poor health.

At century's end, in the era of economic crises, a sharply different pattern of motives appears. Unemployment escalated but welfare and medical benefits cushioned the impact on mature men and women, although stress and disappointment promoted mental depression and marital strains among some. For the first time, young people were prominent among suicides. Many problems of youth were related to schooling, the shortage of entry-level jobs, conflicts with authority, and troubled relationships in the wake of the sexual revolution. In connection with that revolution, it is worth noting that, in the era of economic crises that immediately followed the start of the sexual revolution, the percentages of male suicides who were separated, divorced, or in de facto relationships exceeded the percentages for all other periods (11.6 percent for separated in the period versus 7.5 in all other groups of years; 5.7 percent for de facto status versus 0.4; 2.6 percent for divorced versus 0.8). We cannot say if these proportions differed greatly from the entire population because censuses did not routinely report on all of these "marital states." However, we can report that witnesses and suicide notes in the 1980s and 1990s often portrayed broken relationships in vivid language.[21] There were qualitative as well as statistical

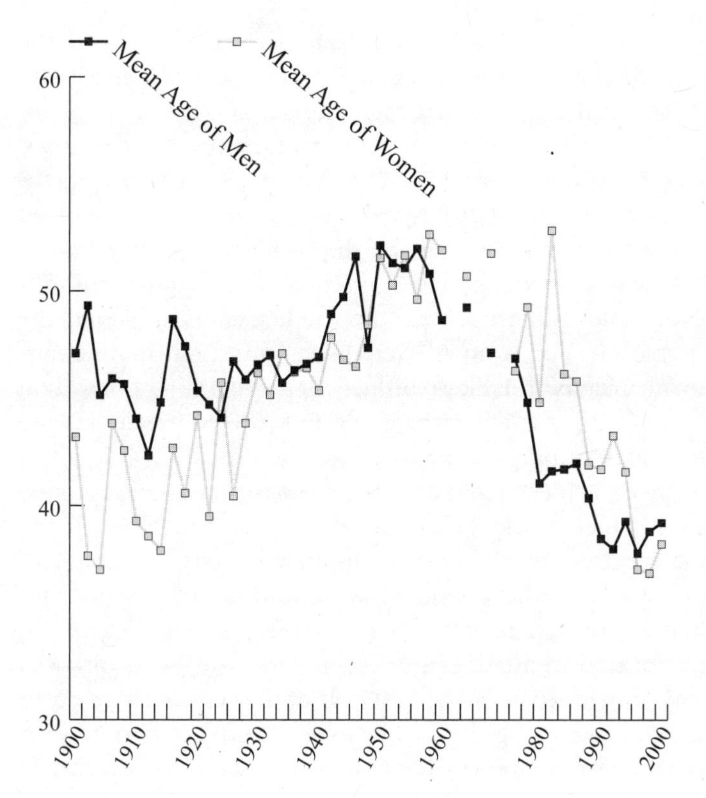

Graph 1.2
Mean ages of men and women, 1900–2000

changes apparent in the make-up of suicides of the late twentieth century. Our impression is that statements by the deceased conveyed more anger and frustration than at any other time. Rage was a coda for a generation.

MEN AND THE WORK ETHIC; WOMEN AND DOMESTIC GOALS

Graph 1.3 captures a persistent and substantial difference between the *completed* suicide rates of men and women. Explanations for this difference often include the caveat that women who attempt suicide greatly outnumber men. Therefore the gap must be approached cautiously so that crises in the lives of women are neither undercounted nor under-appreciated. The gap must not be considered a quantitative measure of relative gender suffering. However, it does call up two observations that, while not perfect answers to the puzzle of gender-based differences in the numbers of "successful attempts," are significant on their own and support important conjectures about the lives of men and women in the twentieth century. First, men and women consistently had recourse to different methods of self-destruction; that difference was meaningful and involved the intentions of the parties and the implements that they had at hand. As we will show in the last section of this chapter, methods express gender roles and property control in households. Second, the relatively static rate for women over the century and the fluctuating rate for men signal the likely influence of something other than intentions and methods. The crucial variable, we contend, was the powerful ideology of paid work.

It is no mere coincidence that over the years the fluctuations in the suicide rate for men track the country's economic fortunes. Work for pay was the great non-biological difference separating the lives of men and women. Many women were undoubtedly breadwinners and many managed households as complex as small businesses, but for most of the twentieth century men corralled the ideology of work for pay and, at least for the first half of the century, many men accepted an accompanying duty to provide. There are two clusters of motives where men dominated, truly dominated, for the whole century: work and finance troubles, and problems with the police and the law. The sheer number of work and finance troubles makes it the more important of the two.

The male duty to provide was never honoured consistently. Details from witnesses' accounts of alcohol abuse divulge negligence, self-indulgence, and self-pity. Abusive alcoholics deviated from the ideology of work and the accompanying duty to provide. Over and over, wives and children made that point at inquests. So too did men in apologetic notes addressed to family members. The data set reveals that the over-representation of men with an alcohol abuse motive was immense during the years of national development, a point we will return to in chapter two. Conventional cultural standards accepted that men could drink to excess. The gender disparity in the alcohol abuse motive narrowed at the end of the twentieth century, by which time gender equality extended to women enjoying a drink among friends, but also to the dubious privilege of alcoholism or public drunkenness. A few male wastrels and scoundrels, who funded their pleasures with the money needed for the family table,

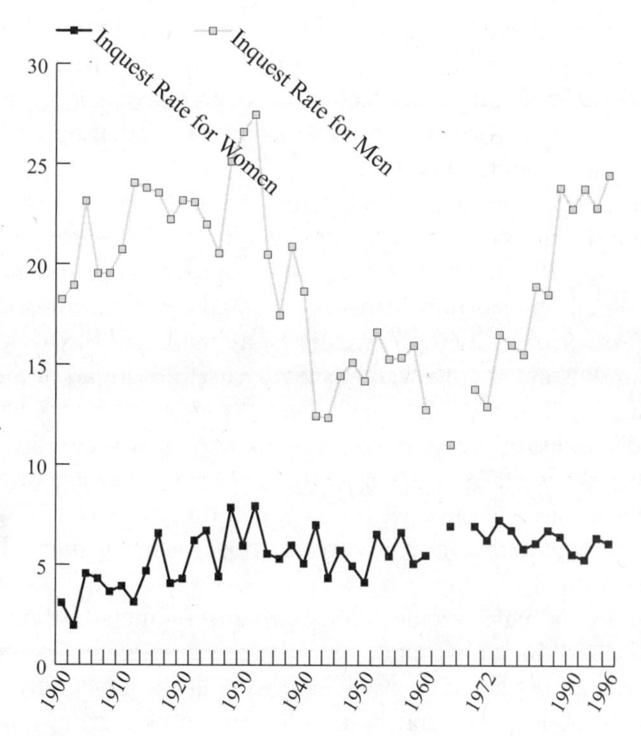

Graph 1.3
Suicide rates for men and women based on inquest files

running out of luck and credit, acknowledged in brief notes their washed-out lives moments before they ended them.

In the later decades of the twentieth century, under the circumstances of a welfare state, work for pay became detached from the old idea of the duty to provide. For many young men of these years, pay meant access to consumer goods, a car, a girl, and vacations. The duty to work did not vanish, for the expression "welfare bludger" persisted. Max Abbott, director of the New Zealand Mental Health Foundation, wrote in a 1982 report on unemployment that "to not have a job is to be an outsider – a social outcast."[22] That still may have been the case in some circles when he wrote, but by the 1980s the duty to provide for a family was not as pervasive or as powerful a cultural value as in earlier times. The duty to work was now believed to be enforced by social norms, whereas its former status as a psychic burden was urgent and implanted in individuals' minds.

Many people had believed in it, although perhaps not the men in menial work with despised bosses. By the 1980s, the welfare safety net and the sexual revolution weakened ideas of personal responsibility. From the 1970s forward, reckless behaviour caught up with younger men, and a few women too.

In the cultural circumstances of a consumer society meshed with a welfare state, in the age of the sexual revolution, work for pay endured as a critical matter for younger men, but less as an obligation to assist others than as the means for personal consumption and gratification. As for older men, the welfare state mitigated the back-to-the-wall circumstances conveyed in suicide case files found in the early 1920s and again during the Great Depression. While work for pay remained a fixation for men, the reasons why men focused on it changed once the welfare state was truly established. The age profile of the men most concerned with it changed too, because young men in the late twentieth century worried about securing that all-important first job.

The percentage of male suicides attributable to financial difficulties displayed a striking consistency over the century. Regardless of the era, nine out of ten suicides involving this collection of motives were male suicides. For women, the two leading motive groups, as proposed by witnesses, were mental illness and romantic or marital problems. The number of men who committed suicide and were deemed to have had a mental illness (n = 1,891) outnumbered women with this motive (n = 1,159). However, this male numerical lead in mental illness was implicit in their general prominence among all completed suicides. More revealing is the expected count of men and women based on the enduring gender ratio of suicides (Graph 1.3). By this standard, the numbers of men with mental illness should have been much greater (expected number = 2,328) than the numbers of women (expected number = 720).

The mal-distributed attributions expressed several culturally constructed elements. Waged labour was principally a male anxiety. As well, witnesses frequently represented women as unstable, emotional, and romantic. Not only were witnesses more inclined to report that the deceased suffered from mental illness, but their descriptions of how the deceased appeared before death matched representations of mental illness. Witnesses described a third of the women (33.6 percent) and a fifth of the men (21.6 percent) as depressed or very depressed. Mental illnesses or disorders may have been under-counted for men, because their conduct in certain specific instances could have been regarded by some psychiatrists and psychologists as expressing an underlying disorder. For example, in each era, men led in alcohol or drug abuse as a motive; in each era, men also led in problems with the police or the law. The assignment of a mental illness motive for a number of women may have captured a bias that credited men with manly deviance and women with feminine irrationality. In some instances, men may have instinctively self-medicated with excessive alcohol consumption for an undiagnosed mental disorder such as melancholia or schizophrenia.

Throughout the book, we note our uncertainty – indeed our suspicions – about an alleged prevalence of mental illnesses as motives. It was common for New Zealand psychologists in the 1990s to dwell on mental illness as an overwhelmingly common motive. Our calculations are more modest than their seemingly unconfirmed conjectures. On the one hand, it is possible that we have under-counted these motives by categorizing some motives as other than mental illness. On the other hand, we maintain that the mental health establishment in recent years has exaggerated the strength of a potential correlation between mental illnesses and suicide. Part of what we believe has been an excessive focus on mental illness is explicable because of the accent that psychiatrists and especially psychologists place on an immediate presentation of syndromes. Often non-medical witnesses at inquests reported an underlying stress motive leading to mental illness, or indicated behaviour that could have been a coping mechanism for a mental illness. Diligent psychiatrists looked past syndromes and sought background crises from what patients told them about their life histories. A lot of suicides originated in circumstances that had nothing remotely to do with a mental illness unless one abandons curiosity, challenges free will on every occasion, and assumes that suicidal conduct in itself is madness. We take an opposite position. Many suicide decisions were well-thought-out and rational in terms of the individual's world view. They could not handle their anguish or they reacted in rage to someone challenging their autonomy, in the case of youth, or their authority, in the case of mature men.

TROUBLES ALONG THE LIFE-COURSE

To organize descriptions of troubles encountered over the life-course, we converted groups of ages into life-course phases: pre-adolescence, adolescence, prime, transitional, and senior. The phases and the ages assigned to them are open to question. What is adolescence? Many international studies, for good reasons, set an upper limit of nineteen. That is what we do in this chapter. We recognize that setting limits is imperfect. There were immature nineteen-year-olds and fourteen-year-olds who, while not emotionally mature, adopted the risky conduct of older peers. Then there is the challenge of defining a senior. On occasion, autopsy reports described deceased men and women as elderly on account of appearances; however, birth certificates and witnesses' statements placed these individuals in their fifties. During the course of the century, life expectancy increased and sixty-five became the new fifty. These changes introduce a problem for comparability. A person considered elderly at a particular age in 1920 was not necessarily labelled that way in 1980. Consequently, we altered marginally the groups of ages that comprised several phases in the life-course. From 1900 to 1940, the phases consisted of the following ages: prime, 20 to 45; transitional, 46 to 55; senior, 56 plus. From 1942 to 1976, they were: prime, 20 to 49; transitional, 50 to 60; senior, 61 plus. From 1980 to 1998, they were: prime, 20 to 55; transitional, 56 to 65; and senior, 66 plus. The designation of pre-adolescent and adolescent remained consistent across all years at under 15 and 15 to 19 respectively. Identical definitions of phases were employed for women and men. It is impossible to fix a single age for the onset of menopause for all women, but the cut-off ages set for the prime of life serve well enough.

Our review of suicide and the life-course looks first at men, and advances from the youngest to the oldest phases. According to witnesses' observations, the troubles that affected male pre-adolescents (n = 60) and adolescents (n = 465) differed radically from the problems that burdened older males. Four out of ten pre-adolescent suicides (41.6 percent) had motives rarely seen among other age groups; they had character and adjustment issues. For pre-adolescents and, to a degree, adolescents, specific issues included disputes with parents, feelings of inadequacy about getting on in life, poor performance at school, low self-esteem, loneliness, and aimlessness. Among adolescents, a number of motives were notably under-represented. These included alcohol and substance abuse; 4.5 percent of adolescent suicides were attributed to this motive as the primary factor versus 7.1 percent for all other males. Additional under-represented motives included work and finance (10.5 percent versus 11.6). More impressive were the differences with respect to physical ailments (4.9 percent versus 18.2), and mental illness (14.0 percent versus 27.8).

Character and adjustment was an over-represented motive for adolescents when compared to older men (18.1 percent versus 4.6), although not quite as dramatically over-represented as for pre-adolescents. A few adolescents tested authority and asserted autonomy, but compared to pre-adolescents, rebellion occurred less often in the family circle or school. Adolescents transgressed in and against the wider community. Their motives thus included encounters with the police (9.0 percent versus 4.0 for all males), and marital or romantic scrapes (18.5 percent versus 13.3 for all males). The latter consisted chiefly of broken relationships rather than marital disputes, for very few adolescents were married. In sum, adolescent problems originated disproportionately in clashes with authority. Chapter seven takes this observation and adds case-based evidence about home and school life, criminal justice, and relationships with young women. Pre-adolescents and adolescents led the way with respect to unknown motives (30.0 and 13.5 percent versus 10.1 for all males). No historical records can establish whether a disproportionate number of character and adjustment problems stemmed from Attention Deficit Hyperactivity Disorder, which is characterized by problems with inattentiveness, overactivity, or impulsivity. It seems likely that this disorder was implicated in a number of cases. Learning disabilities may also have adversely affected some young people to the extent that they knew they were falling behind in the quest for a good life. A few witnesses in the deaths of young people made the connection between a learning disability and loss of interest in life. These individuals did not merely perceive differences between themselves and others; they recognized a real gap that would make a difference in their material circumstances.

Men in their prime constituted the largest group of suicides (n = 5,113); men in their forties had the highest suicide rate of any age-gender group for most of the century, and the prime years were defined in a way that happened to take in many years. As a result of these two factors, a large block of men drives statistical findings. Compared to all other adult male suicides, men in their prime were more likely to be physically healthy. Only 10.8 percent of all male suicides in their prime were believed by witnesses to have had an illness as a primary motive, as opposed to 36.9 percent of the men in older phases of the life-course. Mental health, work and finance problems, problems with the police, and an assortment of minor motives were neither over-represented nor under-represented. Two motives were over-represented when men in their prime were compared with other adult males: alcohol or drug abuse (9.3 percent versus 6.5 of all older men), and marital or romantic problems (17.3 percent versus 3.6). This last observation is important enough to drive an inquiry that occupies most of chapter two.[23]

Men in their prime could get up to mischief and violence, destabilize relationships, and feel injured, shamed, or vengeful when called to account. Marital or romantic problems came in a multitude of shades; the number of specific problems that we listed while reading the case files reached at least two hundred and fifty. The more prominent ones were the following: the deceased was separated and could not handle it (16.8 percent of the troubles in this motive cluster), broke up with girlfriend (9.0), argued with spouse, de facto partner, or girlfriend (6.9), wife left and was applying for child custody (2.8), marital trouble unspecified (2.3), marital or de facto relationship was breaking up (2.1), fiancée had broken off engagement (2.0), deceased was upset when relationship ended (1.5), and deceased was separated from long-term partner (1.4). No explanations for the collapse of a relationship are offered now. No shouts of anger or cries of disappointment are reconstructed at this point. Evidence on these important matters in social and cultural history will sustain the discussions about men and sex in chapter two.

The over-represented primary motives for the suicides of men in transition from their prime years to their status as seniors consisted of work and finance troubles (18.5 percent of the men in this age group versus 13.3 for all men) and physical health (25.0 percent versus 18.2). Many men in this transitional phase of life had acquired responsibilities and debts; when things turned sour they could not envision starting out again. The leading specific problem within the work and finance motive cluster was the burden of debt, because it accounted for 13.3 percent of the work and finance motives for this age group. Men in the transitional years had to worry about keeping pace in physically demanding jobs; the second most common problem was unemployment accompanied by an illness which complicated the situation (4.3). A few had been made redundant (4.3). Some operated a business and worried about its viability (2.9).

For the men in transition (n = 1,138), the list of ailments is not as long as it is for seniors (213 problems versus 316). Also, the leading medical problems varied slightly from those that made seniors despondent, because work was still tied up with the self-definition and self-respect of men in transition, and thus illnesses and employment worries were connected. The major health problems mentioned by witnesses include a stroke and having to quit work (6.5 percent), emphysema and having to quit work (4.3 percent), fear of cancer but diagnosis incomplete (3.2), heart problem (2.1), assorted disabilities and worried about unemployment as a result (1.1), kidney disease (1.1), cancer and feared treatment (1.1), and terminal lung cancer with pain (1.1). The data on health problems and graphic descriptions in autopsy reports remind us of tobacco's health costs to individuals.

Seniors (n = 1,068) were substantially under-represented in a number of motive categories when considered in relation to other adult males. Alcohol or drug abuse, marital or romantic discord, and trouble with police were negligible. Work or financial problems seemed a motive for suicide in a few instances, but the proportion fell below that of other mature men. Thus 7.4 percent of senior males were alleged to have been subject to stresses of this sort; for younger men over the age of nineteen, it was 15.0 percent. Mental health was a less significant motive than it was for younger men (17.0 percent versus 24.2). Witnesses attributed half of the suicides of older men (51.7 percent) primarily to poor physical health. The list of ailments includes the following: no specific problem cited but very old and ill (9.3 percent), strokes (4.1), severe heart problems (3.8), severe emphysema (2.5), prostate cancer (2.4), lung cancer (1.8), high blood pressure, hypertension, and anxiety (1.6), Parkinson's Disease (0.9), and loss of sight (0.9). In chapter five, we return to physical ailments and consider whether certain cases of suicide can be treated as self-euthanasia. Inconsolable grief and unbearable loneliness after the death of a loved one was never a major motive for suicide among men, but understandably it figured slightly more prominently in the suicides of this oldest age group (2.0 percent versus 0.8 for all other age groups).

Men will be considered often in subsequent chapters. It is time to introduce the troubles that deeply upset women. Pre-adolescent girls who took their lives were exceedingly rare (n = 19). Most cases appeared in the 1980s (n = 3, 15.8 percent of the girls) and 1990s (n = 12, 63.2 percent). The sexual revolution played a part, because young girls with troubles at home were vulnerable to the attentions of randy young men. Adolescent women appeared more commonly than pre-adolescents among the century's suicides (n = 148). In relative terms even this number was minor, but each case shocked a community. The cases were concentrated in the 1980s (n = 31, 20.9 percent of the adolescent women) and 1990s (n = 66, 44.6 percent). The leading specific motives for these adolescents could be grouped under the heading of character and adjustment. The specific troubles usually related to violent disagreements about the company they were keeping. Adolescent women who ended their young lives were remarkably susceptible to marital or romantic problems. For nearly a quarter of adolescent women (23.0 percent), the motives were associated with a broken relationship, and the prominence of the related motive cluster of character and adjustment problems far exceeded that found among the older age groups (18.9 percent versus 3.5). Mental illness for adolescents was under-represented compared to older women (24.3 percent versus 45.0 for all life-course phases).

Broadly speaking, women who had taken their own lives were more likely than men to have been described by witnesses as mentally ill or romantically disappointed. There was a life-course bias to these characterizations. Compared to older women, those in their prime (n = 1,556) were over-represented when it came to the motives of marital and romantic troubles (13.4 percent of the women in this age group versus 2.4 percent for more mature women). Mental illness was also over-represented among women in their prime (48.9 percent versus 45.0 for all life-course phases). Women in their prime whose primary motive for suicide appears to have been connected with a mental illness were described by witnesses as depressed (31.0 percent of the mental illness cases), very depressed (5.9), experiencing a nervous breakdown (4.5), deeply depressed (4.3), suffering from an unspecified psychotic illness (3.0), and suffering from schizophrenia and on medication (2.9). There was a slight tendency among women in their prime for greater substance abuse motives (5.1 percent versus 2.9).

Since psychiatry operated in a state of nearly constant adjustment and internal controversy during the century, it is not surprising that an assortment of treatments was reported by witnesses, although roughly one in six women in their prime with a mental illness motive seem to have received no treatment. This estimate is likely low, because of under-reporting on account of shame. Treatment for mental illness frequently came from a general practitioner

(9.2 percent of the cases with mental illness cited), a general hospital (3.2), Porirua Psychiatric Hospital (3.1), or Sunnyside Psychiatric Hospital (2.2). Others in smaller numbers had been attended to at another psychiatric hospital, a general hospital, or a private clinic. By the late twentieth century, an assortment of facilities and specialists were available in the major cities; clinical records depict considerable attention to individuals' life histories, traumatic incidents, and descriptions of how they presented themselves. No single report of appearances, history, diagnosis, and therapy resembled another. An account of mental illnesses and treatment occupies chapter four. Physical ailments were not as prominent as they were for older women. When compared to men in their prime, women in the same phase of the life-course were a law-abiding group. Rarely was an encounter with the police cited as motive.

Women in the transitional phase of the life-course (n = 373) were in stable relationships for the most part. Marital and romantic troubles had been weathered or had not arisen as a crisis in their lives. Mental illness was slightly less prominent as a motive, although witnesses still mentioned it frequently (46.4 percent of the women in this phase). The great difference emerged with physical illnesses. For the great majority of women who committed suicide in their prime, physical health had not been a weighty concern; however, in the transitional phase it accounted for more than a quarter of the motives (25.5 percent). For seniors (n = 338), witnesses and suicide notes designated ill health as a motive in four out of ten instances (41.7 percent).

Troubles altered along the life-courses for men and women. Preadolescents and adolescents were especially prone to rash behaviour when they struggled to find an identity among peers and when rebelling against authority at home, school, and the wider society. A very few took their campaigns for autonomy to an absurd extreme, but an extreme better understood if considered in relation to criticism or punishment in the family and at school. Men and women in their prime had gender-based problems. Some were biological, related to reproduction and sexuality. Some originated in cultural norms. The way the male-dominated culture sorted out work and pleasures along gender lines put men at risk of self-estimations of failure and left a few women feeling worn out, severely disappointed, and depressed. Economic crises made matters worse for people in their prime, although in the last two decades of the century, young people were the group at risk. As men and women advanced into a transitional phase of life and beyond, failing health became a leading motive for self-destruction.

ECONOMIC STATUS

Over the course of the century, the proportion of suicides for many occupational groups showed continuity. For the following groups of occupations, the proportion of suicides committed in each of the six types of years were relatively small and subject to limited fluctuation: elite professionals (fluctuated in a band from 1.4 to 2.7 percent of all male suicides), owners of large businesses (0.7 to 2.2), lesser professionals and high-status white-collar workers (0.6 to 1.3), owners of small businesses (2.8 to 4.9), men in lower-status white-collar occupations (2.0 to 5.1), and skilled labourers (10.6 to 13.3). Semi-skilled and unskilled male labourers were numerous among the suicide cases, but they were also abundant in society at large. Their proportion of the suicides stayed relatively stable over the century (16.1 to 22.4 percent). The New Zealand census aggregated occupations in several different formats over the century; that condition makes it impossible to prepare reliable estimates on the over- or under-representation of a group of occupations among suicides. If poorer status groups were more prominent among the suicide case files, it was likely due to their considerable representation in the populace. We cannot say that the poor were over-represented, but thanks to witnesses' statements and suicide notes, we can show how a loss of work and debts inflicted stress.

Several big exceptions to the patterns of consistency point to dramatic upsets in the structure of the economy. The relative prosperity experienced by many in the era of national development ended with the Great Depression, when farmer suicides accounted for about one in six of all male suicides (15.4 percent). The worldwide slump in commodity prices hit the rural sector immediately following bountiful years when farmers had aggressively financed expansion by borrowing. After 1940, prospects generally improved year after year. Farmer suicides dropped to one suicide in nine (11.0) during the long prosperity. By investing in equipment and rural electrification, farmers reduced their need for casual labour. With a decline in rural jobs, farm workers faded from the scene; once prominent among suicides (15.7 to 13.6 percent of all male suicides though to the end of World War II), rural labourers became the subject of fewer and fewer suicide inquests (4.2 percent in the long prosperity; 2.0 percent in the era of crises).

In the era of economic crises, a number of farmers retired, sold out, or became more astutely entrepreneurial. In this turbulent period, relative to all other male occupational groups, there were fewer farmer suicides than during the long prosperity. The proportion of all male suicides represented by farmers plummeted to 4.2 percent in the 1980s and 1990s. To develop a more complete picture of the impact of crises on farmers, it is essential to keep in mind that this stunning decline in the proportion of farmer suicides relative to all male suicides took place when the country's overall suicide rate was climbing, eventually exceeding the low of the long prosperity by roughly fifty percent.[24] While the relative number of farmer suicides fell, the absolute number rose slightly when compared to the years of the long prosperity. The average number of farmer suicides per year during the long prosperity was thirteen; in the era of crises it was fifteen; in the Great Depression, when the national population was less than half what it was in 1990, the average number of farmer suicides per year was twenty-six.

By the crude measure of farmer suicides, the Great Depression had a far more severe impact on rural New Zealand than the hard adjustments forced in the era of economic crises. Another comparison merits attention. Work and finance motives were moderately prominent among farmer suicides in the 1980s and 1990s (16.9 percent of all motives), but mental illness motives increased notably. These latter motives appeared as the primary ones in 20.5 percent of all motives for farmers in the Great Depression, 20.9 percent in the era of long prosperity, and 35.7 percent in the era of economic crises. At the end of the century, it is probable that economic worries were examined under a cultural lens that focused on emotional and mental health outcomes rather than social and economic stressors. As well, unemployment in an age of welfare benefits led to idle time with opportunities for alcohol and cannabis abuse, with resultant low moods or neural damage. Stress and suicide were being medicalized, not just by the emerging mental health industry but by escapist assaults on the brain. During the period of economic crises the medicalization of suicide applied to more than farmers, the group at risk during the Great Depression. Now young people were disheartened and indulging dangerously.

In the era of economic crises, a rising number of the country's youth and younger adults felt victimized, in the sense that they were not getting a start on the future of their dreams. Economic rationalization extended to more than the farm; the Fourth Labour Government cut back the public sector. As well, by the late 1980s, an Auckland building boom had run out of steam. Older men had ways of coping that had not been there to help their life-phase counterparts during the Great Depression; employees could retire on pensions and some farmers could sell their assets and retire to town. These coping strategies do not mean that all men in their transitional years were pleased about a loss of employment, liquidation of assets, or premature departure from their calling. However, the groups that took the crises on the chin were adolescents and men in their prime. In almost every occupational group, the mean age of suicide fell in the era of crises; the workforce was taking on a different age profile because of redundancies and early retirements. Several facts convey the awful employment situation.

First, redundancy was not the only problem. Getting a first job became more difficult from 1980 to 1990. The number of men who had committed suicide and whose 'occupation' was described as unemployed had always been fairly small; even in the Great Depression it was tiny, because men without work still were identified by witnesses as having a trade. Their trade partly defined them, and they and their families retained the label as a matter of self-respect. In the 1980s and 1990s, an unusually large proportion of men (n = 121) were described simply as "unemployed." In the past, the mean ages of men so described had been around forty-five. During the last two decades of the century, it was twenty-nine.

Second, the number of medical and welfare beneficiaries soared. Since police officers conducting investigations did not always differentiate between the types of beneficiaries, it has been necessary to retain the imprecise but still useful label of "beneficiary." During the long prosperity, there had only been several score beneficiaries who took their own lives. In the era of crises, the number was six hundred and eighty-one. In the past, the mean age of beneficiaries was over forty-five, but in this period it fell to thirty-two. During the era of economic crises, the male population at greatest risk consisted of adolescents and young adults.

Earlier in this chapter, we asserted that "many women were undoubtedly breadwinners." Among women who committed suicide, the proportion in waged labour or working on their own account for income hovered around one in five or one in six until the last two decades of the century, when it reached one in four (24.9 percent of all women in the years of economic crises). One in five was the proportion for the whole century (19.9 percent). In other words, the great majority of women covered in the inquest files were not in waged labour; they occupied other socio-economic categories, including household duties (45.5 percent for the whole century), pension recipient (13.6), beneficiary (7.7), and student (2.8). There were small numbers with other status designations. Household duties included married women described as housewives and single women living at home and caring for a parent. In keeping with many other trends observed so far, a huge shift came in the era of economic crises. As recently as the long prosperity, over half the women committing suicide were in household duties (53.9 percent). In the era of economic crises, the proportion of women in household duties was almost halved (27.2 percent). Other designations grew and included beneficiary (16.2) and student (5.9). The proportion of pensioners fell.

ETHNICITY AND IDENTITY

"Ethnicity" expresses people's roots in what are presumed to be shared experiences. The word's insufficiencies abound when identity has been affected by colonialism. To link ethnicity and Māori is to succumb to colonialism's conceits and marginalize the unique relationship that Māori as a first people have with New Zealand. Nonetheless, as a word that groups peoples outside an ascendant Anglo-Celtic culture, ethnicity serves. Māori accounted for one in fifteen suicides (6.6 percent; n = 768) in the data set. Recent government-sponsored discussions of ethnicity and suicide in New Zealand dwell on current trends for Māori, and properly so. These abundant official reports track trends for Māori suicides over fairly recent years.[25] Our findings roughly agree with these investigations, although we can go back further in time and probe deeper into motives. All sources show that Māori suicides climbed starting around 1980; the most alarming feature has been the substantial portion of suicides among young adults. Toward the end of this section on ethnicity we will consider this phenomenon of Māori youth suicides in relation to occupations, poverty, and motives. Māori suicides are also discussed in later chapters. In particular, chapter seven seeks to explain suicides by young adults in the late twentieth century, and Māori standout during that turbulent period.

We should puzzle over the ease with which writers have accepted the concept of Māori as a stable identity marker for people who committed suicide and for the division of the country's population into ethnic categories. Belief in an actual rate for Māori would be a mistake. The attribution of identity required for time-series comparisons of ethnic rates is questionable, because the concept of Māori at suicide inquests, in death registers, and in the population at large widened to encompass more people over the decades. Self-identification in a multi-ethnic society over a long period is certain to be unstable, altering according to fashion, activism, politics, and benefits. Witnesses' statements covering a century suggest that Māori identity lacked a continuous fixed meaning. Thus rates and percentages of suicides for Māori are partly artefacts of time and place. This warning does not erase the fact that many young Māori, broadly defined, experienced a unique torrent of life-debilitating troubles in the 1980s and 1990s. The official data are not seriously misleading and qualitative information from the inquests convincingly establishes the upset caused by cultural and economic crises in the last two decades of the century.

However, there have been shifts in how individuals identified themselves and how others in turn identified them. These alterations affect ethnic rate calculations. Until the mid-twentieth century, Māori was a narrowly bounded concept. Identity was consistently ascribed and asserted in regions where *whakapapa* was remembered, and that restricted identity had official sanction. The 1908 Births and Deaths Registration Act established a separate registry for Māori deaths that applied to Māori living in particular districts that the governor proclaimed from time to time; additionally, persons of mixed race living as Māori in any tribal situation were deemed Māori. From 1913 to 1961, the government maintained the register and its underlying assumptions about Māori identity as tribal.[26] Urban Māori were out of the picture.

Colonization and displacement during the nineteenth and early twentieth centuries left Māori social life vibrant mainly in specific rural locales, many in rugged and remote North Island settings with marginal economies related to grazing and forestry. *Whakapapa* and identity were maintained there. The existence of decidedly

Māori communities meant that Māori suicides were unequivocally Māori and comparatively rare. Up to the 1970s, these rural suicides disclosed motives common for the entire country and related to hard experiences shared with Pākehā, such as physical and mental illnesses, debt, severe alcohol abuse, war trauma, and relationship troubles.[27] In addition, there were nuances of raging jealousies, infidelities, abuse, matters of honour, disputes, and frictions.[28] As burdens of isolation, these troubles were a derivative of colonialism. Maelstroms in the past affected how people lived in the present.

It is possible that Māori suicide rates for much of the century were low because the count excluded urban Māori of mixed ancestry who lived under Pākehā names and eschewed Māori identity. Probably witnesses thought of these individuals as Pākehā. However, when someone's first and last name was Māori, that person was unquestionably Māori. The locales where these individuals died were often the farms, hamlets, or small towns of tribal regions. If the deaths of people with Māori names occurred in larger centres, these places were close to Māori regions. A sample of small places where Māori suicides occurred before 1970 reinforces the idea that Māori had a bounded rural identity: Aria, Hunghunga, Omatano, Pipiriki, Puniho, Takapau, Tarawahi, Taupiri, Tokanui, Tokomaru Bay, Ruatoki, Waiotapu, and so forth. Larger centres of note add to this picture of Māori suicides taking place in Māoridom, because they occurred in locales such as Gisborne, Rotorua, and Whanganui. A combination of a Māori first name and Pākehā last name also denoted Māori identity. This arrangement of names became noticeable at inquests in 1930s, and sometimes these individuals were deliberately labelled "New Zealander." Except for the instances of double names, identity seemed anything but straightforward to us, although contemporaries readily 'essentialized' people.

More complications arose when the parents of individuals opted for Pākehā first and last names but a witness at an inquest disclosed that the individual was Māori. This identity clash appeared initially in 1914. It came up sporadically until the 1950s. Afterward, the use of a Māori first or middle name was fairly common. Whether these deceased parties would have approved or not, they were categorized for our purposes as Māori. Naming practices pose a challenge for time-series discussions of Māori suicides. The difficulty can best be expressed as a question. How many suicides in any year involved Māori living with Pākehā names and, apparently by choice or perceived necessity, a non-Māori identity? The unknown figure obstructs tidy discussion.

Later in the century, some individuals proclaimed an *iwi* affiliation or Māori identity while retaining both Pākehā first and last names. In the 1970s, Pākehā first and last names were borne by a quarter of Māori suicides; by the 1980s, a third. More individuals than before self-identified as Māori; witnesses reported this identity, which then appeared on autopsy forms and in coroners' findings. No longer did Pākehā first and second names erase Māori identity quite as often as in the past. The places where Māori suicides now occurred included city suburbs, places such as Lower Hutt, Mangere, and Otahuhu. Several larger towns close to Māori regions remained prominent: Hastings, Napier, Gisborne, Whangarei, and Whanganui. Genealogical concealment persisted late in the century and still led to some under-counting of Māori suicides. However, the earlier under-counting is the more significant problem, since the quite low figures that result serve as backdrop to a shocking transformation in Māori circumstances starting in the 1980s. Was the increase real or a derivative of shifts in identity?

Judging from autopsy reports prepared late in the century and assuming that for decades Māori was a bounded identity, Māori suicides from 1900 to approximately 1970 may have been under-counted by at least a third if an open understanding of Māori identity is applied. The "missing Māori" in these many decades were men and women who had taken on Pākehā first and last names; witnesses had not gone into the individuals' ancestry. Should we regard the problem of identity as under-counting early in the century, or as a problem of a late-twentieth-century overestimate of Māori suicides? That latter proposition would apply if we adopted a strict identity threshold in which Pākehā first and last names denoted a family's reticence about Māori identity and removed the individual from our set of Māori suicides. Undoubtedly, there has been a core Māori population. Beyond that, who decides on identity and for what purposes? The complications with an elastic identity mean that Māori suicide rates are imprecise signals. They are signals all the same.

The possibility of under-counting is important. Consider a line of reasoning that dismisses under-counting and endorses the idea of a fairly low Māori suicide rate until 1980 and a soaring rate thereafter. This thesis lends itself to an argument that the support of extended families in Māori communities insulated youth against disappointment, drift, isolation, and recklessness. Statements at inquests supply some corroborating details for this explanation; they will be mentioned in chapter seven. Beginning in the late 1980s, economic crises and painful social adjustments disproportionately affected young Māori. Reports that young Māori were committing suicide in rising numbers indicated a significant development. Two plausible explanations – prior under-counting and the recent deracination of youth – account for the presumed sharp increase in young Māori suicides. By 1980, more people were identified and identifying as Māori, and more than ever, young Māori were affected by economic and cultural upheavals. The identity issue does not invalidate socio-economic explanations, but places them in a tumultuous era where a lot was happening, much of it corrosive for young adults.

With under-counting in mind, we can venture observations. Until the 1980s, the suicides of Māori, according to inquests, ranged from a low of under three percent of all suicides in the 1910s to just over four percent in the 1970s. The consistently low proportion for most of the century may in part be due to identity conventions. These conventions may also contribute to an explanation of what happened in the last two decades of the century when, based on inquests, Māori suicides were more than one in ten of all suicides (a low of 9.0 percent in 1980; a high of 17.2 percent in 1996). Official estimates for the new millennium go as high as twenty percent.[29] The variation between our findings and official counts at the end of the century is slight. More importantly, the relative youth of the individuals in the last decades of the century is a shared observation; official reports focus on the many young adult Māori who took their own lives. Māori encountered in the inquest files for the 1980s and 1990s definitely included many young adults. The mean age was twenty-nine for the 1980s and twenty-eight for the 1990s. The only comparable period was the decade of 1910s when the mean age was thirty. What the official data cannot report is the enduring age spread between Māori and Pākehā. There was a fourteen-year difference in mean ages evident in the 1980s and a twelve-year one for the 1990s. The spread was highest in the 1930s at almost sixteen years, lowest in the 1960s at nine. For the century it averaged fifteen. The spread never narrowed for long.

This difference in the mean ages between Māori and the rest of the population reflected the lower life expectancy of the former, therefore fewer at-risk people in the transitional or senior phases of life. Māori suicides were rare beyond sixty-five. Teens and young adults were relatively prominent among Māori suicides in every decade. Throughout the entire twentieth century, Māori who took their own lives were younger than the rest of the population. Life expectancy is not the sole explanation. Despair overwhelmed Māori much earlier in life than the rest of the population. However, the absolute numbers of Māori affected were not great until the 1980s. During the years of economic crises, Māori young people shared troubles with other young people, but proportionately they had greater exposure than the rest.

Economic circumstances were implicated in this phenomenon of young Māori suicides throughout the century, although the picture is intricate. Across the century, the level of employment among Māori who had committed suicide was about the same as for others who took their own lives, and unemployment *per se* was not a common motive among Māori suicides. However, their occupations were low-skilled and poor-paying; witnesses reported circumstances or conversations indicating that almost half (47.1 percent) of Māori who committed suicide were not doing well financially, while the same plight had affected a third (33.1 percent) of Pākehā suicides. The statements of witnesses and police constables across the century describe miserable living conditions, initially describing families in rural *whare* and later reporting youth flatting in cities. Poverty undermined social and family life. Consequently, the leading clusters of motives were not overtly financial or work-related, but exposed trouble with the law, family altercations, and relationship problems. To be clear, this set of leading motives was prominent for the entire century, although it shifted into the larger towns and cities with a vengeance by the 1980s. At the end of the century during the years of economic crises, unemployment appeared more pronounced than at other times, and this circumstance was expressed in the greater proportion who received welfare and medical benefits compared to Pākehā. From 1980 to 2000, over one in four (26.1 percent) Māori suicides was a beneficiary; for the rest of the population the proportion dipped to less than one in ten (8.7 percent).

There are two other non-European groups represented in significant enough numbers in the even-numbered years to merit attention, namely Chinese immigrants (n = 76) and Pacific Islanders (n = 126). Their contrasting situations add to the case for studying suicide historically. As a result of immigration restrictions that for many years made it difficult for women to emigrate from China, the individuals who committed suicide were exclusively male until 1960. By and large until the 1960s, they were pensioners and older laundrymen, gardeners, and alluvial gold seekers. Their ages and marital status as single men explain the leading motives for their taking their own lives: physical illness, mental illness, and work or money problems. Relationship troubles and encounters with the law were quite rare. Islanders were readily identified on account of recent immigration and name retention. Over nine in ten suicides (91.5 percent) among this population occurred in the 1980s and 1990s. Unlike individuals from East Asia but similarly to Māori, they were young adults and their work status or occupations comprised a short list. Beneficiaries, labourers, and students accounted for half. Their economic plight in the 1980s and 1990s was not much different from that of Māori. Well over half were not doing well financially, but the leading immediate motive was marital strife. Māori and Islanders will receive more attention in chapter seven.

TECHNOLOGY, INTENT, GENDER, AND METHOD

Trends in suicide methods during the century shifted in association with technology, including chemistry and pharmacology. As well, recourse to a particular method depended on the individual's determination and on access to the necessary material. Two traditional methods, hanging and drowning, were widely accessible (Graph 1.4). Drowning was also a cause of many accidental deaths each year.[30] Some individuals chose it because of the possibility of a coroner's finding of accidental death or an open verdict. Hanging often meant an excruciating death by strangulation; individuals did not always comprehend how to achieve a swift death. Occasionally friends or family discovered individuals who were "brain dead." In the late twentieth century, a few were placed on life support systems.[31] It comes as a shock to observe this archaic method on the rise during the last quarter of the twentieth century. When the proportion of hangings increased, the mean age of those who employed the method dropped from the mid-forties to mid-thirties. Rash young people turned to a crude death. A number of hangings each year throughout the century occurred in a police lock-up or prison, but when the whole century is considered, the overwhelming proportion of deaths

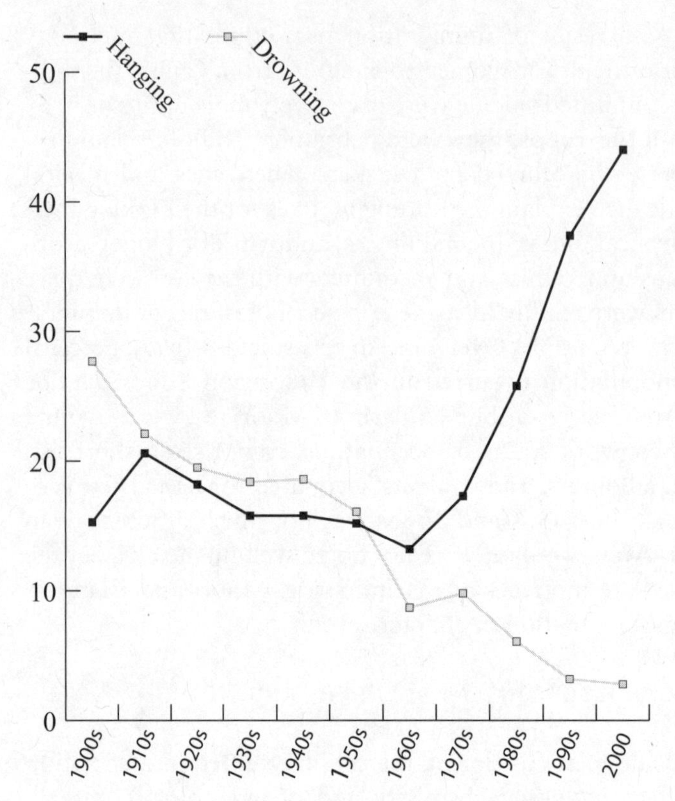

Graph 1.4
Major non-technology-based methods by percentage of deaths, 1900–2000

in custody by hanging transpired in the 1980s and 1990s. Out of seventy such hangings, over three-quarters (77.1 percent) took place in these decades. In these same decades, young women (ages 9 to 24) who committed suicide turned to hanging as never before. What can explain this combination of the young and the crude?

Like drowning, hanging had for decades been a method of self-destruction favoured by people with restricted access to firearms, automobiles, and poisons. Prominent among these individuals were pensioners (10.3 percent of all hangings), housewives (10.2), labourers (4.8), and farm labourers (4.2). Hanging was a method of the powerless and poor. It accounted for a steady fifteen percent of all suicide deaths, but abruptly, in the last two decades of the century and especially during the 1990s, it soared into prominence among secondary-school and university students. The rise in youth suicide contributed to the leap in suicides by hanging. The mean age of men and women who employed this method remained consistently in the mid-forties in all decades until the 1980s and 1990s when it fell (40.4 in 1980s; 34.4 in 1990s). Of the two hundred and fifteen students who committed suicide in the sample for the 1980s and 1990s, almost half hanged themselves (n = 99, 46.0 percent).

The sudden escalation in hangings by students transpired in cities. Urban students at the end of the century who considered taking their own lives had relatively few techniques available. Their choices narrowed if action followed an impulse, which was the case for many young people acting while intoxicated or in a rage. In rural New Zealand, guns and agricultural poisons were at hand, although by the early 1960s the Ministries of Health and Agriculture had intensified management of restricted herbicides and pesticides.[32] In the first three decades of the century, a common rodent poison, Rough on Rats, was readily available and used in at least one suicide a year (Figure 1.2). In the countryside, there were alternatives to hanging even if access to them had become better controlled. In the cities, older people had choices too, including access to medication. From around 1950 until the mid-1970s, barbiturates were favoured by seniors. Adults also had greater access to vehicles and thus death by carbon monoxide poisoning. Not all suicidal young people in cities were restricted in their choices, but sufficient constraints applied in enough instances to shift upward the numbers of hangings by preadolescents and adolescents.

There are also conjectural explanations for young people employing hanging. First, hanging did not leave a mutilated body. A streak of narcissism in young men and women or a concept of life after death within the current body-form may have deterred a few young people from mutilating their bodies or subjecting them to decay or attack in rivers or the sea. Drowning remained an older person's method. For the elderly, the body had less appeal in its state of decline. Second, in a few cases the intent of some young people was not to die. They hoped for discovery, rescue, and sympathy; in the estimation of some coroners, a few adolescents had set up the hanging to manipulate a relationship but had expected a rescue and apology.[33] Strangulation by hanging allowed intervention, but the margin between discovery and death was tight, a circumstance that might not have been well calculated (if considered at all) by young people in a flush of anger.

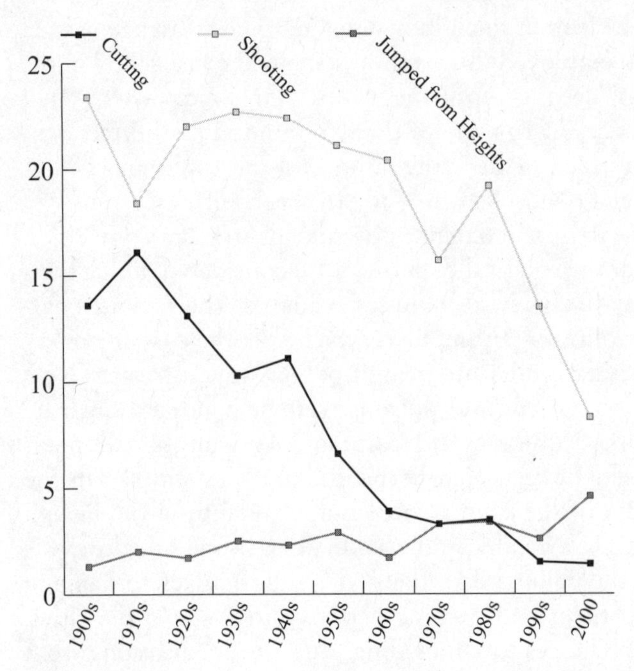

Graph 1.5
Major violent methods by percentage of deaths, 1900–2000

The remaining unsophisticated methods, namely cutting, shooting, and jumping from heights, inflicted the greatest violence to the body of all frequently used methods (Graph 1.5). Throughout the century, men had greater recourse to them than women. These violent methods involved minimal technology, although cutting to achieve swift death required knowledge of anatomy that many individuals lacked.[34] As a consequence, a few men and women had lingering deaths in hospitals; a few succumbed to septic pneumonia rather than to the loss of blood.[35] The decline in cutting that occurred from the 1910s to the 1960s expresses the growing popularity of the safety razor. For the entire century, the straight razor accounted for nearly sixty percent (n = 438; 59.4 percent) of the cases of self-destruction by cutting. This often-used instrument was passing from the scene by the 1950s. From the 1930s forward, the straight razor appeared mainly in the suicides of men in their fifties and sixties. Women infrequently chose the straight razor; the ratio of men to women was nine to one across the decades (over 88.9 percent to 11.1 percent).

Firearms were commonplace; however, non-accidental self-inflicted shooting deaths (n = 2,081) occurred with greater frequently in rural and remote rural areas (33.4 percent of all such suicides) and in small towns (18.2 percent) than in larger towns (17.4 percent) or city suburbs (15.3 percent) or inner-city areas (7.0 percent). Of all suicide deaths by firearms, nearly six out of ten involved a rifle (57.5 percent). Māori had a preference for the shotgun (44.3 percent as opposed to 26.8 percent for Pākehā). Pistols were useless for hunting and thus handguns appeared primarily at suicides in towns and cities. Only two Māori suicides in the entire data set involved handguns.

Several technological innovations that reached into households had lethal potential. The first was coal gas (Graph 1.6). With New Zealand's pattern of gender roles that positioned women in domestic work for much of the century, it comes as no surprise that coal gas, prominent as an urban cooking fuel, was a major method for women. Over a third of coal gas suicides (38.7 percent) in the century were by women, but women altogether accounted for less than a quarter of the century's suicides (23.6 percent). As households converted their cooking and heating equipment to electricity or natural gas, coal gas deaths fell away. Other 'soporific poisons' appeared. The most important was automobile-generated carbon monoxide. This odourless and colourless gas, produced by the incomplete combustion of carbon fuels, forms a strong bond with the iron atom in haemoglobin, impairing the oxygen-carrying capacity of blood.[36] Increasing automobile ownership influenced domestic architecture, thus affecting the locales for suicides. Largely on account of the carbon monoxide method, the garage after World War II became the second most common site for suicides (9.7 percent), following the house (28.2 percent). During the 1990s, the garage assumed greater prominence; it became the scene for one in five suicides (21.9 percent). Carbon monoxide poisoning led the list of garage-based deaths, but hanging followed closely, particularly in the 1980s and 1990s (Graphs 1.6 and 1.7). The decline in the proportion of suicides by carbon monoxide detected in 2000 will accelerate as an unintended outcome of automobiles having catalytic converters that reduce carbon monoxide by 75 to 90 percent.[37]

A dreadful explanation for the late-century prominence of garage hangings emerges from the period's much remarked-upon rise in suicides of young people. Some despondent young people who took their lives had a limited choice of means; hanging was uncomplicated. Furthermore, quite a few very young people in the 1980s and 1990s acted impulsively after arguments in the home. The garage offered a convenient location and, for some young people, a location that could have resulted in a hoped-for discovery and rescue. Intent, age, resources, knowledge, and the precipitating circumstances influenced the method and location of self-destruction.

The status of men as heads of households, thus as car owners and licence holders, explains carbon monoxide's appearance as a male technique. Males accounted for 85.7 percent of all carbon monoxide cases. It was entirely a male method in the 1940s, and nearly so in the 1950s (90.6 percent) and 1960s (90.1). During these same years, barbiturates became a predominately female method (54.8 percent of barbiturate deaths) with peak use in the 1960s (57.5 percent). Women turned to barbiturates with uncanny timing; as coal gas declined, barbiturates took its place. Then, quite suddenly, in the early 1970s the number of barbiturate suicides collapsed (Graph 1.6).

In the 1950s, 1960s, and 1970s, the Department of Health, as well as local medical officers, circularized doctors in an effort to get them to cut back on prescribing barbiturates. At first, general practitioners took little heed and prescriptions rose. As one defensive doctor put it at a suicide inquest, "even if barbiturates could be made unavailable, there would still be suicides. There is nothing to stop such persons from buying far more deadly poisons, from any grocer, seed merchant or florist." He conceded that access could be controlled by limiting prescriptions.[38] The national consumption of barbiturate sedatives climaxed in 1972 at roughly twenty-one million doses; in 1974 it had slackened to just over fourteen million.[39] On 1 December 1976, the government struck barbiturates off the list of medications available at pharmacies free of charge under social security.

Official alarm about addiction, overdose deaths, and suicides culminated in a "Barbiturates Conference" in Wellington on 23 February 1977 attended by twenty-two leaders of medical groups. The slide in barbiturate suicides had already begun.[40] Conference participants, wanting to accelerate the retreat in addiction, overdoses, and suicides, recommended that doctors be pressured to reduce their prescriptions and that personnel from the Department of Health visit practitioners who prescribed significant quantities.[41] Prior to the

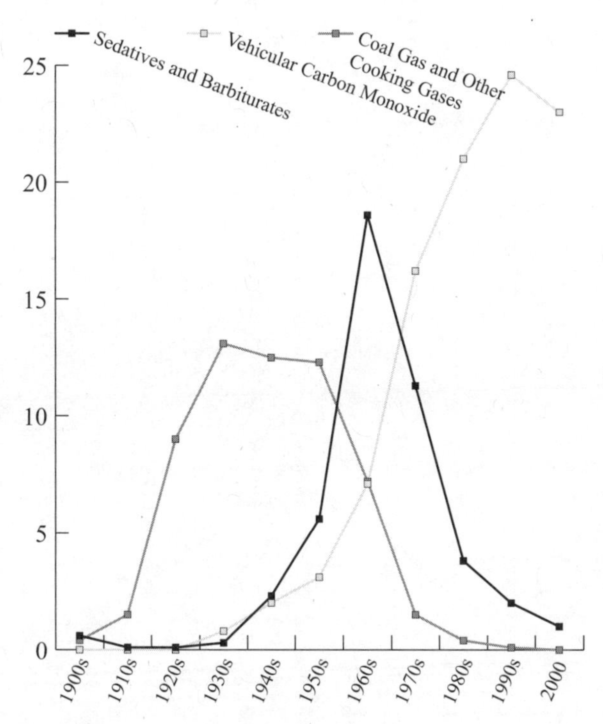

Graph 1.6
Major sleep-inducing methods by percentage of deaths, 1900–2000

conference, in a plea for autonomy, doctors claimed that "very few practitioners admit to having instituted barbiturate therapy in recent years except for the use of phenobarbitone in some cases of epilepsy or as a temporary measure in times of stress or grief of bereavement."[42] Since the introduction of safer sedatives, the elderly were deemed the principal users of barbiturates; some of these older long-time users had developed a dependency.[43] This age claim is borne out by the mean age of the women and men who deliberately took fatal overdoes. During the last half of the century that figure was fifty years or more.

By the 1970s, each death from a narcotic overdose, suicidal or accidental, received substantial attention from the police, health officials, and coroners. Inquests took officers into the squalor of the urban illicit drug scene. Evidence about addicts' living conditions, paraphernalia for injections, a drug subculture, and crimes committed to secure drugs came to light in a few inquests. Coroners also disclosed the naiveté of several doctors whom police believed

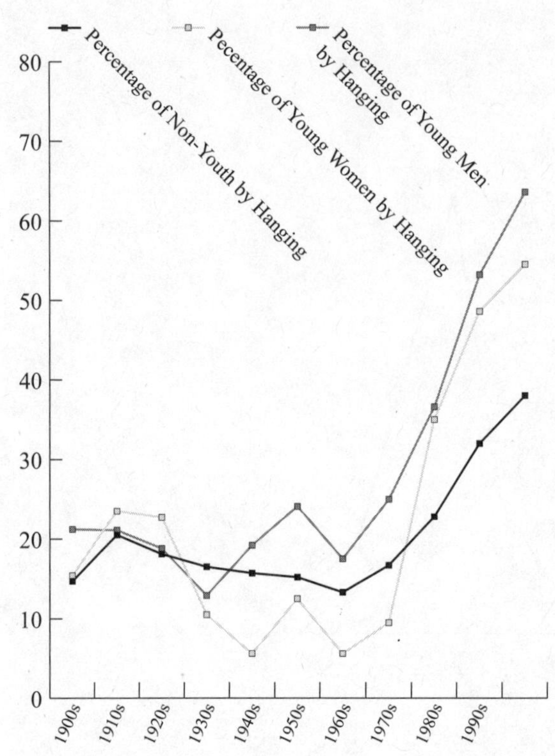

Graph 1.7
Return of hanging in the late twentieth century, 1900–2000

had recklessly prescribed methadone.[44] In terms of suicides, however, there was abundant smoke but little fire. For the entire century, we found fewer than a hundred cases of suicide by narcotics (n = 95), even when we added cases of an overdose that a coroner found accidental but, after reassessment of evidence, we considered deliberate. This relatively modest figure includes methadone poisoning. Narcotics seldom topped one percent of the methods in any decade (Graph 1.8). Half (47.4 percent) of the deaths by narcotics and methadone occurred in the 1990s. Dr D.M.F. McDonald, superintendent of Carrington Psychiatric Hospital, explained the relative scarcity of narcotics as a method of suicide in 1974. "It would be easier to commit suicide with a combination of barbiturates and booze," he explained, "than it would be with narcotics."[45] Individuals who took barbiturates to end their lives frequently had an adjacent bottle of scotch, gin, or sherry. Dr McDonald added that his

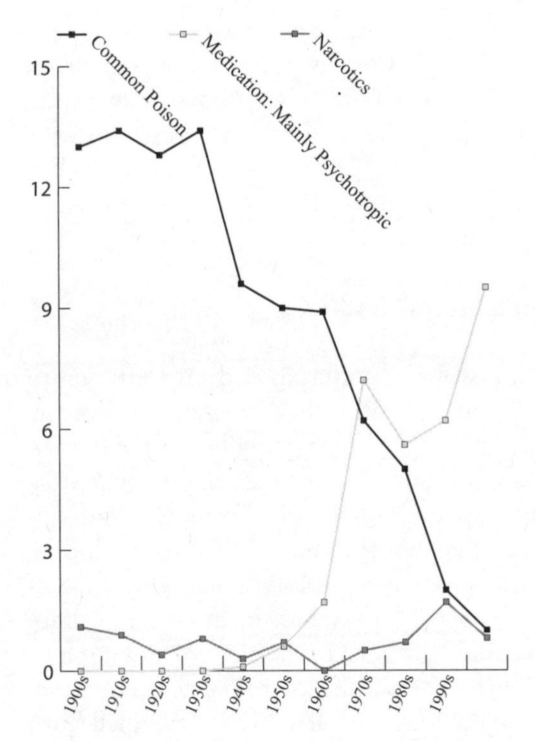

Graph 1.8
Chemical means: Poisons, medication, and narcotics by percentage of deaths, 1900–2000

experiences made him more concerned about alcohol abuse than narcotic addiction. He suggested that a perceived threat to order and property from drug abusers had panicked the public, who then ignored the greater social harm of alcoholism.

Women favoured poisons throughout the century (34.1 percent of all poison suicides). During the first three decades, swallowing the disinfectant Lysol had been a fairly common and painful method. The fluid burned the throat, oesophagus, and stomach. It did not kill quickly, and for that reason police constables were able to interview some of the men and women who took it.[46] Its use dropped as did the overall ingestion of toxic substances, many of which had produced prolonged painful deaths.[47] Women's preference for suicide by toxic substances persisted with the appearance of psychotropic drugs late in the century. For women, there was a definite succession spanning the century, beginning with household toxins and then moving to coal gas, barbiturates, and finally including new psychotropic drugs. The majority of overdoses of these later drugs involved women (59.0 percent of those who used this method). The figure had risen at the end of the century (62.6 percent in the 1990s). Each of the new generation of drugs used as a method of self-destruction – Amitriptyline, Doxepin, Dothiepin, Nortriptyline, and Prothiaden – was an antidepressant.

CONCLUDING REMARKS

This chapter introduced a history of suffering and rage attuned to continuities and changes during a century and over the life-course. An associated objective was to emphasize the fragility of the human spirit, and to point out how conditions in New Zealand's economic and cultural development impacted this spirit. To understand suicide, it is essential to be familiar with a society's history, including economic fortunes, types of employment and self-employment, demography, and technology. Prior to the establishment of the welfare state, many male suicides could be traced to the rigours and insecurity of employment in a particular setting of primary production. After the late 1930s the opportunity to work, when coupled with the safety net of the welfare state, turned a land of plenty into a land of contentment. This generalization works as a reasonable summary of the era of prosperity. When global conditions undercut employment and precipitated the era of crises, burdens fell disproportionately on the young and on individuals early in their prime of life, but the welfare state assisted men in their prime who had experienced some contentment in previous years. The young had no adult experience with such a period and worried about the future. Mental illness was a major motive for men and particularly women throughout the century. However, use of terms such as mental illness, mental disorders, and mental health requires vigilance, because their definitions were short on objective measurements. As well, due to a late-twentieth-century clinical focus on checking off symptoms and prescribing medication, mental-illness diagnoses could be detached from any interest in the precipitating root troubles of economic setbacks. In addition to mental illnesses and anxieties rooted in economic stress, troubled relationships and sex were sources of upset. We now turn to these latter problems, and particularly to the conduct of men. The following chapter overflows with rage.

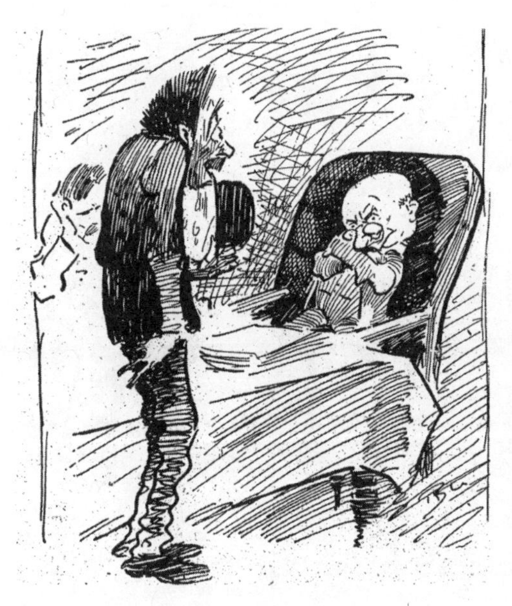

Figure 1.1
"Coroner: 'Now, witness, I caution you before you answer, remember it is a grave matter, and to withhold any information in front of this Court of His Majesty the King is too awful for me to explain. Now, sir, you say you know what the motive the deceased had in committing suicide? Answer at once.' Scared witness: 'Yes your honour, he wanted to kill himself.'" The tautological answer was only slightly less enlightening than end-of-century academic explanations that noted that suicidal people had a mental disorder that made them perceive that life was empty. The image was scanned from the *Observer*, 19 February 1910. Courtesy of Alexander Turnbull Library, National Library of New Zealand, Te Puna Mātauranga o Aotearoa.

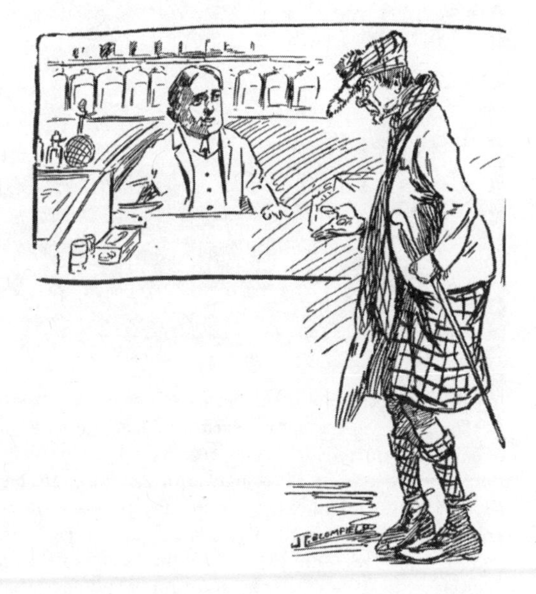

Figure 1.2
Ethnic jibes were once a common feature of humour and the Scots of the South Island were not exempt. "Customer: 'Twa penny worth o' Rough on Rats.' Chemist: 'We only sell it in sixpenny packets.' Customer: 'I'll no commit suicide.'" Rough on Rats was a poor person's means of a cheap and miserable death. The image was scanned from the *New Zealand Free Lance*, 8 September 1906. Courtesy of Alexander Turnbull Library, National Library of New Zealand, Te Puna Mātauranga o Aotearoa.

Figure 1.3
Employment insecurity meant that workers needed friends or relatives to help them through hard times. Single immigrants had a difficult time. "Mr Merchant: 'You mustn't talk of committing suicide my man. Why should you take this step?' New chum: 'Well, sir, I've been here every day for the last three months and I haven't got a job yet.'" The image was scanned from the *New Zealand Free Lance*, 9 September 1905. Courtesy of Alexander Turnbull Library, National Library of New Zealand, Te Puna Mātauranga o Aotearoa.

TOUGH TALKING WATCH-DOG NOT REAPPOINTED —NEWS
HIT AND RUN WOULD BE MY PRELIMINARY FINDING...
GARRY EVANS CORONER

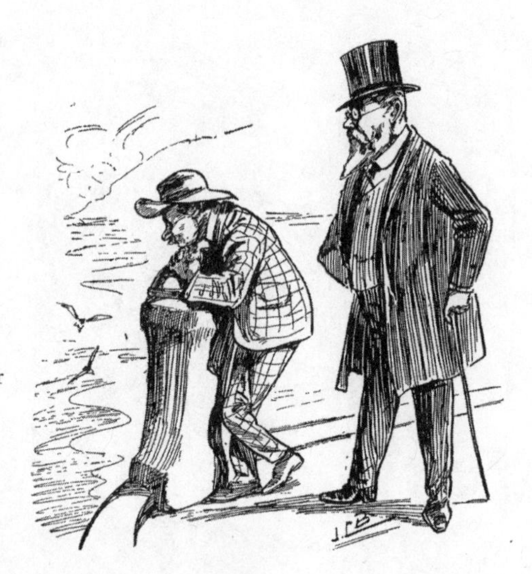

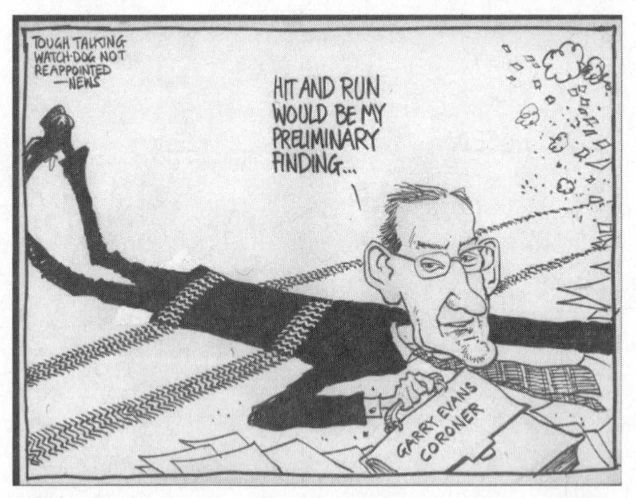

Figure 1.4
In former British colonies, the office of coroner evolved in distinct directions. In New Zealand, they were usually magistrates; legal rather than medical training was and remains a characteristic. Some coroners, taking the view that they should work to prevent violent deaths, unflinchingly criticized hospitals, doctors, prison officials, and people's conduct. Following a re-organization of the service to create a corps of full-time professionals, one "tough-talking watch dog" was not re-appointed when a government minister took exception to his stand on the right of the press to report suicides. Coroner Garry Evans was subsequently appointed and promptly entrusted with some of the country's more difficult inquests. The cartoon appeared in *The Dominion Post*, 8 June 2007. With permission of the artist, Tom Scott. Courtesy of Alexander Turnbull Library, National Library of New Zealand, Te Puna Mātauranga o Aotearoa.

2

Relationships: Sex, Alcohol, and Violence, 1900–80

A higher rate of *completed* suicides for men than women appears in the suicide data for a multitude of countries. New Zealand's inquest files suggest that this pattern has persisted for a long time (Graph 1.3). Discussions of this gender difference must begin with a firm warning. Any explanations for the male lead in suicides must take into account the greater number of "unsuccessful" attempts by women. The gender gap in completed suicides does not measure relative gender suffering. In fact, a fair number of inquests into male suicides expose men who abused women; the alarming capacity of men to bring harm to themselves and others figures all too often at inquests. Why should this have been the case? Why is it still the case?

We can begin looking for answers in the world of waged labour, a realm of daily social interaction and self-reflection dominated by men and intrinsic to ideas of masculinity. Work for pay was the great non-biological separator of men and women. Many men accepted an accompanying masculine duty to provide; however, as we are about to see in graphic detail, a few men rejected this obligation to family. Men raged when courts imposed maintenance orders directing a delinquent husband to support his wife, or wife and children, after legal separation. These orders precipitated some vengeance suicides, because men challenged by their wives had a fundamental belief that their wages earned them complete ownership of everything in the residence and command over all within.

Late in the century, under the conditions of a welfare state fused with a consumer culture, work for pay had less urgency and immediacy in relation to the duty to provide. At this juncture, more than ever before, income for younger men meant access to a car and a girl. In a consumer society under-girded by a welfare state, in the age of the sexual revolution, work for pay became a critical matter for younger men. For many older men, a job was less urgent than it had been in prior decades when to be out of work was to face destitution, to carry the burdens of a household, and to tremble at the shame of bankruptcy. Men and remuneration remained inseparable during the entire century, but late in the century the shrinkage of entry-level jobs dealt younger men a body blow. The employment crisis for youth that persisted through much of the 1980s and into the 1990s was a rude and momentous upset; it changed the age group most affected by the creed of work for pay. No pattern in suicide data is explicable without a consideration of the times, and the late twentieth century stands out as a difficult time for young men and for a few young women, who now more than ever were also seeking waged labour. The unusual economic and cultural tides of change in the late twentieth century receive special attention later in the book when youth suicide is a focus. Therefore, this chapter by and large deals with trends up to 1980. However, the persistence of some behaviour means that illustrative cases have been selected into 2000.

In addition to changes over time, especially those that affected employment, there was a timeless factor implicated in the preponderance of male suicides. An evolutionary-biological drive, in concert with pervasive cultural formulations of masculinity, contributed throughout the century to male possessiveness and macho histrionics that occasionally spiked in violent confrontations and self-destructive acts. As one man expressed it, "he couldn't stay alive and see his partner and children with some other guy."[1] Men in their prime were prone to emotional turmoil when a girlfriend or spouse left, but also became violently upset because these women challenged their husbands' primacy by seeking a legal separation or maintenance payments. The loss of control over earnings enraged men. Across the century, over one in eight suicides by a male (13.3 percent) involved a romantic rejection or marital break-up. For men in their prime, the proportion rose to one in five (18.9 percent). For men and women, considered together, marital and romantic motives were surpassed in number only by cases where witnesses mentioned a mental illness as a likely primary motive.

LOVE DENIED

There are several ways to express the distribution of romantic or marital problems among male suicides: their prominence in particular eras, the stages in life when the crises occurred, the outward emotional state of the parties, and the leading types of upset. From 1900 until the 1970s, the romantic and marital motives were under-represented, but thenceforth they were associated with more suicides than would have been predicted if the proportion from prior decades had prevailed. The expected count for the marital and romantic motive cluster in the 1980s was one hundred and ninety cases, but the actual count reached two hundred and forty-six. In the 1990s the expected count was two hundred and seventy-five, while the count itself reached a shocking four hundred and fifty-two. Another end-of-century shift appears alongside this explosion of suicides connected with relationships and sex. Decade after decade, from the 1900s to the 1970s, the mean ages of men and women who committed suicide principally on account of a terminated relationship fluctuated from thirty-five to forty, but in the last two decades of the century it dipped to the low thirties. These figures plus the words of the deceased and witnesses suggest that, while the sexual revolution that began in the mid-1960s spared some people from unhappy binding relationships and multiplied guilt-free sexual encounters, the greater freedom to experiment fostered incidents of betrayal, sexual exploitation and hurtful infidelity, premature partnerships, and unanticipated marital responsibilities. Immature men and women handled these multiplying situations badly.

The number of romantic and marital upsets increased remarkably at century's end, and yet the types of emotional turmoil stayed consistent. Troubles increased, but they were the same old troubles. During a smoke break, Will Turner asked a workmate, "what would you do if your missus was cheating on you?"[2] The great change was that now break-ups afflicted younger as well as mature couples. Judging by witnesses' statements, two broad states of mind arising from vexed relationships put men in their prime at risk of self-destruction. A break-up plunged some into depression. Across the century, witnesses described men who committed suicide over a marital or romantic crisis in the following terms: depressed and disappointed (15.9 percent of romantic and marital cases), upset (10.1), very depressed (2.2), upset and crying (2.0), broken-hearted (1.7), upset and depressed (1.2), and very miserable (1.0). An assortment of other descriptions conveyed the idea of depression; men were described as downhearted, moody and unhappy, melancholy, morose, and glum. Other men reacted with rage.

Witnesses' accounts in these circumstances distilled into descriptions of men as upset and angry (8.8 percent of cases), violent and nasty (2.5), bad-tempered and angry (1.7), and jealous and unbalanced (1.0). These were the leading summary descriptions, but other expression indicated anger too. Men appeared jealous and vindictive, bad-tempered, quick-tempered, and excitable and impulsive. Psychologist Thomas Joiner attempts to dismiss anger as an explanation for suicide; "suicide is not primarily about anger or revenge; it is sadder than that, in that those who die by suicide have concluded that they are bereft and that their deaths will be a service to others."[3] The language is slippery. Of course suicide is not primarily about revenge or any other particular motive for that matter, but revenge may certainly be a component. Anger was evidenced on many occasions.

Connecting "bereft" to suicide, as Joiner does, is vague, overreaching, and tautological. We have more to say about language, psychologists, and suicide studies in chapter eight, but here we can state that in numerous cases of male suicide, the idea that the deceased embraced death as a service to another person is ludicrous. Scores of suicide notes cited in this chapter indicate male selfishness and vindictiveness. However, we certainly do not claim that these are the only attitudes. It is the individuality of the acts that must be proclaimed.

Romantic or marital distress took many forms, some mentioned in chapter one. For the sake of a quick review, we need only mention that they included the end of intimate relationships by girlfriends and boyfriends who were seeking new partners, formal and informal marital separations, and divorces. However, even a detailed breakdown of the general motive cluster of romantic and marital troubles would fail to convey the authenticity of the crises, the depth of the bitterness, the assortment of reactions, and the crashing sounds of dismay or rage. Witnesses' statements and suicide notes disclose passions and moods; this chapter presents the rawness of these moments. It would be easy, but wrong, to downplay the trauma of failed relationships. They can be dismissed by third parties with the usual consolation that there are many fish in the sea; however, inquests capture the crazed hurt that renders this well-meaning advice trivial to the tormented. The last time Paul Dowland saw his friend Murray Thomas, the nineteen-year-old "was crying and very upset." His seventeen-year-old girlfriend had told him "it was the finish and she would not go out with him again."[4] When Pauline O'Hara was jilted, a good friend consoled her. "I tried to reason with her but she finished up by telling me to get out of the house."[5] There was little place for reason in moments of deep disappointment. In chapter seven and the final chapter, impulsiveness is considered in greater detail.

Most instances of romantic upset, as opposed to marital trouble, involved young people. For much of the century, Romeo-and-Juliet tragedies were rare, reflecting the fact that parents kept a tight rein on girls and even boys until the years of the sexual revolution, when star-crossed lovers turned up with much greater frequency as subjects of suicide inquests. Parents exercised greater supervision and control over children in the decades before the 1960s. Patricia Fowler's mother warned her in late 1930 to stay away from a certain young man. "I told her if she made her bed she would have to lie in it." She took strychnine and lived for twelve hours.[6] When a young Māori man discussed his marriage plans with his family in 1960, his mother objected forcefully on the grounds that he could not afford to marry and she wanted him to marry someone else.[7] In another instance, a heartbroken young Māori man had fallen for a white girl but "it ha[d] always been impressed on him by his parents and other members of the tribe that he must marry a Maori girl."[8] The number of broken romance cases soared in the last quarter of the century.

The place of freer sexual activity and a related rise in romantic suicides late in the century is worth introducing now, although it will be more fully explored in chapter seven. The proportion of youthful suicides brought about by a failed relationship rose late in the century. Indeed, in 2000, for the first time in the century, relationship troubles at 25.0 percent of incidents (n = 124) overtook mental illness at 23.6 percent (n = 117) as the most prominent suicide motive according to our assessment of case files. However, the dynamics of the situations that devastated young men and women were substantially the same in all eras. Young women broke away from boyfriends for a variety of reasons and delivered the message in assorted ways. Young men did the same, and the jilted partners continued to reject advice that they should move on. When a relative told Graham Craig in 1988 that there were other girls, "he took exception to this remark and a minor fight developed."[9] Youth was itself a basis for winding up relationships. Mary Brown ended her engagement to nineteen-year-old Henry Cormack because she reasoned that they were too young to be tied down.[10] Occasionally parents intervened for this reason, or because of social disapproval. Farm labourer Eric Murphy, a quiet man with "a rather high strung temperament," was heartbroken when the parents of a sixteen-year-old girl barred her from keeping company with him.[11] Smitten by a girl, young store clerk Henry Parkinson tried over and over without success to contact her after a rupture in their romance. To a friend, he confided, "I am so depressed I could do myself in." His parents described him as a little impulsive.[12] Impetuousness accompanied youth.

Young women let men know that a relationship was over by simply going out with other men, refusing to answer telephone calls, leaving a social event with another person, asserting a firm no, or returning engagement rings. At a New Year's ball, George Higgs got the message that Maud Horton would no longer be his girl when she announced she would dance with another man for the evening.[13] When Reginald Lord discovered that his girlfriend was two-timing him, he telephoned her. "Are you going with him again?" Hearing her answer he slammed down the receiver.[14] In the envelope with her parting note to August Jensen, Evelyn Ferguson enclosed a ring. "You will think me a nice one to be keeping it so long. Your loving friend." A witness observed that when Jensen read the note, "he stood as though he was riveted to the spot for about five minutes."[15] The day Pauline Desmond refused the offer of a ride home with her former boyfriend, he shot himself.[16] Alice Patterson thought that the rupture with her nineteen-year-old fiancé had gone as well as could be expected from her perspective. She felt that they had agreed that she was too young to marry; he would sell the ring and split the proceeds. He could then pay the money he owed for his bicycle.[17] Seeing his girlfriend with his best friend was more than Wayne Tuckett could stand.[18] And so it went, over and over throughout the century.

Suspicious men had their fears confirmed in ways that unhinged mental stability by depriving them of sleep or piquing their temper. Locomotive driver Hugh Alexander wrote that his wife "has made up her mind to clear away from home and he [her lover] is to follow her. As I am off my mind I can't rest for one minute night or day. I have not had sleep. I can't do my work ... It can't last much longer."[19] The discovery that a recent boarder staying with them was having an affair with his wife made Andrew Benson furious. The row extended over days, with Benson threatening to shoot others and then himself. A police sergeant finally intervened and thought that he had settled the fracas until he was called to the scene of the suicide.[20] "I caught her at the Church doorway [with another man]," wrote Thomas Fountain. "How I kept from going mad I don't know."[21] When Eric Pelkonnen discovered his wife with another man in a public park, he went immediately to a police station and sought advice. A constable recommended a counselling service and told him not to do anything rash. "It appeared to me," the constable later reported in tones of understatement, "that he had many worries on his mind."[22]

Some means of breaking the bad news were intended as gentle ruptures. It was Velma Dejong's opinion that after she broke off her engagement, "we were always on good terms but we never kept company again."[23] Men and women dismissed the other party with the kind yet hurtful line that "we should part good friends."[24] To an insecure young man who felt repulsive, a girl's refusal to kiss him because, she alleged, she wanted to keep the relationship on "a friendly basis" confirmed his acute sense of inadequacy.[25] At the end of the century, a physically mature fourteen-year-old girl – "on the pill" – was told by her boyfriend of seven weeks that "he wanted to be friends as before."[26] The continuity in message and impact over many decades is noteworthy.

Other messages were sharp, decisive, and missing the olive branch. "I broke off the engagement at 7 pm," recalled Clara Hardy. Her ex-fiancé seemed to accept her decision and told her "that he would leave here on the 15th by the early train." Instead, he hanged himself the day after the break-up.[27] Alma Wilson spurned the advances of her brother-in-law: "he asked me on Monday to leave Joe and go with him. I said no."[28] Decisive too was the waitress at a boarding-house who told a coroner that "it was a week today that I told the deceased that I would have nothing more to do with him."[29] Farm labourer Henry Norman had been seeing the same girl for three years and finally asked her to marry him. She rejected his proposal, stating that marriage was a serious step and she did not love him enough.[30] The fifteen-year-old girlfriend of farm labourer Samson Lawrence recounted their last conversation. '"Joyce don't you want me any more? Won't you have me back, I have been a good friend to you?' I replied saying 'No.'" Later he said, "well Joyce, if you won't have anything more to do with me you will hear where I have gone."[31] A distraught Cameron Maxwell phoned his mother-in-law to say, "by the time you get here I will have made her [his recently separated wife] happy."[32] Some suicides, then, were perverse "I'll make you pay for it" acts.

Impulsiveness followed rejection. Henry Norman immediately resigned his job.[33] A friend described Ted Wall "as very much down in the dumps on the night of his death." His girlfriend had just turned him down.[34] Following news that his fiancée was breaking off their engagement, Harry Reeves went on a drinking spree for many days.[35] Well-to-do farmer Eric Clarke reacted to "word from the lady to whom he was engaged cancelling the engagement" by riding all that night to come to his parents' farm. Deeply hurt, he told people he would be better dead.[36] When Charlotte Dalby declined sex, her boyfriend "left in a huff." Later he telephoned to ask if "the spark's gone." She replied, "well, yeah." He had told friends that "he didn't know what he'd do if they ever split up." He killed himself shortly after Charlotte ended the call.[37]

For Andrew Barker, a recent rejection contributed to an overall sense of failure. Concerning a young woman, he wrote, "I thought that I may one day Marry Her but I failed again."[38] His insertion of "again" accents the emotional blow of this rejection, one of many. Repeated rejection similarly obsessed twenty-year-old Mark Kerry, who wrote to his father, "I can't stand living without a girlfriend. Its driving me mental. I know I can never get a girl because I have inherited your ugly face. I have been mad on girls for years."[39] "Love," wrote one man as he slipped into unconsciousness, "is one off the wast pain you can get."[40] Love could be imagined and the fantasy shattered. A workmate mentioned that young Paul Gibson told him "that he didn't have a girlfriend but he would like one." Paul had a crush on Sarah, but when she showed up a party and introduced her new boyfriend to the group, Paul fell silent. "He ate little."[41] The frozen reaction was common in these situations.

A few men threatened to kill themselves unless a woman consented to marriage.[42] We will soon see comparable threats from married men who threatened themselves as a mode of coercion. In chapter seven, this practice of threatening to retain a relationship persisted and likely even increased in frequency on account of the sexual revolution. Emotional blackmail was applied then to a greater extent by immature men swept up in the adventures of the sexual revolution but trapped in a horrific period of youth unemployment. This sudden outbreak of youth threats did not displace but accompanied the ongoing pleas and threats of mature men.[43]

Women shared the pain of rejection.[44] Romantic upsets and marital breakdowns could put some women directly into a suicidal frame of mind. Thrown over for another woman, Hilda Macdonald left a note that, like some written by men, was calculated to punish. "Tell Jack," she wrote, "I said goodbye to him and I loved him to the last. Perhaps when he sees my dead body brought up from the river he will be sorry for the way he treated me on Saturday."[45] The coroner who looked into the drowning of Bridget Quinn concluded that "the drinking habits and cruelty of her husband so played upon her mind that at the time she committed the act she was in such a mental state as not to be responsible for her actions."[46] This statement can be read as a courtesy finding that kept the death from being labelled a suicide, but it also contained a condemnation of male abuse. Not only did a few women succumb to outrages, but they were subject to unwanted pregnancies by irresponsible boyfriends or undeserving spouses.

Inquests into the suicides of men often parenthetically describe women's suffering, but also a few acts of exasperated resilience to the abuse. When we turn our attention to mental illness, however, the background occasionally shows domestic hardships leading not to resistance but to depression and suicide. In cases of resistance, men were affronted by challenges to authority and a loss of wages exacted by maintenance orders; in cases of depression, women were physically worn down by managing a household and emotionally devastated by a spouse's misconduct. Mental illness commonly appears as a motive for suicide among women, but in the background there were sources of stress such as an abusive husband or the strains of raising a family in poverty or amidst violence. On a few rare occasions, women were rendered suicidal by beatings and abandonment. Late in the century, when the work ethos and masculinity were less closely allied than they had once been, incidents of domestic violence exposed raw obscene control. A burglar out on bail, a member of the Head Hunters Motorcycle Club, grabbed his wife by the hair and punched her repeatedly with a closed fist. "You fuckin mad bitch, what are you doing?" She had questioned his promiscuity. She took her life the next day.[47]

In common with young men, young women could be pushed into despondency by well-intentioned parents. According to her father, eighteen-year-old Ida Dodge "was keeping company with a man named Turner which my wife and I did not approve of. She generally resented what I said about this matter, and she did so this evening."[48] Disapproving of the way her step-daughter dressed for school, Mildred Burgess ordered her to change her boots. "She was very cross." An argument erupted over whether the step-mother had "a mother's feeling for her."[49] Mary Hart's mother told her not to bother coming home after she learned that her daughter was seeing a private in the medical corps.[50] The brief lapse of time between a confrontation and a rash act in these instances is a feature worth keeping fixed in mind. On many occasions, young men and women disciplined by parents reacted without careful assessment of the years remaining relative to an immediate setback to pride and budding autonomy. As well, for women before and even after the sexual revolution, there was infamy and the censure that landed on them when they were seduced, pregnant, and abandoned.[51] In the first decades of the century, employers dismissed maids who were unwed and pregnant.[52] In all eras, parents kept alive the idea of disgrace. It served the purpose of limiting unwanted mouths to feed, but presented as a moral standard it risked promoting feelings of shame and disgust among women 'in trouble.'

The most shocking instances of a suicide precipitated by jealousy were murder-suicides and attempted murder-suicides.[53] These very often involved jealousy or domestic strife. Out of ninety-four suicides by individuals who had either attempted a murder or carried one out, eight in ten (83.0 percent, n = 78) were committed by men. In the overwhelming number of attacks (75.6 percent, n = 59), the victim of the attempt or the murder was a woman, usually a wife (55.1 percent, n = 43) but girlfriends were prominent too (20.5 percent, n = 16). Young unmarried men assaulted their young girlfriends; older married men attacked their wives, although some married men had girlfriends whom they assaulted. Other fatal attacks that led to the perpetrator's suicide were against parents, employers, and police constables.

It is impossible to analyze statistically the exact events leading up to the attacks involving a relationship, in part because sexual activities and romantic entanglements were complicated and the uses of suicide to exact vengeance were diverse, refracted as they were through the minds of enraged individuals. Some inquests discovered straightforward motives and disclosed preceding acts of jealousy or a series of clear threats. To stop what he felt was his wife's infidelity, a Māori man brought his wife to a different village.[54] When Gilbert Marshall suspected that his de facto had deceived him, he said he would get even.[55] James Holt was so jealous that he read his de facto's mail.[56] More complicated were the events leading to the suicide of farm labourer George Taylor, who ran off with his employer's wife. The husband pursued them and persuaded his wife to return. Taylor then ambushed the husband, took the wife back, and later killed her and himself.[57]

In some cases, the marital relationship had been notably strong; and from a distorted sense of love a mentally unbalanced husband would assert that he could not leave a wife behind.[58] There were instances too when a married man decided not to die alone but to take a mistress with him, not out of malice toward his girlfriend but from the crazed idea of a suicide pact. The women in question were not necessarily willing participants. William Urquhart's girlfriend put up a struggle. His note indicated that he hoped to get back at his wife, who had refused him a separation. "You will get the shock of your life," he wrote. To affront her, he wrote an eighteen-page letter elaborating on his affair with the other woman.[59] In some cases, women were fortunate that a husband's violent tendencies led to his suicide rather than her death, because there had been a history of prior assaults and threats.[60] In response to her complaints about his gambling, George Rockton threatened, "I've come back to settle you and then I'll settle myself." They clashed in the kitchen. He attacked with a cleaver and she defended with a frying pan.[61] Alice Pippin told a coroner that "a number of times I had considered leaving him, but each time I said I was, he would threaten to kill me."[62]

Women who committed a murder-suicide seldom killed a spouse; more commonly, when they decided to end their lives, they resolved to take a child or children with them. There were several rationalizations. Some believed in an afterlife where they could keep one another company. Some thought that they were sparing a child or several children a life of misery. "As I see it," wrote Beatty Wood, "it is a case of having to go. I am taking the children with me."[63] When Mary Stevens heard that her boyfriend had become engaged to another woman, she killed her infant daughter and then herself, explaining in her note that "I am taking Betty with me because this is not a happy world at the best of times and it would be a shame to leave her to face it alone."[64] One mother felt that by giving birth she had "proprietary rights" in a custody case and was not going to let her ex-husband see the children even when they asked.[65]

A handful of young lovers whose parents had attempted to put an end to their relationship decided to die together with the woman's consent and on a rare occasion with her leadership. When a girl's mother attempted to stop her from seeing a labourer, the pair co-operated in a double suicide with a symbolic message. The pair stood back to back while he extended his arms backward around her; she then tied his wrists together and they threw themselves into a river. Her skirt was missing.[66] A few older couples having an affair died together in the belief that one of their spouses was making life unbearable. Several quite elderly couples, having lived long together, decided to die together.[67] A small number of same-sex double suicides were noted, but only one involved a definite sexual relationship and because one party was a minor, the case is discussed later with instances of illicit sex and shame.[68] Altogether, a dozen double suicides were identified in the years studied. We move on now to consider a far more common situation, the separation of married couples.

COURT ORDERS AND BITTER MEN

Separations could be informal but permanent. David Dean's estranged wife met him at their son's cricket match and delivered the news that "the separation was likely to be permanent."[69] Separations which involved a formal complaint before a magistrate, who could order separation and maintenance payments, enraged men because of the assertion of independence by a woman, the intervention of third parties who then knew about their conduct, and perhaps most of all because of the transfer of some wages by the maintenance order. A separation order struck at male control of the household and signalled the unlikelihood of reconciliation. Gladys Masters told her husband she had had enough and would leave him and, in her words, "make him keep me." Rather than do that "he told me he would jump in the sea." He did.[70] A co-worker reported that Leonard McFarland had recently lost his property and half his wages due to a separation order and "he appeared to be obsessed with this matter when under the influence of drink."[71] On the day before he was to see a solicitor about his wife's application for maintenance, farm labourer Mark Poranga shot himself.[72]

The humiliation of a court proceeding was more than Henry Watson could stand. His wife refused reconciliation. In his attempts to win her back he said "he could not face the disgrace."[73] Levelled by the prospect of legal action, some men insisted on having the last callous word. In his suicide note, Matthew Dunn blamed his wife for his pending death. "I had a home for 35 years," he wrote, "so I do not wish to knock about the world by myself. Let God be the judge between you and me."[74] After writing in his last letter to his wife, to tell her that he would not appear in court to contest her petition for a separation order, Murray Douglas threatened her. "There is a higher tribunal above where we shall meet one of these days and wrongs will be righted." He was not finished. Insisting that he had been true to her and her alone, he wrote, "I only hope one thing and that is that my face, the face of a true and devoted lover may haunt you to your dying day."[75]

Confident women who refused to put up with drunkenness and violent attacks saw a magistrate or, if they could afford it, went first to a lawyer. After she left her alcoholic husband, Louise Charles dealt with her husband solely through a lawyer. "I instructed my lawyer," she testified at an inquest, "to write to him on the subject of our differences. I wished the lawyer to try to bring him to his senses."[76] This type of intervention was rare; the cheaper course was to bring a formal complaint of abuse directly to a magistrate. Such forceful independence infuriated men. Under the terms of their separation, farmer Will Bragg had to ask his wife for funds. She granted an allowance if he stayed away.[77] At an inquest into the death of her husband, Bertha Patrick recounted that she "was taking proceedings to obtain a separation order; the deceased wanted the proceedings withdrawn." When she refused to comply, he started to poison himself in front of her.[78]

Here and on other occasions, a man was determined to inflict a nightmarish memory on a spouse or girlfriend.[79] A retired miner told his wife that "someday she would find his bones at her door."[80] Myrtle Powell recalled, after rebuking her husband for his drunken state, that "he said he was going to write a note and putting the blame on me. He called out 'goodbye.'"[81] Jealousy after a separation triggered a few suicides. Martin Pacey had been separated from his wife for two years, but his landlady observed that "lately he has seemed subject to depression of spirits … Certain rumours he heard about her seemed to be preying on his mind."[82] Farm labourer Howie McBeath wrote to his wife that "you can stick to your Boy Friend and I hop he doos as much for you as I have Don may God pardon me for all my sines and allse your to."[83] William Fowler's note expressed jealousy and vindictiveness. "I met you as a prostitute in the De Lux Pink and seems like you have gone back to your old ways. I hope you when you read this you and that Bastard Engineer has the most miserable remainder of your lives that anybody could wish upon you."[84] Certain that his wife would not take him back, Tim Prentice left a note expressing his love for his children and "I leave it to you to explain to them."[85] The ways of laying the foundations for guilt were manifold. In his note to his wife, Jim Baird said that "there is no more disgrace in what I am doing than in your step in going to a lawyer."[86]

Formal separation proceedings jeopardized the autonomy of men and, from time to time, they undermined a reputation for looking after 'the missus' romantically and sexually. In case after case, recourse to a magistrate occurred following multiple broken promises to quit drinking or refrain from violence. Explaining her decision to seek a separation, Enid De Bryun bluntly informed a coroner, "I had put up with him for years."[87] Martha and Samuel Ryerson had fallen into a pattern respecting his drinking bouts. She would leave; he would promise to mend his ways; she would return; he would resume drinking. After many years, she departed and determined never to return. He ended his life a fortnight later.[88] James Mallory's wife left him on five occasions due to his habitual drinking. On the last occasion, this former barrister was forced to live in a boarding-house. Knowing the circumstances of his separation and shocked by his decline in social status, family and friends had nothing to do with him.[89]

A doctor reported that Richard Miller had frequently beaten his wife; he knew this for a fact because he had treated her injuries. She eventually took her husband to court, but then withdrew charges when he promised never again to "molest" her. When he resumed his old ways, she left him for good. Unemployed, without savings, without his wife, and owing her maintenance, he drank carbolic acid.[90] Martha Cunningham and her boy fled her abusive mate. She left no trace of where she had gone. The last straw had been when he "threatened to do away with me and himself too."[91] "We were afraid for our lives," another woman told the court. After she took steps for a formal separation, her spouse shot himself.[92] The self-critical testimony of Ellen Wallace gives a harrowing account of a hellish life: "John used to hit me quite a bit. He was a very jealous and possessive person, and the arguments used to start between us over very small things. The worst times were if either of us or both of us had been drinking. The arguments used to start over money or the children, or things like that. We split up many times."[93]

Arrested for assaulting his wife while "suffering from the effects of drink," Allen Dutton took his life in the police station.[94] With a stunning frequency across the century, men threatened suicide to control a wife. According to Lillian Robbins, for years her husband had said "if I left him or got a separation order, life would not be worth living on his own and he may as well not be here."[95] "When I was leaving," testified Aileen Munroe at the inquest into her husband's death, "he told me he was going to kill himself."[96] Police reports on Charles Douglas in the 1990s stated that his wife would threaten to leave him "and he would threaten suicide in order to make her return to him."[97] One-sided summaries of domestic arguments understandably lack the witnesses' replies when confronted by such intimidation. We can ask: in a state of passion, did women dare a boyfriend or spouse? "Go ahead." "I'll be better off without you." Would a witness admit to making such a taunt? "I thought it was just another cry for attention. He had done this sort of thing before, dictate things."[98] The full script of an explosive exchange can never be known, but some rash acts were likely unthinking and perverse comebacks by men to show who was in charge.[99] A constable who attempted to prevent a suicide reported his conversation with the young man. His former wife "told him he was a hopeless father and he found that very hurtful and hard to take."[100] Enough testimony survives to speculate plausibly about the exchanges in domestic warfare.

The ages of suicide victims from battling couples declined toward the end of the century, partly because of the trend toward younger relationships. Another factor was that most women could find refuge in shelters and from there confront spouses without waiting until the children had grown up. Shelters opened at Christchurch in 1973 and Auckland in 1975. There were twenty-five by 1983 and approaching fifty by 1988. From 1987, the police were instructed to consider an arrest as a first option when responding to domestic violence.[101] Feminist campaigns were manifest in these developments, which influenced some women's actions, although as before there were men who reacted with a vengeance suicide. In 2000, Indo-Fijian bride Deviani Ghosh entered a women's refuge with access to legal counsel and later took out a protection order against her violent husband, who had a history of failed relationships. Rather than meet with her lawyer, he took his life.[102] On the one hand, due to women's shelters, more women like Mrs Ghosh acted sooner than their counterparts had in prior decades. On the other, some women continued to tolerate and suffer abuse because of complex intimate family dynamics. At the inquest into her husband's suicide, a young Māori woman mentioned that she and her spouse had had domestic rows over the years "but only twice had the police been called." "When his voice changes, it is time to leave. In the past he got punchy with me." On one occasion, she made up her mind not to return but relented when "the kids moaned at me that they wanted to go home to see their dad."[103] Other women laid charges, but we will see soon how badly a number of these actions went down. In every year, a separation order or a court summons brought on fits of male despair or rage, and led to further trouble.[104]

The time between a legal action and a fatal act was often short. Living apart from her husband "for some considerable time," Elvira Fleming finally decided to secure a separation order, at which point her husband poisoned himself. In his note he exclaimed, "I have died for love."[105] Usually, the triggering event was closer. James Meade told an acquaintance that "he was in great trouble and could see more trouble coming." A few days before that conversation, he received both a letter from a lawyer and a court summons.[106] When a lawyer brought the separation agreement to Alexander McKay's house for his signature, he refused and left a suicide note that stated, "dearest wife, you are too cruel."[107] The estranged wife of "silent drinker" Alex Talbert reported at an inquest that she had sought a legal separation; the legal proceedings were "set down for today."[108] Shortly before his death, labourer Thomas Pollard received at his boarding-house room a summons in a case initiated by his wife. An autopsy disclosed that he had pulmonary tuberculosis. Legal action struck this individual – others too – with a bounty of troubles. Pollard could not imagine how he could pay for his wife's maintenance plus his room and board.[109] Farmer Ole Johansen shot himself the day after a maintenance order was served. He had no money and was out of employment.[110]

A deterioration in marital relationships could originate in financial insecurity that promoted a sense of failure as a breadwinner and increased solace-seeking in bouts of drinking. In a downward spiral of fortunes, financial circumstances worsened for all parties under the conditions of a maintenance order. Court orders could not address the inequality of men and women in a labour market where men occupied the better-paying positions, such as they were. Used to the management of household income, men under court orders sought ways to retain control by disappearing or ending their lives. The stress of farm management with a debt load, an enduring feature of New Zealand life, contributed to irritability. There were violent outbursts followed in a few instances by self-destruction. A young farmer recalled how his dairy-farmer father used to "take to Mum in the cowshed. Once it was with the high pressure hose, soaking her and he took to her with an alkathene pipe or lump of wood." Reacting to police intervention, the father swore, "I'll get you bastards, you'll pay." The son reported a common refrain: "Mum refused to lay charges." However, the police did. The father's vengeance on his family was suicide.[111]

This mentally unstable dairy farmer made his fatal move the day after a court order. Other men also acted soon after reading a document that changed their standing. Alan Robison's wife demanded he move out of the house and the day that "their separation papers had come through" he shot himself on the property.[112] Only several days separated the moment when Fred Davis received a summons to appear in magistrate's court for failure to provide maintenance for his wife and five children and the moment when he took his life. Described as "a habitual inebriate," Davis was a thin, miserable-looking man. The summons precipitated his decision to escape multiple troubles.[113] Several days separated when Phillip Perkins received a letter from his wife's solicitor and when he shot himself.[114] Called to settle a domestic dispute, a constable took notes that John Colville's wife intended to leave him and would be seeing a magistrate. Colville swore that "he would sooner go to gaol than pay for her."[115] A few men went to the grave to defy a court order. The receipt of legal orders that constricted their authority and threatened their spending triggered existential crises. In his suicide note, Claude Armstrong ranted about the injustice of a maintenance order calculated on his maximum earnings with overtime. In a bitter postscript, he asserted his sanity. "I'm not Insane – In fact I am as sane as the Magistrate who Imposed the maintenance Order on me when he Separated us."[116]

Following separations, police constables delivered court orders compelling the payment of overdue maintenance and prohibiting "molestation."[117] Officers also intervened to break up disputes in progress. These intercessions infuriated men who felt aggrieved or cornered by the law but also by their poverty. Walter Tippet was literally cornered. With no work or money, drinking heavily, and threatening his wife, he locked himself into a room when the police arrived. At that point he cut his throat.[118] A warrant had been issued to arrest financially distressed land agent Ernest Williams for failure to support his wife for eight months.[119] Florence Costello had initiated proceedings against her husband Henry for breaching a maintenance order and, as she put it, for "having molested me." "Seeing you are not going to come back to me," Henry wrote in his last letter, "I am going to take my only way out of misery and trouble."[120] Short of money and behind on his maintenance payments, Peter Littleford had to borrow from his employer, who commented at the inquest that Littleford ran out of money because "he was addicted to drink."[121] "A heavy drinker of spirits" according to police, John Pollard had just been prosecuted for ignoring a maintenance order. His faltering business had recently been assigned to creditors. In a self-exculpatory note to children, he wrote, "my Darlings think kindly of Daddy, robbed of his home and business."[122] Directed by court order to leave the house on account of assaulting his wife, Paul Maxwell returned the next day to threaten her with a shotgun. When the police turned up, he took off and killed himself.[123] After her husband "bashed her about," Anne Rule applied to the magistrate for a non-molestation order. Shortly after it was served on him, he ended his life.[124] The feeling of victimization by a cruel wife occasionally originated from a loss of access to children. Many men missed the money, but some also wanted their kiddies.[125]

Besides court orders and the appearance of police constables, other related precipitating events set men in motion, men who had brooded over a failing relationship. For Bryce Firth, the night following the marriage of a good friend turned into a period of restless self-evaluation. Explaining that he had "had a gutsful of everything this life can give me," he went on to observe how he had brought people together. They were now happy and "that's what it's all about." However, his girlfriend's parents had barred their association and destroyed his chance for happiness. In a confused state of envy and vindictiveness, he told his girlfriend, "don't blame your folks."[126] The note sowed discord while he played the martyr. Vindictiveness could be powerfully expressed, and on rare occasions it was women, not men, who sent the message. On the photograph of her three children, Elizabeth Maltby had written, "please look after my three Darlings. Now you will have the freedom you wanted."[127]

Alcohol broke up more marriages and led to more remorse than infidelity, but there certainly were instances when married men were discovered to have additional relationships; wives initiated legal proceedings for separation and maintenance on these grounds too. As one witness put it, "my brother was having domestic problems at home through drink and other women." Rather than pay for his wild ways in maintenance to an ill-treated wife, he took his own life.[128] Young farmer Desmond Walker arranged parties to which he invited a number of women. "Some of the women," his wife testified, "were known to my late husband but not to me." On a recent Saturday night, she continued, "my husband had a few drinks that night and later I tackled him as to something going on between him and one of the women." He admitted it and she decided to leave and take the children. It is impossible to say whether it was shame or remorse that led to his rash deed, for he left a blunt confession stating: "I was never any good and after what happened on Saturday night you will likely find out a lot more. Try and keep the place going for the boys."[129]

During the first three or four decades of the century, the resolve of married women to stand up to husbands wavered due to dependence on the husband's earnings and a willingness born of hope to grant a multitude of second chances, if not for their own sake then for the benefit of the children.[130] A case in 1936 foreshadowed a new independence that broke from the round of forgive and forget. Financial necessity compelled a wife to work to help support the couple in the Great Depression. Her employment put a strain on a marriage.[131] After three weeks of marriage, Anne Day secured a job that required her to live apart from her twenty-four-year-old husband. She paid him occasional visits. Feeling that she had let her position take precedence over her wifely duties, Dermod Day was very upset. Alone in his boarding-house room, Day composed a note to his wife before taking his life with coal gas. "Goodbye Anne," he wrote; "I only had owne [sic] thing to live for – that was you – I loved you as I never loved before."[132] Early in World War II, a young soldier and his wife had quarrels that led to her declaration that she intended to go out to work. In her words, "he had not agreed to this and we finally came to a decision to separate."[133]

Marital breakdowns that began with a dispute over where to reside and that ended in a suicide were rare, but they applied to the wider crisis of male dominance. When David Prince's wife opposed their moving so that he could pursue a new job, he threatened that "if you don't go, I will and I won't come back." To get her compliance, he had also told her that "he would jump in the river." His skeletal remains were found there months later.[134] Joe Connolly threatened to kill himself whenever his de facto left to visit her legal husband and children. "I told him that this was not helping me to reach the right decision."[135] Instances where men threatened self-destruction to coerce compliance could lead to a masculine existential bind, for if their bluff failed, they lost face, and then what? John Fritch's wife slept in a separate room, and he used to threaten, "if you don't come to bed with me I will blow my brains out."[136] For a few men, a threat evolved into a course of action to save face, make a point, or inflict pain.

The collapse of a marriage usually seems to have been the fault of the husband. However, on occasion, women found a more appealing partner and skipped out.[137] When his wife ran away with his brother, a young labourer broke down and cried in front of his next-door neighbour.[138] A young Māori farm labourer could not get it out of his mind that his wife "was carrying on with another man" after they had quarrelled and separated for two months.[139] When his wife began to share her bed with another man, Murray Williams wrote about his pain. "We have been lovers for 25 years and now to be turned down for a damned scoundrel is more than I can bear."[140] When his second marriage failed, Robert Clifford became despondent in the estimation of his nephew.[141] Convinced that his de facto wife had been unfaithful, Alfred Curry said he would get even with her.[142] When his wife refused to pay his gambling debts, David Hopkins told her she would suffer until the day she died.[143] In a suicide note addressed to his wife, David Peel wrote, "You lose or do you. I think you lose."[144] Vengeance suicides that aimed to embarrass and impoverish women were spread across the century.

Occasionally, a wayward husband acted from remorse. Regret overwhelmed alcoholic Thomas Shearman. On a spree for weeks, he confided to a publican that he grieved over broken promises and a full life that could no longer be achieved.[145] According to a friend, war pensioner Alfred Ellis "was passionately fond of his wife and brooded a good deal over her leaving him.[146] Accounts of suicides and relationships would be incomplete without mentioning that there were men whose life companions died and left them devastated. As some of them put it, they could not go on alone.[147] At the other end of the spectrum, there were individuals whose character and circumstances contributed to rancorous violence and even multiple deaths. Pete Czerwinski beat several women. In his final note he wrote, "well it is nearly four years since I was convicted for what I did to Cathy. No one will ever believe me that I never intended to hurt Cathy. Now four years later I am in the same boat."[148]

ILLICIT SEX, SEXUAL OFFENCES, AND SHAME

There were suicidal men whose self-destruction followed exposure for committing sexual offences. We are interested here in how men reacted to a police investigation into their sexual conduct. Sexual offences that shamed men into suicide involved sex with minors or rape. Charged with rape, Fred Reeves jumped in front of a train.[149] Almost one in five suicides arising primarily from a criminal justice investigation, charge, or conviction pertained to a sexual offence (19.0 percent, n = 82). Men accounted for eighty instances. The ages of the suspects varied from seventeen to eighty-three, but with a mean age of forty-nine, many suspects qualified for the label 'dirty old man.' By the late twentieth century, a few male sex offenders were put on testosterone-reducing medication.[150]

Sexual relations with underage girls violated the law, and when discovered, men were distressed by the shame of exposure, or if unrepentant, were determined to avoid imprisonment. One young man wrote to his parents that "once you are accused of something like this your life is ruined whatever the outcome. I did not do anything to those girls."[151] According to the father of a twenty-year-old Māori man, his son used a shotgun on himself because "he had been misbehaving himself with a young girl, a near relative, and having been found out, died by his own hand through shame."[152] A man in his late teens wrote that "I died for the love of Sarah Malone." An investigation exposed a complicated affair. The deceased "had been very intimate" with "a Maori girl" who was thirteen and both sets of parents had opposed the relationship.[153] After Thomas King, a farm labourer, entered the bedroom of his employer's fifteen-year-old daughter against her will, he was ordered to pack his belongings and leave.[154] His violation perhaps amounted to no more than holding her hand. Far more egregious acts were encountered.

A few instances involved fathers, step-fathers, and other males with authority over children.[155] A seventeen-year-old girl had an argument with her father who was estranged from their mother; a fifteen-year-old daughter had possibly disclosed abuse to her older sister. Following the altercation, the older daughter sat down to write a letter. What are you writing? her father asked. She replied that "she had not written anything out of place." He flew into a rage and killed the younger girl and then himself.[156] Released from a three-year prison term for having intercourse with one daughter, an unrepentant and abusive man had sex with another daughter, aged fourteen. Telling police that he would not be accompanying them, he fled and later shot himself.[157] A fifty-two-year-old man, charged with "attempted unlawful sexual connection" with the fifteen-year-old daughter of his de facto, managed to convince the latter that the daughter had been at fault. To get the daughter to drop her complaint, the mother threatened suicide, but when this failed, the two adults committed suicide.[158]

The police were about to question a sixty-seven-year-old man about an indecent assault on a nine-year-old girl, but he pre-empted the investigation by taking rat poison.[159] A local butcher and family man stood accused of indecent assaults on girls.[160] The custodian of a local swimming pool was charged in the presence of his wife after parents complained of indecent assaults.[161] Facing charges in family court, a self-confessed paedophile wrote that a "private shame is very different to a public shame."[162] Just as legal intervention had triggered suicides in the instances of some men whose wives were seeking separation or maintenance orders, a pending court appearance for sex offences determined the timing of suicides with these motives. An Auckland man "charged with indecency with another male" on 8 July 1980 disappeared on 9 July and was found dead on 10 July.[163] Ethnicity was mentioned on autopsy forms routinely in the 1980s and 1990s. It was not commonly reported until then. Therefore, it is not possible to tell if any one group had more of these offences during the entire century, although late in the century no one ethnic group stands out, nor does any class.

During the years when same-sex relationships between men could lead to a criminal prosecution, police arrested a few men, and on very few occasions the suspect took his life.[164] During the first half of the century, statements at inquests about sexuality were indirect.[165] Cases were rare. Early in the century an unmarried music teacher of fifty-two, "a man of culture and refinement," was "arrested on a certain charge" and shot himself.[166] Sexual relations between an adult man and a boy, if reported, could lead to police investigations and suicides.[167] In a bizarre 1918 incident, local men, suspicious of their schoolmaster, spied on him, caught him in the act, and allowed him an honourable way out.[168] A veteran of World War I defended himself by saying that "he had seen 2 or 3 boys doing certain things which had been fairly common amongst men in the trenches and that he had not tried to stop them."[169]

Over the years, several teachers faced sodomy allegations.[170] The father of a fourteen-year-old, suspicious of his son's thirty-four-year-old boss at a weekend job, found confirmation of a sexual relationship when he read the boy's diary. The older man confessed to a friend that he could not break off because "he had gone too far and loved Bob too much." Questioned by police, he feared a prison sentence. The two committed suicide together, but the boy's distraught father disputed the coroner's finding, arguing that his son was not responsible but acted under the influence of the other person.[171] Discovery could result in wounding censure from a suspect's family or friends. A twenty-six-year-old man sat in silence and then left his girlfriend's home after she asked "if he had made a suggestion to a nineteen year old boy."[172] At the end of the century, a forty-year-old alcoholic drug-using fisherman faced criminal charges for "touching up a boy." His father stated that "we don't see eye to eye or really see him ever."[173]

THE DEMON IN THE BOTTLE

As we have seen, instances of marital breakdown occasionally involved the husband's abuse of alcohol with ensuing loss of money, recriminations, arguments, violence, remorse, promises, promises broken, a spouse's recourse to a magistrate, and a male's impulsive act. The essential question is, how often did alcohol contribute to the breakdown of a relationship and then to a suicide? On the one hand, we cannot be certain of the proportion of marital troubles leading to suicide that originated in drink, because investigating constables and coroners did not ask witnesses a common set of questions. On the other hand, constables who investigated suicides wanted to demonstrate competence and displayed their knowledge of community goings-on. If the deceased was well known to the police, they mentioned why. "From my knowledge of the deceased," stated one constable, "I know there had been matrimonial trouble in the family brought on by the deceased's excessive drinking." At the time of his death, the man had been drinking sherry mixed with kerosene.[174] Based on reports such as these, alcohol abuse and domestic violence seem related, as one might expect, but gleanings cannot clarify the scope of the association. From the statistical side, we do have information on marital status and also on the presence of alcohol abuse as the leading motive for suicide, which is not the same as knowing the proportion of men with romantic or marital problems who drank to excess or were alcoholics. However, we must take what we can from the sources at hand.

One striking observation is that alcohol abuse was essentially a male motive for suicide. In roughly one in twelve male suicides (7.9 percent, n = 644), we judged alcohol the primary factor.[175] Women were less prominent (3.5 percent, n = 91), but the effects of addiction were just as shocking for the atypical women; across the century, there were tales of addiction, hallucination, marital collapse, destitution, and incarceration.[176] For men who committed suicide in the twentieth century, separation was a notable marital state for suicides, especially when we consider that an overwhelming number of all adult men in the country were either single or married. About one in eleven men who took their own lives (n = 732, 8.9 percent) were separated. Of these individuals, roughly one in eight (n = 95, 13.0 percent) had committed suicide due to an alcohol abuse problem. The expected count was fifty-eight. Excessive drinking and marital failure were connected; possibly foetal alcohol syndrome played a part in the suicides of a few young people at the end of the century when school performance and training assumed greater importance for employment. Thus, alcohol abuse had an indirect influence on some suicides; as well, alcoholism as a disease was a motive on its own, since it promoted self-loathing among a few individuals. Attributing suicides to a motive of alcohol abuse, as with assigning mental illness as a motive, amounts to an expedient that has greater validity in some instances than in others.

International studies report that the proportion of suicides – men and women – who were alcoholics has varied from fifteen to twenty-seven percent of all suicides; one study estimated the suicide rate of alcoholics at 270 per 100,000.[177] During the twentieth century, roughly one in thirteen suicides in New Zealand could be related firmly and directly to alcohol abuse. If other forms of substance abuse are added – narcotic addiction, prescription drug misuse, and solvent sniffing – the number rises slightly to one in twelve. Extreme drinking leading to physical, psychological, and social problems was largely a male problem in every group of years. However, not every group of years showed a similarly high proportion of alcohol-related suicides, and thus recent international studies must be treated warily as snapshots lacking the ever-important historical context. By far the worst years for alcohol abuse problems were those of national development, a prosperous time when men, if married, controlled family income and when the drinking of spirits was far more common than in later years. On account of the deleterious influence of excessive drinking on finances and domestic relations, the attribution of alcohol as the leading motive in suicides is probably under-counted.

The contrast between the prevalence of alcohol abuse reported in the era of national development and that reported in all other eras supports our attribution of alcohol-related troubles in specific cases, because errors in judgement or bias would have been carried through all eras and depicted a steady trend in alcohol-related troubles. Statements in alcohol abuse cases from the era of national development were so vivid and shocking that few mistakes were possible. When a constable was called out to Tommy Osborn's house, he found him "mad drunk" and his wife was being protected by some local workmen.[178] A neighbour of farmer Bill Perkins testified in an inquest that "the eldest Perkins girl came to my house and told me that her father was very drunk and knocking her mother about." Sick of his conduct and alcoholism, Perkins took prussic acid.[179]

In *Be a Man*, Peter Stearns proposed that industrialization challenged men to bolster masculinity in a new environment which minimized their property and reduced their control over work. Men assumed that in return for the burdens of heavy toil, they could claim rewards. For married men, these included the status of breadwinner, control of the household budget, and domestic authority.[180] As we noted when looking at separation and maintenance orders, control of money mattered to men. Another reward was alcohol, although men who defined themselves partly by the bar's sociability disadvantaged themselves as breadwinners and family heads. Empirical studies have verified a connection between male socialization, frequent drinking, and suicide.[181] In New Zealand, over half of male suicides who had alcohol-abuse problems (52.7 per cent) were unemployed or self-employed and having trouble. By any measure of financial well-being, men with alcohol abuse problems fared worse than other men. A young New Zealand swagman captured a philosophical outlook when he wrote in his diary, "drink, for tomorrow we starve."[182]

The presence of itinerant labourers on grazing stations, in mines, and on public works projects promoted a masculine camp culture that escalated reward-taking and increased subsequent health and social problems. This culture likely peaked in the late nineteenth century, but continued on into the twentieth. Physicians in mid-century diagnosed some alcoholics with what they called dipsomania, a condition described as leading to oversensitivity and an inability to cope with difficulties, humiliations, setbacks, and stress. Still others had chronic alcoholism; these individuals were sociable and emotional at the bar but irritable at home. Men with alcohol-related problems were plagued by unemployment, marital breakdown, and debt.

Why did men drink a substance known to be addictive and unhealthy? First, the ambiance of the pub appealed to men who otherwise had no opportunity to entertain and show they belonged. Boarding-houses, bunkhouses, and construction camps lacked recreational setups. For socializing and entertainment, the countryside offered little other than the pub. A second reason was that drinking has long been associated with anxiety and depression. Men may have self-medicated by chance and thus, in a tragic irony, aggravated their depression.[183] Alcoholic women were less evident.[184]

As early as 1900, witnesses at inquests described alcohol-dependent males as depressed; they also used terms such as "confused," "strange," "excited," "off their head," and "impulsive." Family members saw these men as belligerent, violent, nasty, quarrelsome, and complaining. Marital breakdown figured often in alcohol-associated suicides. Single alcoholic men were more prone to suicide than their married counterparts. Some alcoholic labourers were unmarriageable, but others had been married, had fled court-issued support orders, and preferred anonymity. Witnesses at inquests for labourers included fewer family members than did those at inquests into suicides by middle-class men with alcohol-related problems. Single, divorced, and separated men were at greater risk of suicide than married men.

The most dramatic symptoms of alcohol abuse in New Zealand, well-known to constables and men on pastoral stations, in timber camps, and at public works, deserved to be labelled "the horrors." Delirium tremens was a phenomenon that men in work groups came to know well. Hallucinations involved animals, insects, and devils.[185] Recent research on suicide peaks after holidays supports the proposition that withdrawal is a risk-laden period for people with alcohol dependence.[186] The inquest records show that hallucinations during withdrawal drove men to bizarre conduct. Witnesses early in the century were used to seeing men with the horrors. Familiarity is not surprising in view of the levels of consumption. Consider Augustus Bergman, whose erratic life was not unique. A co-worker remarked that Bergman "was a man who worked steadily for a few months at a time and then usually had a drinking bout for a few weeks, shifting about from district to district."[187]

Witnesses recounted marathon binges. Farm manager Lachlan Caldecott told a coroner that his cook had been in the habit of overindulging and had recently gone on a six-week spree. "Since he returned he was dodging about the hut, suffering recovery."[188] Deckhand Roberto Angelo had known Tony Agate, a former fisher, well enough to say of him, "I think he suffered a good deal while recovering from drink."[189] Dr David Johnston treated Alexander Rose for alcoholism over three weeks in 1914. "Whenever he took alcohol he became an absolute lunatic."[190] A blacksmith who saw thirty-six-year-old farm labourer James Chapman after a spree "concluded at the time that the deceased was off his head." Chapman's employer was precise: "I would say the deceased when I saw him last was suffering from delirium tremens."[191] A friend of labourer Richard Lindale described him as an excessive drinker whose "mind was perfectly unhinged."[192] Constable John Murphy had charged a man with "being a lunatic at large, but the medical evidence went to show he suffered from drink."[193]

A type of paranoia affected men with the horrors, and it is possible that the delusions were symptomatic of alcoholic psychosis. Such clinical language appeared in only a few accounts. One doctor reported that his patient, a heavy drinker, was "suffering from marked depression of spirits and showing signs of delusions of suspicion."[194] Acquaintances described events memorably. Farmer Timothy Neill drank whisky with nips of Chlorodyne. A farmhand thought Neill had "a touch of the delirium tremens" because he imagined "the police were after him and going to arrest him."[195] The men who worked with Scott Waltham in 1912 had sleepless nights because from the bunk he screamed that "they are after me." Following a spree five months earlier, phantoms had pursued Scott into the bush. His mates on the most recent occasion tied him to a bunk and told him to shut up.[196] Adele Curtis observed that her carpenter brother "seemed to think that people were watching and following him."[197] Widowed clerk Terrence Armstrong downed a fatal quantity of carbolic acid in front of a witness, exclaiming, "Thank God, it is all over. The Indians will not chase me any more." He left a note: "I am prepared to suffer by my own hand rather than suffer the tortures I have seen."[198] Mariner Peter Renkowski spent on drink the money he had saved to outfit himself as a gum digger. During withdrawal, he worried "about people looking fiercely at him."[199] When trooper Horatio Bishop went into withdrawal in his tent in early 1916, he believed that other soldiers thought he was a spy.[200]

The horrors drove men mad. Richard Fulton, an unemployed farm labourer, had been drinking for a week. An acquaintance gave him a ride in a gig. Twice on their journey Fulton said he saw men on horseback following him. He jumped out on a bridge and threw himself into a gorge. He often asked, "Who is that?" but there was no one.[201] Fifty-two-year-old Southland farmer Daniel O'Brien would disappear from his home for a week at a time. He spoke of "seeing things at night and even in the daytime." Several days after drinking bouts he became depressed.[202] Māori teamster Matene King was only twenty-six when withdrawal symptoms convinced co-workers that he was "out of his mind." A friend stated that Matene woke him about 4:00 a.m. the day before "and asked me to say prayers as he saw a lot of people outside the house."[203] Shortly before he took his life, Edward Vince experienced nightmares. A co-worker "heard him express wonder why people were going to hang him as he had never committed murder."[204]

Men helped workmates through bad periods. A casual acquaintance of withdrawal sufferer Daniel Hoolihan fed him steak and put him in a bunk.[205] Fencer William Innis noted that a friend had been unwell with delirium tremens for a week. "As a friend I was looking after him."[206] Police constables arrested drunks but also furnished food and modest medical attention and sometimes contacted family. Constable Dennis Byrne spoke to James Wayne's co-worker Abraham McBride, asking that he "keep him off drink." McBride complied and scarcely left Wayne for a fortnight.[207] Employers could be tolerant. The foreman of a public work project delivered one of his labourers by buggy to the nearest police station because the man had delusions – "they seemed to be in reference to his mother."[208] A justice of the peace recognized delirium tremens and remanded him to the local prison for medical treatment. Farmer William Barron let one of his men have the day off because "he was slightly the worse of drink." Barron prepared the man's meals while he recovered.[209] William Walker, a licensee at Bluff, dismissed twenty-five-year-old barman James Whitman for drinking and neglecting work. Unwilling to send the young man packing immediately, Walker gave him a room and helped him through the attack.[210]

The acts of civility are touching contributions to a picture of homo-sociability, but there were ugly properties of the drinking culture. The squandering of pay by married men led to neglect of family and much worse. Janet Hardy made a disastrous decision when she remarried. Her new husband stole her money, went "drinking about the town and shouting for all who came about with her money." She was "down in the dumps" and gassed herself and her eight-year-old daughter.[211] She was not alone in feeling wronged by a drink-centred masculine culture. If there was no more money, desperate men sold whatever they could. Returned soldier Andrew Keith sold his boots and clothes "to by some boose."[212]

The celebration of drink and matesmanship focuses on pub life, but a number of serious drinkers isolated themselves. Their rough, self-destructive behaviour went unseen. Blacksmith Thomas Davies slashed his throat in a hut filled with bottles. "It smelt of whiskey. Judging from the number of bottles I should say he had been drinking heavily."[213] "When I first went into the kitchen," said Mary Donaldson at the inquest into the suicide of her de facto husband, "I saw a lot of empty beer bottles lying on the table."[214] According to his wife, John Bowman kept a shed for his retreat and "often retired to this room to do his drinking, and I suspected that he had been drinking and was probably sleeping it off." She added, "I fear my husband when he has been drinking."[215] The constable who investigated the death of Brian Blake found that "some empty and some full bottles of wine were in the deceased's room suggesting that he had been indulging in a drinking bout previously to his death."[216] When farmer George Shields drank whiskey and kerosene, his wife fled with their children.[217]

The impositions of dependent drinkers constituted at best irritating burdens and at worst terrifying upsets to others. Acquaintances, friends, and employers could berate a noisy sufferer, walk away from the problem, or shunt the man along to the authorities. Managers of institutions that furnished shelter for workers or the destitute tolerated some drinking, but they had to be firm for the sake of others. The overseer of the Lyttleton Seaman's Institute turned out mariner Stephen Gilliam "owing to excessive drinking."[218] Wives and children suffered because they could not eject a chief income-earner without simultaneously inflicting hardship on themselves. When women did act, it was often after many years of enduring their spouses' drinking. Charles Tindale recalled that his father had had an attack of delirium tremens, and his mother had taken out a prohibition order against her husband and then finally left him.[219] Men so barred were common enough to be known as prohibited men.[220] Lucy Walker refused to go out and fetch more alcohol for her husband; drinking was undermining their stake in a farm. She also could see the effects of drink on his mental health. "At all times, other than when a depression occurred after a drinking bout," she said, "he was most agreeable."[221] Many forgiving wives said the same: "He was all right when he was off drink. He was a good husband."[222] "If he wasn't drinking he was a splendid man."[223] Not every suffering wife would concur. After a drinking binge, Arthur Parr committed suicide and left a note for his estranged wife: "I remain your disobedient Husband."[224] Alcohol, separation, unemployment, and violence were associated. Wives endured a lot.

Males other than husbands could disrupt households. Pensioner and widower William Street came to his son's house in a drunken state and threatened people. "We tried to pacify him as we had a music teacher in the house giving the girl [his granddaughter] lessons. We had to ask the teacher to leave the house on account of the language."[225] Woman had a distinct perspective on the misconduct of drunken men. Bertha Houston, daughter of a boarding-house keeper, had to fend off William Creswell. "I smelt liquor on him. He said would I go out with him? I said no I would not. With that he hit me on the face and head with his fists ... He had said previously that he would do for [kill] me if I did not go out with him."[226]

Abuse of alcohol affected mental health beyond the horrors. During the hours when he was not drinking, the habitual drunkard was ill-tempered, discouraged, depressed, taciturn, and incapable of concentrating. Kathleen Monahan recalled her efforts to bring her husband to his senses. "I prevailed upon my husband to leave hotels about six weeks ago in order to save expense, and in an endeavour to keep him away from associating with drinking companions ... During that time my husband was endeavouring to obtain a business, or employment, and his failure to obtain either was worrying him badly. He was drinking heavily, and was wasting his money, and was worried about it."[227] The association between alcohol and depression are complex. Nevertheless, it is striking how frequently witnesses before World War I used the expressions "depressed in spirits," "depressed," and "depression." A doctor in 1906 remarked that "it is a very common thing for persons a few days after they have left off heavy drinking to become melancholy and suicidal."[228] Boarding-house keeper George Hill noted that wharf labourer Humphrey Franks had been drinking heavily of late and became "more and more depressed."[229] A constable ascertained that Alfred Ball had been "drinking to excess over the past two years and when on these drinking bouts he became very depressed."[230] Whether depression came before or after a pattern of heavy drinking is less important, we think, than noting the overall corrosive effect of habitual drinking to excess.

Witnesses described prodigious drinking. William Prior, only twenty-nine when he jumped in front of a train, had been drinking heavily for five weeks.[231] Before he threatened to shoot his wife, Alfred Ransley had been "drinking on and off for three weeks."[232] Labourer John Finn, separated from his wife, had "been drinking heavily for the last fortnight."[233] Blenheim constable Dennis Byrne knew James Easton well enough to report that he went on sprees that could last a month.[234] Shopkeeper George Manson went for a five-day binge in 1914 and on his return "was very excited as a result of drink."[235] Emil Pederson told a friend that he could not work because of the effects of drink. Pederson had just come from a ten-day spree.[236] In early December 1914 Daniel Dugan, employed at a public drainage works, took a drink. Unable to stop, he drank for at least three weeks and could not resume work. An overseer said that "his only trouble was drink."[237] Charles Thomson claimed that his father "had been drinking from the beginning of May till about the 4th of August."[238]

A depressed boot-maker, William Bonham, had been drinking for over two weeks when he killed himself. According to his brother, "he used to break out on the burst every three months." Between sprees, he consumed two cases of whiskey every three months. "My brother got through a good amount of whiskey when he got going."[239] Unemployed during the post-war recession, Henry McEwen nevertheless joined his mates for drinking bouts, when "they practically lost count of days and nights or time."[240] For some men, a craving was so great that when family or the authorities secured a court order to put them on the list of prohibited persons or when they had run out of cash or credit, they descended into abject misery. At age fifty, farm labourer Richard Chisholm remarked that he was getting too old to follow his usual line of work, but to make matters worse, the licensee "had stopped his drink and life was not worth living."[241]

Drinking caused or exacerbated health problems and aggravated isolation. A patient of Dr John Paget had an attack of the horrors. Paget worried that heavy drinking would affect the man's brain and heart. If he was insane when he committed suicide, said Paget, "it would probably be the result of chronic alcoholism."[242] Post-mortems occasionally added incidental information about heavy drinkers. Master mariner Henry Jepson was forty when he took an overdose of Chlorodyne in 1910; the post-mortem showed damage to the stomach from alcoholism.[243] The report for John Renton, who died in 1914, stated that "the liver showed old standing and chronic alcohol cirrhosis. The heart was unhealthy and showed disease of the aorta."[244] Alcohol-plagued men were more likely than others to be emotionally isolated; they were more likely to be unmarried, divorced, or separated. Men with alcohol-abuse problems were more likely than other men to have committed suicide in hotels, boarding-houses, huts, tents, workers' barracks, and bodies of water rather than in a house.[245]

The most abundant of the shocking accounts of alcohol abuse and suicide originate in inquests held before 1920. The number of cases dropped sharply after World War I (Table 2.1). During the first two decades of the century, a period roughly coinciding with the years of national development, bars possessed a social attraction for men who by and large benefited from years of economic growth and construction. Compared to the post-war recession and the Great Depression, the pre-war years seemed a time of optimism and spending. Serious drinkers during this era consumed distilled spirits. Temperance initiatives and belt-tightening financial conditions, beginning with the post-war recession, could have diminished the volume and character of alcohol consumption. Alcohol's soul-destroying potential had only abated, not disappeared, in the 1980s and 1990s. Loss of work, family, and self-loathing continued to be the burdens of addiction.[246] The use of other intoxicants was now on the rise.

Sad biographies of alcoholics surfaced to the end of the century, although less frequently than in earliest decades. Robert Steele, who died in 2000, started drinking in his teens, turned to substance abuse, tried a Salvation Army detoxification program, returned to drink, took up meth, and became psychotic. Toward the end, "he just seemed to have lost the will to fight."[247] Fully aware of the costs of alcohol abuse, governments had a restricted scope for action. Prohibition, of course, was out of the question, but government policy long subsidized abusive consumption. Under the principled standards of social security introduced in 1938, individuals could be granted an invalid benefit on account of their alcoholism, accepted as an incapacitating illness, even though it was "recognised that there are problems associated with payment of benefit monies directly to beneficiaries who are alcoholics." Payments conditional on treatment were rejected.[248] The Fourth Labour Government addressed the enduring problem with a competition for new funding for treatment programs. With well-established work in the field, the Salvation Army was a leading recipient.[249]

In the closing decades of the century, straight alcoholism as a motive for suicide was certainly encountered and possibly increasing at the turn of the millennium (Table 2.1), but there was also poly-addiction. Poly-substance abuse had started to hook teenagers. In the 1980s, as we show in chapters five and seven, cannabis was becoming a popular intoxicant, especially among young adults. However, adolescents too young for work or to receive benefit payments experimented with the cheaper alternatives to cannabis and tried "huffing" butane, petrol, glue, hairspray, and fly spray.[250] The expression "poly-substance abuse" surfaced with alarming frequency in medical reports to coroners in the 1990s. There was a marked cultural shift as adolescents and young adults turned to diverse forms of substance abuse. Fresh health challenges arose on account of increased numbers of drug-induced psychoses. There was as well an unprecedented need for counselling and detoxification facilities for teens.[251]

Table 2.1
Percentage and number of suicides in which alcohol abuse appears as the leading motive: Types of years and gender

	Years	*Men*	*Women*
National development	1900–18; 1924–26	18.5 (*n* = 202)	8.3 (*n* = 18)
The Great Depression	1928–38	8.6 (*n* = 87)	1.5 (*n* = 4)
War recovery years	1920–24; 1946–48	9.8 (*n* = 96)	3.6 (*n* = 11)
The Long Prosperity	1940–44; 1950–74	6.9 (*n* = 109)	3.9 (*n* = 26)
The era of economic crises	1976–98	4.5 (*n* = 170)	2.8 (*n* = 32)
Recovery begins	2000	11.0 (*n* = 40)	9.7 (*n* = 10)

CONCLUDING OBSERVATIONS

Most cases illustrating this chapter's themes occurred in the years before the late-twentieth-century economic crises. This selectivity expresses our impression of extraordinary changes in cultural values that began in the 1960s and that overlapped with a breakdown in economic opportunities originating in the 1970s. These alterations continued with force into the 1980s and 1990s. The shifts in cultural values and the collapse of economic prospects for young people go a long way toward explaining a late-century escalation in youth suicides. Discussions of relationship cases from the 1980s and 1990s are therefore largely postponed until chapter seven. In the current chapter, we have evidence of a different time.

These earlier decades provide a baseline that shows marital strife and women's entrapment. Against that baseline, we detected both continuity and change. From the perspective of troubled relationships, the late-century economic crises had some firm associations with the past. Certain features of male conduct continued; men resented separation orders and they postured and threatened. However, on account of a greater recourse to de facto connections and a decline in formal marriages, by the end of the century break-ups displayed greater informality in more instances. That informality arising from the sexual revolution meant that many more intimate relationships were fluid; moreover, the perilous events in many of these late-century relationships occurred much earlier in their inception than what has been seen in this chapter. For most of the century, women in bad marriages endured violence, drunkenness, and squandered money until middle age or later. The inquests after 1980 disclose a greater proportion of youthful break-ups.

It is striking that women during most of the century had endured abusive mates for many years before taking legal action. Separation and maintenance orders did not always protect them. Some men and women represented in the inquest files stayed together for a long time despite irreconcilable differences. Liberalized divorce laws and wider acceptance of de facto relationships may have improved the lives of many. However, an impression left from reading thousands of suicide case files for the last decades of the century is that the men and women, often boys and girls, who formed and subsequently ended relationships were extremely immature. In earlier eras, there were precursors of such individuals and events, but not in great numbers. In prior times, as we have seen in this chapter, suicidal men with relationship troubles usually were married. In this chapter, too, we remarked on the passions of jilted boyfriends and threats by men of diverse ages to kill themselves if a woman did not stay with them. Threats of suicide not only persisted but increased with the sexual revolution, when adolescents and young adults resorted to this manoeuvre. By at least the mid-1970s, psychiatrists referred to such an incident as "a suicidal gesture."[252]

This chapter does not showcase admirable conduct from men. Violence and threats of violence are prominent. The National Collective of Independent Women's Refuges had good reason to advocate, as it did in 1985, that "male violence needs to be recognised rather than a victim-oriented only approach which is the easy way out."[253] Alcohol abuse runs as a substantial theme in the first two decades of the century, and thereafter seems a modest one, although other substances came into play late in the century. Men remained alcohol's foremost 'victims.' In addition to reprehensible aspects of male conduct that may have been built up in a culture and thus were susceptible to education and reformation, there is evidence of a biological element in men's lives. The sex drive in its variations continued from adolescence into the prime years and beyond. This drive was evident in suicide cases where the motive was rejection, before marriage or during a break-up. The drive surfaced in a few cases of sexual abuse. These episodes, ending in suicides, could have been discussed in relation to law and order. A few individuals, once again primarily men, took their own lives rather than face the shame of a courtroom appearance or rather than endure punishment for having committed a theft or an assault. Sexual offences were and are distinct from other offences and can be considered with other modes of conduct that partly originate from a sex drive. We found eighty men and two women who committed suicide as a result of an investigation into a sex offence. The problem that opened this chapter, the difference in the suicide rates of men and women, can best be explained by case-based inquiry.

Intent and method played a part in the persistent difference in male and female suicide rates. There were differences in the patterns of motives for men and women. Some motives and the associated intentions of the individuals led to deliberate choices in the method of self-harm. More so than women, men aggravated life's troubles with alcohol and violence. They created difficulties for themselves respecting relationships and the law. Some men who took their own lives on account of these motives had conceived of a solution that had to be nothing less than complete self-destruction, because in their minds death alone would deeply wound another party or end feelings of shame. An unsuccessful attempt was insufficient for these objectives. A mere attempt could signal suffering and elicit help, but these were rarely the desired goals of men at the moment of decision. Impulsiveness characterized many of the men. They were impatient with their girlfriends or wives; they set ultimatums; if rebuffed, they had to deliver on the threat and blight the life of a spouse or girlfriend. They made rash decisions shortly after an incident that upset them. In the next chapter, we consider how the ideology of work produced further crises for men.

3

Dark Days and Golden Weather: Despair and Work, 1900–80

An assumption that downturns in business cycles increase suicides has driven attempts to correlate suicide rates with measurements of economic health. We can present our data to show a simple relationship between economic conditions and suicide rates; roughly speaking – very roughly speaking – good times brought low rates, and bad times brought high rates (Graph 1.1, Table 3.1). On their own, inferences connecting bad times and rising suicides are unremarkable. To confirm and clarify associations between people's economic circumstances and suicides, it is necessary to look directly into real-life circumstances. Economic troubles enter individuals' lives by diverse paths, not only through hardships attending the shocks of economic recessions. Other circumstances include insecurity due to labour market practices, personal conduct, and sheer misfortune. It is important to note political changes as well as the phases in the business cycle. For example, social welfare measures tempered the impact of economic downturns, while legislation on labour relations improved the lot of workers. Over the century, government altered the world of work in ways that improved everyday life, but not always for everyone. For men who had a job, a pension, or disposable assets such as a farm, an economic crisis could be weathered. For young people, the crises of the 1980s meant a delayed start in life. These considerations and many more to follow, all derived from case files, suggest the thinness of arguments based on correlations of aggregate data.[1]

In addition to paying attention to grand scale economic events, political action, and demography, it is essential to observe the interaction between major events and personal responsibility. Some financial reversals originated in addictions and misconduct. Men went deeply into debt, lost jobs, suffered reductions in status, or failed in business on account of alcoholism and gambling; many went through costly domestic troubles of their own making. Yet not every self-inflicted laceration to pocketbook, masculine pride, or morale can be disentangled from the business cycle, the economy's structures, or the state of social welfare. Men were known to drink to excess to escape momentarily their financial disappointments and career regrets; they were known to throw violent fits in black moods of defeat when their constricted autonomy had been challenged further at work or in the home. When their words and deeds are before us, it is difficult not to censure unseemly conduct, but we must spare a thought for their lives at work. Case histories show the hard realities of work and finance in everyday life.

WHERE DO ECONOMIC TROUBLES END?

This chapter on suicide and the economy opens with statistical overviews based on two variables in our data set that allow us to connect suicides directly to economic circumstances. That sounds promising; however, working with these variables raises the crucial problem of separating economic motives from many others. Whether or not money was the root of all evil, its absence figured as the root of much unhappiness. Did unemployment or financial difficulties precede or follow other prominent motives for suicide? Case files show that certain motives interacted: work and finance troubles undermined relationships; they upset mental health; alcohol abuse undermined work and finances; physical ailments resulted in a loss of work. It is apparent that many men in the workforce who committed suicide had struggled to make ends meet, and that persistent effort cost them peace of mind.

The second way of connecting suicide and the economic circumstances of men is to consider the deceased's state of employment or financial circumstances. Police investigations and witnesses' statements nearly always yielded information on the employment status or financial condition of the deceased. For adult men in the workforce who were neither retired nor too young to work, this information surfaced somewhere in virtually every file (92.6 percent of all male cases, n = 5,463). This number excludes retirees who committed suicide (15.7 percent of all male cases, n = 1,313); their files

Table 3.1
Estimates on suicide rates of men and the proportion of male suicides (men in the workforce) that involved work or finance problems, 1900–2000

	Range of suicide rates for all males	*% of cases with a pronounced work or financial motive*	*% of cases with a reference to work or financial trouble*
National development	18.2–23.8	17.2	58.9
The Great Depression	17.5–27.5	20.1	57.0
War recovery years	14.5–23.1	17.4	57.1
The Long Prosperity	11.0–16.0	13.4	32.4
The era of economic crises	16.0–24.5	10.6	52.4
Addendum (2000)	18.5	9.3	43.4
All cases in the century (excluding 2000)	11.0–27.5	13.8	50.9

Table 3.2
Employment or financial status of all males, 1900–98

Employment or financial status according to witnesses	*N of cases*	*% of cases*	*Percentage with Economic Troubles*
Employed	2,325	27.7	
Unemployed	1,067	12.7	12.7
Self-employed, doing well	123	1.5	
Self-employed, not doing well	1,229	14.7	14.7
Self-employed, no added information	426	5.1	
Not in the work force: student, inmate	603	7.2	
Beneficiary	705	8.4	8.4
Retired	1,313	15.7	5.0 (est.)
Private means and other	23	0.3	
Unknown	574	6.8	3.4 (est.)
Total	8,388	100.0	45.8

did not routinely contain information about financial security. Half the men in the workforce and about whom we have pertinent information experienced work or financial troubles (50.9 percent, n = 3,001). An unknown number of retirees surely had economic troubles; the status of students, inmates, and others is outside the calculation, so perhaps economic difficulties extended to forty percent or more of men of all ages who committed suicide (Tables 3.1 and 3.2). Economic information for women rarely appeared in the case files, because constables and coroners commonly used the labels "housewife," "spinster," "girl," or the expression "domestic duties," which

Table 3.3
Employment or financial status of all females, 1900–98

Employment or financial status according to witnesses	N *of cases*	*% of cases*
Housewife or home duties	948	36.4
Employed	387	14.9
Unemployed	252	9.7
Self-employed, doing well	3	0.1
Self-employed, not doing well	103	4.0
Self-employed, no added information	29	1.1
Retired or pensioner	365	14.0
Not in workforce: student, inmate, patient	223	8.6
Beneficiary	157	6.0
Private Means	25	1.0
Unknown	112	4.3
Total	2,604	100.0

conveyed nothing about economic circumstances but presumed dependence (Table 3.3).

By adopting a narrow conception of material circumstances, captured in the motives variable, we can say that one in eight men committed suicide due to a serious work or economic problem. By applying a looser conception of economic trouble, reflected in the economic status variable, we can say that perhaps half of adult males were affected by poor economic circumstances. The two approaches confirm that loss of work and financial setbacks were suicide risk factors. To learn more about the actual connections among economic conditions, individual reasoning, and suicide, we must explore beyond these estimates and consider the structure of the labour market, the burden of responsibility for failure that the culture placed on individuals, and the isolation of people in need. On occasion, we can get close to the thoughts that mediated people's material circumstances and their mental states.

There were groups of years when connections between the health of the economy and suicide rates were patent. Rates soared for awhile during the Great Depression. The case files help explain this connection by showing precisely who suffered, how, and why. Witnesses explained the specific plights that overwhelmed the deceased; that degree of detail, which accents the importance of identifying populations at risk, could never have been extracted from aggregate data. If we follow the logic of an inverse relationship of suicide rates to economic growth, then during the years of the long prosperity we would expect to find rates falling. They did decline. However, in addition to these two confirmatory sets of years, our data exposed two anomalies.

First, during the years of national development, a simple connection between economic expansion and a presumption of low suicide rates could not be unconditionally accepted. Suicide rates were moderately high in those years, although most of the years covered were ones of relatively good if uneven economic growth. There were a considerable number of suicides by adult men with economic or work-related troubles. Testimony at the inquests shows more exactly how poor working conditions adversely affected men and their families during these years. As well as the economy's overall performance, its structure is significant. Second, case files in the years of economic crises at the end of the century disclose an important inconsistency: there was a surge in witnesses mentioning economic troubles, but also an abundance of non-economic motives, particularly mental illnesses. The soaring references to the latter pulled down the proportion of economic motives. Disastrous economic conditions do not directly explain the rising suicide rate in the last quarter of the century. Complications attending efforts to connect the economy and suicide are clearly challenging, but they can be untangled to reveal the workings of historical change and the interaction of people's material expectations and mental states.

To better understand the connections between suicide and employment or finances, this chapter assembles statements from witnesses and suicide notes from the years of national development and the Great Depression. Statements have been sorted by themes within the sets of years in order to reconstruct the constraints that afflicted people and, where possible, to show the fusion of the material and mental realms. The two eras just mentioned show commonalities in terms of the types of people who were economically vulnerable: small farmers, farm labourers, and general labourers. Yet the Great Depression was a distinct period. Not only was the proportion of suicides associated with work or financial troubles high, but it attained its peak for the century. The exceedingly complicated era of economic crises in the last two decades of the twentieth century could have been considered in this chapter. However, that period involved enormous and diverse economic challenges that overlapped with important cultural, demographic, and medical changes. Therefore, it requires a chapter of its own, chapter seven. Finally, for the sake of contrast, the current chapter looks at the long era of prosperity.

The four sets of years mentioned in the preceding paragraph represent more than distinct phases of economic health. They track the evolution of the state's management of the economy and the setting-up of social welfare. During national development years, some important large-scale state ventures such as the railway with its stations, manufacturing shops, and housing estates came to maturity. There were additional indicators of national material development including the construction of schools and hospitals, and the noteworthy creation of mental hospitals. A modern community was being built in bursts of construction, often with public funds. As well, in 1898 a modest old-age pension funded from general government revenues was put in place. Tom Brooking reasonably describes the pension as "mean and limited."[2] The bulk of economic activity and popular thought about work and society occurred in a laissez-faire setting; the country's presumed natural abundance was supposed to minimize requests for welfare assistance.[3] A culture of individualism thrived without effective countervailing pressure from a labourers' political party. That situation began to change during World War I, although governments that catered to farmers and the middle class dominated until the Great Depression.

The Great Depression exposed problems arising from individualism. In 1938, toward the end of the slump, the First Labour Government introduced social welfare safety nets in the form of benefits for the unemployed and the sick. State economic planning and control was launched.[4] A convergence of the mature welfare state and a strong demand for the country's exports produced material contentment. During the years of prosperity, the fall in the suicide rate and a fall in the proportion of male suicides attributable to economic motives show another side of the association between suicides and the economy. Over a long period of mainly prosperous years, a generation presumed all was well. When the overseas markets for agricultural exports crumbled for exogenous reasons, the managed economy could not be sustained in its entirety and the years of crises began. Welfare and medical benefits remained in place for the poverty-stricken during much of this trying period. However, young people by the early 1980s looked to the future with foreboding as never before, because of an abrupt disappearance of entry-level jobs.

LAISSEZ-FAIRE ANXIETIES

We have characterized many years in the early twentieth century as ones of national development. Nevertheless, the economy during those many years experienced boom and bust turbulence. Organized labour gained ground, although rival unions expended considerable effort in conflicts among themselves over whether the best strategy for extracting more decent awards was through arbitration or the strike. Legislation allowed both options but unions had to choose how they would register. Divisions within the labour movement and determined opposition from the government checked union radicalism during a series of strikes in 1912–13. Labour in politics developed a good-sized following during the war. For the time being, however, unevenly distributed prosperity and high unemployment continued to make life difficult for wage-earners. As Tom Brooking points out, "up to 10 per cent of the work force was probably unemployed in an intermittent and seasonal manner in the years preceding the First World War."[5] Their difficulties surfaced in the economic motives for suicide cited in witnesses' depositions and in constables' reports on their routine investigations into violent deaths that accompanied inquests. In his report into the 1906 death of an unknown labourer, a Christchurch constable stated, "I think he was of the vagrant class."[6]

Unemployment and the sense that workers were falling behind when the country was prospering, or falling behind after the country had prospered in the 1890s, help to account for labour militancy in the mines and on the docks in 1912–13.[7] Our case-based account of economic motives for suicide can begin here, because a handful of suicides connected with strikes capture intimate scenes of workers denied easy choices. Married men worried about supporting their families. A union official directed blacksmith Harvey Nichol to walk the picket line; he refused and desperately wanted to get back to work, as he had serious financial problems and an injured son who needed medical treatment.[8] Some men crossed the picket lines and suffered for it. After the end of a coal mine strike, a union refused to put one such miner on its membership roster on three occasions, thus keeping him out of employment. On the first occasion, he had "a nervous breakdown." After the third rejection, he wrote: "Seeing I have so much trouble with work concerns. Being turned down. And having to leave the place. I have made up my mind to end my life rather than shift the family about."[9]

Miners, seamen, and wharfies were in dangerous trades. As James Belich aptly describes, they were ambivalent about the risks and toil; they resented bosses, but the work helped define them.[10] When not working, they could become depressed. The dockworkers' strike put sailor Alfred Spencer out of work "for some considerable time."[11] Hardship and disappointment extended to strike leaders. A union organizer went without work for weeks, became violent when things did not go his way, and sat brooding in the dark.[12] Organized labour's struggles claimed a few victims. The more common problems described below show the inequities and hazards of *laissez-faire*. Some sources of hardship would never have vanished without combative opposition. In justification of labour's skirmishes with capital, it is important to document what kept many workers impoverished and drove some to self-destruction. Through the extreme example of self-destruction, the inquests show that workers paid a price in mental anguish for their stands against employers.

In the years of national development, fanciful schemes for getting ahead endured and so did the reality of the power of a few over the many. The structure of work relations left wage earners vulnerable. Days of reckoning collided with the rainbow myths of private lives. At times, individualism burst out in the romantic hopes of the poor, in their dreams of escaping poverty by finding gold or by saving all through a winning wager. Accountant Jim Pattison "lost all his savings a year ago by gold digging speculations."[13] Hope did not spring eternal. In the material world, defeats had to be acknowledged, debts paid, and loans extended. In 1870, John Dowling had deserted HMS *Conqueror* and joined the Otago gold rush; a single, destitute alcoholic by 1916, he ended up penniless.[14] Hoping to find gold but bringing only hard times to his family, Stuart Scott shot himself near his diggings.[15] Poor and without work, Andrew Gratton went to the races in hope of getting some money and failed.[16] An otherwise "most correct living young man" was further described by a constable as in financial trouble due to "his gambling mania."[17] Clerk George Rivers had misappropriated funds, "the result of betting."[18] A few who gambled and lost accepted personal responsibility. Douglas Reid, who had no relatives in the country, had speculated on gold mining shares in the 1870s and their failure caused him ongoing difficulties. A friend remarked that Reid "declined help and said he could get through."[19] After three days of losing at the race track in 1906, Walter Newland told a chum that "he was tired of this life and never did like work."[20]

Individualism fostered dreams, the inverse of which was the shame of personal failure. John Lindsey's debts depressed him, but his inability to keep the matter out of the newspapers crushed his pride. According to his brother, "he was very sensitive as to his name appearing."[21] Shame arising out of the ethos of personal responsibility and the almost bankable asset of reputation could overwhelm men in financial trouble or men who had fallen in status. Reflecting on the events that led to Andrew Collingwood hanging himself in jail, a constable testified that he had been summoned to a farm. "I took the deceased's swag and strapped it on my saddle and told him I would arrest him as an idle and disorderly person." Collingwood refused to give his name, because, he said, "I do not want my parents to know I have come to this."[22] The constable arrested the young man because farmers enlisted the police to remove lingering discharged labourers. A few men internalized explanations for their fallen status.

The era's often one-sided labour management practices could intimidate men who feared a boss's displeasure. Anxious about their livelihood in a setting of high unemployment, workers took it seriously when bosses knocked them back. John Brunton, a heavy smoker and a nervous man, had little sleep or food when he worked on a particular farm because, his wife remarked, "he thought he was going to be discharged."[23] Young men seeking a trade entered apprenticeships that placed them in the hands of craftsmen who appraised their skills and development. Reprimanded by a cabinet maker, apprentice John Fellows feared dismissal. His father remarked that "he is inclined to be sensitive and would feel hurt if spoken to sharply by anyone in authority."[24]

Larger farmers gained from cheap labour. By hiring boys and young men, a few farmers secured workers whom they could bully and exploit. Sixteen-year-old William Pettit immigrated to New Zealand under the auspices of Flock House. Funded by sheep farmers, this organisation brought out roughly 760 orphans, mostly sons of United Kingdom seamen killed in World War I. The organization allocated juveniles to participating sheep stations. The coroner inquiring into Pettit's death remarked on the lad's "lonely solitary existence" and what this would have done to "a shy and reserved boy who found it difficult to make friends with the very few people available [on the isolated station]." The magistrate criticized a "taciturn, unapproachable and close-fisted" employer, and condemned farmers "whose chief interest in the Flock House scheme is that they may return them a fair proportion [of former prosperous times] by way of cheap farm labour." Pettit was not only being exploited – two-thirds of his wages went to Flock House – but Flock House representatives at the inquest had pressed to obtain an open verdict to protect this scheme's reputation.[25] On other occasions, farmers criticized young labourers for failure to heed instructions. The employer of twenty-year-old Ralph Gibbs stated that he "was leaving my employ as a result of my desiring him to work differently." Gibbs shot himself.[26] Hierarchy and an expectation of deference permeated this laissez-faire culture.

Workers were vulnerable and fearful because they saved little if anything; some men who died by their own hand in this era consumed their pay in alcohol. Their unsteadiness led to complaints about the quality of their work. Insobriety resulted in the suspension of telegrapher Percy Burton, whose position demanded reliability and accuracy.[27] Horse trainer Edward Hale, out of work and out of money, took poison. He did not die immediately and so was questioned by a sergeant of police who asked how he lost his money. "I spent it." On drink.[28] The old-age pension helped cover boarding-house expenses for the many retired workers who did not live high on the hog.[29]

Among the men who committed suicide and who were out of work at the time, support from family members was rare for a multitude of reasons. A lot of men were single and new to the country. Friends assumed that being unmarried left a bachelor free from financial troubles, when it could as easily have been assumed that an extended family of in-laws might have rallied to support men in distress. A mate of unemployed James Simmons put the supposed benefits of bachelorhood this way: "he had no monetary problems as he was an independent man." In fact, Simmons worried greatly about losing his job.[30] However, the comment that single men had no financial worries does call attention to the cares of raising a large family. Responsible for supporting such a family on a failing sheep farm, George Fredericks "seemed to be suffering from depression."[31] A Danish newcomer with five children faced eviction when the owner of the small plot the family occupied would not renew the lease.[32] The overriding point is that labourers traversed life on a financial tightrope where every step was perilous.

If they fell, who would come to their aid? What would happen to men, like those observed in chapter two, who had forfeited family respect? Misconduct meant that families wanted nothing to do with them.[33] A court order for arrears in family support pushed the financial circumstances of many men into a chronic state of debt or sent them packing.[34] The government placed responsibility for the maintenance of wives and children on men, no matter how impoverished. This legal reminder of men's duties supported individual responsibility, and contained government welfare expenditures. Evasions of court orders – often seen in case files – disclose the flaw in the practice, just as the inquests disclose a few of the strategy's victims.

Men could lack supporting social networks for numerous reasons, among them transience, marital disputes, downward mobility that cut them off from former friends, and recent immigration.[35] Lack of income overwhelmed single immigrants who landed in the country without local family ties. Welshman William Jones, a swagman and alcoholic whose money had run out, had no relatives in the country.[36] William Adams had emigrated from Scotland where he had been an engine fitter. Without a patron and unable to follow his trade in New Zealand, he drifted as a casual labourer.[37] Another recently arrived Scot found himself without work or prospects and entirely alone.[38] Carpenter Eric Brown, from the Hebrides, had only been in the country seven weeks when he was let go without prospect for work or relatives to assist.[39] Miner John Franklin from the Newcastle coalfields had barely settled into work at Huntly when a strike by coal miners left him without earnings. Lonely in his Salvation Army lodgings, he often mentioned his mother back home. "He seemed in extreme mental depression."[40] According to an acquaintance, Transvaal newcomer James Chatham said that "he had no work and appeared to be miserable."[41]

Isolation was one thing, hostility another. Joe Lee Chin felt that people stopped taking laundry to his establishment when "European women" started a business.[42] Shortly after the start of the war, Austrian labourer Frank Fischel – "chased and cursed by some Englishmen" – despaired of getting work on account of his origins.[43] It was not ethnic-based hostility that hurt a Melbourne theatre manager who had arrived in the country, but attitudes close to home. When he encountered business troubles, his brother-in-law lectured him: "Shake yourself together. Be a man and move yourself ahead in the world."[44] Individual responsibility pervaded the culture, but people's troubles often had social origins too big to face alone.

In lieu of a robust welfare system and in view of the hostility or absence of a family, emergency assistance had to be secured from other connections. Publicans, boarding-house keepers, friends, lodge brothers, and pawnbrokers advanced cash.[45] Pawn tickets turned up in the pockets or at the lodgings of the deceased. Constables assisted men down on their luck.[46] Tobacconist John Ryan helped out old labourer Michael Scully by holding his earnings and doling out money "to keep him from unwise spending." Ryan also lent him money. On their last meeting Scully "[b]urst into tears and said he was disappointed at not getting work."[47] There came times of reckoning when accounts fell due and credit ended. Late in 1930, the village butcher turned away Lucy Paige, whose common-law husband had no work. "He stopped our credit," she told a friend, "and will not let us have any more meat."[48] Impoverished Wilhelm Schmidt was evicted from his boarding-house for overdue accounts; his former landlord "was surprised to learn that he had 3d on him when found as [he] did not think he possessed any money at all."[49] Once work dried up, the last pence were gone, and informal sources of credit had been exhausted, destitute workers fell back on charitable bodies, the foremost being the Salvation Army. In all years of the century, men 'between jobs' stayed with the 'Sallies.'[50] In Auckland at the outset of the Great Depression, men without work shuttled between the Salvation Army's Working Men's Home and city-run "Shelters at the Domain."[51] Unemployed seamen "lived in the Sailors' Home."[52] A few hard-pressed families put their children in orphanages or convents.[53]

New Zealand's old-age pension gave eligible recipients more support and thus greater freedom than was granted to elderly counterparts in most places in the economically developed world. Still, individuals who expected more than bare survival, and especially those who did not qualify, had to save for retirement years or be supported by children. A few white-collar workers and businesspeople who invested in shares or real estate discovered that their retirement investments had been ill-chosen.[54] Workers in the agricultural and mining sectors had little chance of saving and struggled to work even when too old to handle the pace or load of manual work.[55] At sixty-eight, miner Edmund Field was out of employment and "this seemed to worry him." "I see no future for me," he told his son.[56]

Sixty-five-year-old French immigrant Louis Vernier worked at anything he could get.[57] Aged seventy-three and incapacitated for two years due to a painful rupture, farmer Reginald Francis felt useless.[58] Another man of the same age "did odd jobs" to stave off poverty.[59] "A feeble old man" with a drinking problem lost his employment as a market gardener and slipped into destitution.[60] At sixty-four, widower and itinerant labourer Harry Walters wrote that "I am getting too old for it now so the best thing is to end the penny section [a reference to getting off a street car at the end of a section of a line]."[61] Aging thrust manual workers into precarious circumstances and family members were not always eager to assist; some tried to place the men against their will in charity hospitals or old men's homes.

Old age in this era could be defined by the rigour of work. Shearing wore men out at an early age. When Richard Whitson, a shearer in his late forties, returned home at the end of the season, he was thin, run-down, and despondent about facing work the next season. His doctor said he suffered from nervous exhaustion.[62] On account of illness or injury, men of all ages could have trouble coping with an employer's demands. There was no social insurance to cover a portion of wages lost when ill or disabled. Farm labourers, urban labourers of no fixed trade, miners, and "wharfies" were numerous and their chores hazardous.[63] Men in these occupations turned up often in the files. Injured in a fall and also suffering from a heart condition, farm employee Richard McKinstry had not worked for six months.[64] A rupture that required a truss impeded Danish immigrant Hans Petersen, who had been working as a farm labourer.[65] According to his doctor, farmer Thomas Burke "remarked that he was annoyed at losing so much time over his sick leg."[66] A back injury kept James Pike unemployed. With a large family to support, he experienced "fits of depression and was frightened."[67] Other men similarly felt "depressed when out of employment."[68] A link between unemployment and depression could originate in sheer anxiety about survival, but there is evidence too that men of property who had found purpose in their work coped poorly when they stopped. So it was with Douglas Archibald. At the age of sixty he visited his doctor, because "the work on the farm was heavy." He could not accept advice to sell out, because his life was tied up with his farm.[69]

The interludes of recession inflicted an assortment of painful experiences on men. In the years of national development, many were caught in the recession after the South African War; next came a construction downturn that began just before World War I, and then a worse crisis after that conflict's end.[70] When the post-war recession took hold in 1920, Alexander Johnston lost his business, became a labourer, and feared eviction from his house.[71] During these periods when real estate speculation and construction faltered, carpenters appeared as a prominent occupational group among suicides. They and kindred tradesmen such as bricklayers rode the peaks and troughs of the business cycle.[72] When housing demand fell, creditors pressed; work dried up; their own properties held on speculation lost value.[73] A young building contractor lost all his money on a contract during the post-war recession.[74] Around the same time, another contractor suffered from worry-induced despondency because he could not obtain the materials needed to complete a contract.[75] Retired builder Melville Buckley lost his savings in housing investments.[76] In the estimation of his business partner, Ernest Harper "had been somewhat depressed of late" and "had been worrying unnecessarily about slackness of business."[77] Early in 1930, builder Walter Morris exhausted his overdraft coverage at the bank and, according to a friend, "he owed money to many people."[78] During the recessions of the early twentieth century, crushed pride, fear, and sleeplessness overwhelmed the country's small entrepreneurs, including its farmers.

The sheer number of farmers in the country made theirs the most numerous occupation cited at the suicide inquests; their prominence in these records also derived from the challenges they confronted. Farmers carried the double burden of hard physical labour and the ordeals of managing a business. They had to make crucial decisions about selling or retaining livestock, and investing in improvements and land. Established farmers had an easier time, but men who expanded or opened new farms to take advantage of the dairy and frozen meat booms had difficulties.

Some small farmers who committed suicide were overwhelmed by a belief that they had made a grave mistake. At different times farmer Charles Lang "said how sorry he was to have bought the island wool property."[79] He considered that business worries had unbalanced his mind. To a friend he confided that "the way things were going it would drive him to the asylum."[80] Klaus Reinhardt wanted to improve his family's situation by acquiring a sheep run, but discovered too late that the land selected was abysmal. Living alone in a tent on the tract, while his wife stayed in town, he thought that he had made a huge mistake.[81] Worried to the point of insomnia, John Green could not decide on the best strategy to benefit his children. He needed the greater revenue of a larger farm to raise them, but liked his current property.[82] Young farmer Ralph Herrington "worried about making the wrong decision." His parents were dead and he had to manage the estate for his brother and sisters; they made him feel ashamed for having sold the family farm. "It was our home as well as his," said his brother, "although he owned it."[83] This trace of recrimination may have been sharper, louder, and hurtful when Herrington was alive.

A work culture that emphasized individual responsibility and an economy that called for cheap physical labour put workers in spirit-crushing circumstances. The young could be bullied and isolated; the newcomer could drift without assistance; the ill and injured could plummet into destitution in a trice; the old could spend their last years sliding from their struggle with unsustainable work into poverty. Harsh working conditions, diverse uncertainties, and personal decisions established complex relationships between suicide and the economy. The hard circumstances persisted into the Great Depression and were magnified for a time in rural New Zealand.

DESPERATION IN THE "SUGAR-BAG YEARS"

In New World settlement societies, there were commanding myths about farming's importance to initiative, independence, and happiness. These Arcadian myths sustained nostalgia about rural contentment and internalized the work culture that contributed to feelings of guilt or inadequacy among farmers and wage earners when ends did not meet. Up to and beyond the Great Depression, New Zealand governments subscribed to these myths. An occasional work of fiction depicted the harshness of rural life. Some historians have deflated the notion that rural life was more wholesome and integrating than its urban counterpart. The case-file evidence reviewed earlier in this chapter describes abysmal conditions for rural labourers and less established farmers. The rise in the suicide rate during the Great Depression suggests that for more people material circumstances had become worse, and with that spread of poverty and worry, mental health crises increased (Graph 1.1). The fall in food consumption, notes James Belich, is a good indication that the "'sugarbag years' when the unemployed made clothes out of hessian sacks from the Chelsea Sugar Refinery" were truly dreadful times.[84] Far from being bucolic, it seemed that rural living had become more gruelling than life in the towns and cities. To test this impression of hardship and suicide in the countryside, we endeavoured to calculate rural suicide rates for the first half of the century when the country was rural to the core in its national myths and productive output.

In order to calculate the crucially important suicide rates for the rural sector, reliable counts of rural suicides had to be extracted from the data set. But what is a rural suicide? There were at least four possible ways of counting rural male suicides. It proved even more difficult to count women, because witnesses and officials seldom gave them occupational labels that placed them in the country. Since a woman in a rural or urban setting was described as a wife, a housewife, a girl, or a spinster tending to household duties, it was impossible to neatly separate farm women from other women. For men, the presence of occupational information, locales, and incidental facts allowed several means of separating rural men from others. We could have included men selected by the following criteria: (1) all who committed suicide in rural settings; (2) all with an agricultural occupation; (3) all who both lived in the country and had a rural occupation; (4) all who had a rural occupation plus a prorated assignment of cases with an unknown occupation on the basis of the location of their suicide, rural or other.

The first method of selection, simply by rural location, yielded 742 rural suicides by males from 1900 to 1950. It is worth noting in passing the distribution in other locales: male suicides in small towns numbered 709, in large towns 1,192, and in cities 642. A handful of suicides occurred at sea. Since a substantial number of farmers (n = 149) and farm labourers (n = 199) killed themselves in urban places, there is a sound reason for including all cases where the deceased had a rural occupation. By selecting purely on the basis of rural locales, we would have passed over the travels of farmers into towns for business or a visit to the publican, ignored the proximity of many farms to small towns, and missed the itinerant character of farm labour. Typically, the urban locales where farmers and farm labourers committed suicide were small centres. During the years under consideration, much of New Zealand was a land of *urbs in rus*.

The problem with the second means of establishing rural-sector suicides, sorting by occupations, is that in 370 instances of the 3,337 male suicides from 1900 to 1950, no occupation was stated. That left 1,066 men who were assigned typically rural occupations by witnesses: "The body is that of my brother. He was 38 and a farm labourer"; or to cite another illustration, "my husband had been milking on shares." The 1,066 men included farm labourers (433), farmers (431), retired farmers (30), gardeners (29), station cooks (19), station managers (16), rabbiters (10), well drillers (9), horse trainers (8), share milkers (7), and a smattering of men in each of over thirty additional occupations. The third method, constraining rural sector suicides by requiring both a rural location and a rural occupation, produced 571 men. In common with the first technique for determining a rural suicide, this method excluded men who worked in the rural sector but happened to die in an urban place. The final way of selecting rural sector men – using rural occupations and adding men of unknown occupation whose bodies were found in the countryside – would have added fifty cases to the 1,066. Some men could have been in the country while in transit between urban places, so the addition of these fifty cases would also be an imperfect solution.

We decided to consider all individuals with a rural occupation. In several parts of the discussion, farmers (n = 431) and farm labourers (n = 433) are compared. The concentration on these two groups seemed reasonable due to their great prevalence. There were many gradations of farmers but witnesses seldom disclosed the size or nature of the operation. It was impossible to ascertain all farm women in the data set, although we identified 130 women who lived in rural locations and another thirty-five whom witnesses called farmers' wives. The shortcoming of the first number is that we can assume that some farm women visited urban centres and a few lived on the margins of hamlets. The number of rural women is under-represented at 165 cases. On the basis of the four-to-one gender ratio for all New Zealand suicides, the number of rural sector women who took their own lives from 1900 to 1950 should have reached 250 or more. Our discussion of their circumstances is limited to qualitative evidence. Farm labour combined with family rearing no doubt drove many women to despair – we have seen this in case files – but the burdens of rural living might have weighed more fatally on men, and there is little doubt that masculine conviviality at the bar put alcoholism into the mix. Women largely escaped that affliction.

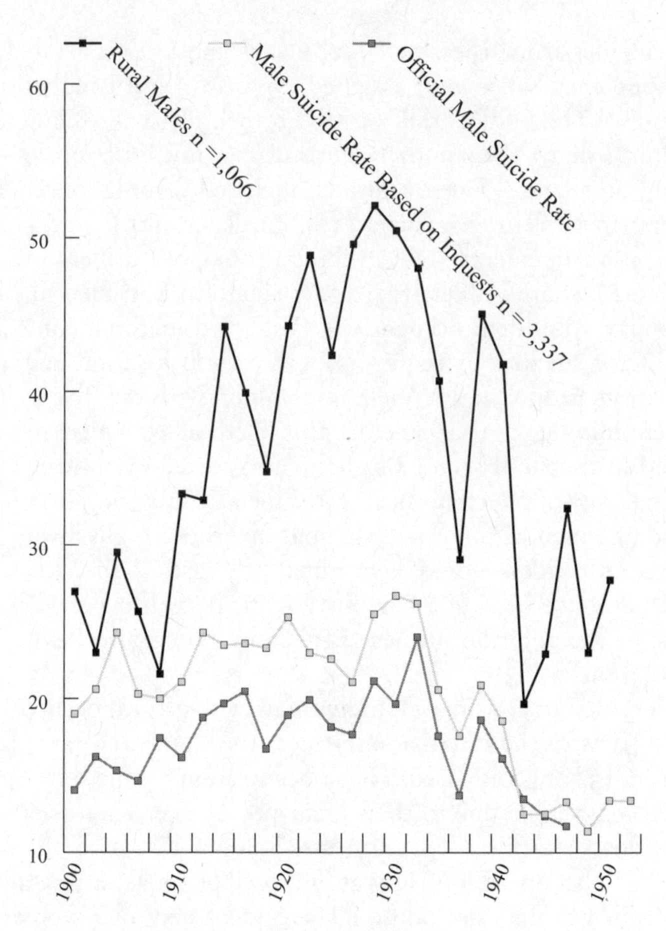

Graph 3.1
Rural male suicide rates compared with other male rates, 1900–50

No calculation of a suicide rate for a sub-population can avoid imprecision. To find the divisors needed for the calculation of a rural rate, we scoured New Zealand censuses. New Zealand conducted censuses every five years except in 1931 and 1941. Linear interpolation was conducted to estimate the rural sector working population in years between censuses. The computation of rates shows that the male suicide rate was higher for the rural sector than for the male population generally (Graph 3.1). The trend had begun before World War I, and widened during the war and again in the early 1920s.[85] Post-war price deflation among farm commodities was underway immediately after the war.[86] On the surface, there appears to have been a connection between the economy and rural suicides. Of course, there were other motives. On occasion, a farmer would mention that he could not abide isolation. Mercury Bay farmer William Harman, single and thirty-seven, told people he was "lonely, sick of the place."[87] By no means, however, was rural isolation a prevalent factor in suicide. Nearly three-quarters of all rural sector men who took their own lives from 1900 to 1950 resided near a railway line, harbour, town, or city.

Lower returns for greater toil discouraged farmers. Falling global prices for primary products may have started to affect farmers before 1930, because the suicide rate for males working in the rural sector peaked in 1928 at 52.1 per 100,000. Since land values soared during World War I, fell in the early 1920s, and collapsed further in the 1930s, many farmers who had acquired land before 1920 carried mortgages above the market value of their land. Loans for supplies from ubiquitous stock agencies piled up debts. Between 1931 and 1936, successive governments provided mortgage relief and a guaranteed price for dairy produce, but these measures were only partially successful.[88] In 1939 a Lands Department field inspector for rural Otago summarized a basic dilemma when he appealed for the government to implement a farm subsidy to revivify rural life. "On average prices for produce it is impossible, after allowing for reasonable labour costs, to allow more than a pittance for the farmer himself, who has all the responsibility of managing the place. Either the labour or the management must suffer, and as the farmer himself desires a decent standard of living it is natural the labour is skimped."[89]

Economic scrapes affected young and old men differently. Unless they were from established farming families, young farmers carried debts for recently purchased land. In the estimation of William Frise's father, the twenty-five-year-old was "very depressed and worried lately over money matters relating to the farm property."[90] Young rural men, like their counterparts in the city, experienced romantic rejection. However, farm labourers were especially at risk for romantic disappointment. The arduous and sometimes isolated nature of farm work, combined with poor wages, uncertainty of employment, and the lack of legislative protection, meant meagre prospects for social mobility.[91] Dismissed from his job, farmhand Herbert Ellis could not support his wife, so she moved in with her parents. Ellis felt that his in-laws were coming between him and his wife.[92] Thirty-five and unemployed for several months in mid-1934, Henry Crocker could not afford married life, broke off his engagement, and in a state of depression jumped off a wharf.[93] Part-time work or relief work allowed young men to survive, but some could not see a fulfilling life ahead.[94]

Relationship troubles overlapped with economic crises. As reported in chapter two, a maintenance order added to the predicaments of being out of work. William Schaeffer's wife initiated proceedings against him for separation and maintenance; he had taken to the road to flee a maintenance order and find farm work in a distant locale. He was found with his sugar-bag swag and a suitcase near a tent where he had stayed the previous night.[95] Women undoubtedly had a hard time when compelled to separate. For a woman, a man's refusal or inability to pay maintenance made a bad situation worse. Freda Hancock, whose husband kept moving to avoid contributing to her support, tried to run a boarding-house, but when she fell into arrears the authorities cut off her electricity.[96]

As in the past, a handful of elderly men committed suicide when they could no longer support themselves. George Roland worried about being unable to obtain work and having to live with his sister.[97] Dairy farming was regarded as "a young man's business, and he must be fit to make it pay."[98] Often dairy farms were owned and operated by different individuals and the operator, the share milker, carried enormous burdens in poor economic times. Any debilitating illness jeopardized a family's well-being and that could precipitate an emotional breakdown. These circumstances affected George Brown, a forty-nine-year-old share milker who took an overdose of a sleeping draught in June 1930. "Owing to illness," his wife testified, "he has not done any work this last six months."[99] In the same year, farmer Thomas Sadlier hanged himself in a field; a friend stated that "he had no worries other than farm troubles and ill health." Sadlier's wife indicated that they needed a loan to retain the farm and "if the money could not be raised, we would have to sell out."[100] At the inquest into the death of farmer Paul Carment, his wife remarked that he "has worried over the property for the past two months as he thought he might lose it."[101]

Upcoming clearance sales of property greatly upset farmers.[102] All types of agriculture suffered from the bind of depressed prices and fixed debts. To this fundamental difficulty were added hazards that could occur at any time, but were economic or work troubles nevertheless. A 1936 storm destroyed an orchard owner's crop; his wife recognized his state of depression and made him promise not to do anything "unbecoming."[103] Wet weather in some locales in 1938 guaranteed a bad season for farmers who were demoralized by the natural obstacles to working the land and then for only a small return.[104] Livestock dealers, machinery agents, and mechanics shared the farmers' hard times.[105]

The physical stress of farming took its toll. A sudden illness or persistent ill health affected one's ability to work the land, as did the onset of declining physical powers. Sixty-five-year-old Charles Eden, according to a neighbouring farmer, had troubles in connection with working his farm.

> He could trim the fences and do odd work & look after the sheep but he wasn't capable of working the tractor. I then offered him the loan of a six horse team to help him with his work through the winter & he accepted the offer & appeared very grateful, but at the same time he appeared very despondent. I again met him on my own farm ... he went over old ground with me ... He told me he was worrying about his financial position & that he had seen Mr Hunter about selling the farm & that Mr Hunter had informed him that there was little prospect [of that] at the present time & when he left me he was completely down hearted & when I heard of his death I was not surprised.[106]

In a few instances, old men simply had nothing to fall back on. Seventy-three-year-old rabbit-shooter James Rowntree spent his pension on drinking sprees, disappearing for several days. He was single and had been living in the same hut on the same farmer's property for almost half his lifetime. His estate came to twenty-one pounds ten shillings, almost half of which was realized from the sale of his radio. He had two pounds in the Post Office Savings Bank. The rifle with which he shot himself sold for one pound ten shillings and his old horse fetched a further one pound and was butchered for dog tucker.[107] Drink and gambling ruined stock breeder Christopher Muir, who took his own life a few days before "a meeting of his creditors."[108]

Mental illness among worried farmers, expressed as a nervous breakdown or mental depression, increased during the Great

Depression. Living with his wife and two young children in a two-room house, a desperate twenty-five-year-old farmer shot his family. His brother-in-law testified that "he used to say he could not see how he could make the farm pay. When he got in this state of depression he used to sit down and meditate."[109] Witnesses' descriptions over the years included remarks about men sitting in silence, hanging their heads, becoming reclusive, seeming pensive, and so forth. These were portraits of men likely to have been in the throes of crisis-induced mental depression. They were more than briefly saddened; they were in states of protracted mental distress. Farmer Otto Jorgensen worried about the taxes he owed and had had several nervous breakdowns.[110] Farmer Michael Goodwin's wife proposed that "the trouble was due to worry on the farm on which things have been going badly lately. He has been very depressed."[111] Economic worries brought out other problems. Jorgensen had not enjoyed good health since his return from the war. A number of returned soldiers who farmed were now acknowledged as medically unfit. They faced falling commodity prices but rising medical costs, and thus they risked losing farms after clearing virgin land that had cost them years of unremitting toil. A 1935 report on soldiers' settlements attributed some of their failures to the war. "Age and the latent effect of war service are affecting the constitution of the men. A re-action on the health of quite a number of men, previously fit and good farmers, has now set in, and in order to keep their farms going it is now necessary for these settlers to employ outside labour. Medical, hospital and similar expenses are becoming constant and material charges against farm revenue."[112]

Recurring themes in rural suicides are the burden of debt and strain of running a business. The worry of making a living, providing for one's family, and paying bills all featured in farmers' suicides during these years. Problems streamed into one another. In 1932, fifty-four-year-old Arthur Crowder swallowed strychnine when notified that the power was to be cut off on account of overdue electricity bills. As his son pointed out at the inquest, eighty cows could not be milked by hand day in, day out.[113] Towards the end of the Great Depression, eighty-year-old dairy farmer Alfred Smith wrote in his suicide note that he did not intend to continue "making butter fat below cost. I'm too old to take responsibility any longer. Spent £3000 on improvements to farm over past 32 years not realising the present prices would com – coming winter will be the worst NZ has ever had – had enough."[114] Age, financial strain, and a feeling of futility had combined.

Farmers had their particular troubles; farm labourers had theirs. The low wages paid to farm labourers made the repayment of small debts seem insuperable. Twenty-eight-year-old John Smith "did not know how he was going to get out of debt again."[115] Sixty-seven at the start of the Great Depression, John Pollock had been three months without work; he slept in woolsheds and farm huts.[116] Men surviving on relief work wore the countenance of defeat. Describing a labourer who took his own life, a witness reported that "he said he was hard up and on relief work. He seemed weary and fairly knocked up." As if to stress the responsibility of hard times and not a man's failings, this witness added, "he was perfectly sober."[117]

During the Great Depression, the rate of rural suicide was exceptionally high, but the crisis had victims in towns and cities too. Labourer Travis Watson's wife described him as very nervous, "worrying over bad times and being unable to work."[118] Anxiety affected professionals, educators, and businessmen. They lost status as well as income. A university demonstrator who had hoped to study at the University of London felt there were few prospects in university teaching.[119] Young farm labourer Robert Crofter's "chief worry was that he having a good education was unable to secure suitable employment to put it to its best advantage."[120] Tailor Todd Edgar had to give up his trade and survive on relief work.[121] Cobbler Andrew Gabowsky told his housekeeper that "he could not make a living at it."[122] An auto dealer repossessed lingerie salesman Gerald Jacob's vehicle; he was "financially embarrassed."[123] Mechanic Fred Anderson could only get casual farm work.[124] A former insurance agent sold coal door-to-door.[125] According to his son, jeweller Samuel Moller "had serious financial worries and ... at times he was mentally very depressed."[126] Young merchant Terrence Kent wrote, "I am in debt and cannot see my way clear so this is the only way out. It is no doubt a coward's way but there is some I hope who will remember that I tried to live a decent life."[127]

Trouble from the police surfaced occasionally, and it could have an economic twist connected to the severity of the times. A former officer in the Taranaki Regiment killed himself in early 1930 when the police arrived to question him about his issuing of valueless cheques in several cities.[128] Harold Smallbone had been unemployed for four weeks in 1932 and was due to appear in court for theft of money and clothing.[129] Police wanted to interview an unemployed alcoholic for redeeming relief work vouchers for work not performed and to speak with a bread deliveryman about stealing the money collected from households on his route.[130] Department store salesman Bert Harvey, caught stealing three neckties, pleaded in vain to keep his job.[131] A secretary of a citrus fruit growers' association embezzled funds.[132] Transgressors in these instances had seized an opportunity during hard times; they were not habitual or professional criminals, hence their shame when exposed. In each of these instances and many more besides, the Great Depression had not just impoverished people but diminished their stature in their eyes, and they could not envision a way back up. It required a positive turn in national economic fortunes to provide that.

A VIEW FROM THE SUMMIT

Edmund Hillary's ascent of Mount Everest in May 1953 symbolizes the years of the long prosperity. New Zealanders had scaled the standard of living and reached a world summit by the early 1950s. By no means were the years from 1940 to the mid-1970s free from economic crises, nor were they lacking in social and racial problems. Historians looking critically into the 1950s have remarked on an absence of political creativity, condemned the assault on civil liberties that accompanied the Nationals' crushing of the 1951 wharf workers' strike, and bemoaned the far from avant-garde cultural scene. To many who remember these times, they were "dowdy, boring, grey." A rounded assessment indicates, however, that despite brief economic crises and the fact that the good times depended on favoured treatment in distant markets, the country experienced "golden weather." Serious woes were ahead, but at the time people experienced a "long, slow boom." "A boom is a boom," writes Bronwyn Dalley, "and it lay behind much of the comfort of this period."[133] The comfort goes some distance to explaining the comparatively low male suicide rate. Tom Brooking labels the period from 1951 to 1967 "the last good years."[134]

A drop in suicides had begun during World War II. An explanation for that phenomenon must take into account the fact that many individuals at risk, namely young adult males, were out of the country. Suicides by service personnel in the field were not included in the published mortality tables and were not subject to a coroner's inquest back in New Zealand. These suicides remain unknown, but the suicides of returned soldiers were investigated. In chapter four we report on the markedly high suicide rate for returned men. The Depression reached its nadir in 1933, but the war truly ended it. As measured by the two variables on work and finances, good economic times appear to have depressed suicide rates. Qualitative information supports this proposition. Fewer men were found to be unemployed, having financial difficulties, or dealing with offensive employers; on all fronts, economic motives for suicide faded.

Farmers during the war prospered from supplying the United Kingdom and the American military in the Pacific, so the exceptional stresses experienced in the 1930s on farms dissipated.[135] In the 1940s, the number of farmer suicides declined by thirty percent when compared with the 1930s, and the number of farm labourers who committed suicide plummeted. A scarcity of labour may have worried farmers, but it was a boon for most rural labourers. Still, old habits persisted and casual rural labourers were all but anonymous. Farmer Alvin Fowler, who hired a general bush hand in 1954, testified at an inquest that "I know nothing of his antecedents nor of his place of birth, nor do I know what his age was."[136] Urban workers did well. If we accept that good economic circumstances depress suicides, at least at the margins, we can understand why the numbers of suicides of skilled and semi-skilled labourers were much lower in the 1940s than in the 1930s. When we select only the cases of men who committed suicide for an economic motive, the numbers of farmers, farm labourers, and other workers are rare. The war produced its own motives which are assessed in chapter four, but economic motives were scarce in wartime. The exception that illustrates the rule is the 1940 case of Meyer Feldberg, a refugee German Jew, who could not pursue his old profession and who wrote, "My profession prospects are very bad and just a poor living for oneself is not worth doing it."[137]

In the years of national development and in the Great Depression, there was no shortage of cases to illustrate hardship and no scarcity of witnesses decrying the bad times; in the 1940s, these hard-times cases and comments thinned out. For farmers, a few inescapable economic troubles remained; beyond falling commodity prices, a lot could go wrong on a farm. During the 1949 general election campaign, future prime minister Keith Holyoake described a farm as a "piece of land surrounded by mortgages. A farmer is a land worker surrounded by troubles. Weather, prices, costs and pests."[138] Toward the end of the war, fifty-eight-year-old farmer Peter Percival worried over his management of the family property while his brother was in the army. He could not cope with the modern implements and suffered heavy stock losses due to "worm trouble among his sheep."[139] In early 1950, Jim McCain's wife noticed that he made a point of telling her about the challenge of keeping the farm going. Current work was completed, "but he could see a lot of work ahead and was worried that he might not be able to carry it out. He did mention that he might sell the farm and that this seemed like an admission of defeat."[140] Farming remained a stressful business. And yet, to leave a farm could precipitate intense regret.

The once-plentiful reports of older men worrying about their capacity to withstand more grinding labour declined but did not vanish. Employers still dismissed men for alcohol abuse. There were still destitute men without means of support; banks foreclosed on farms, and business partners and investors threatened legal action. When two business associates of Walter Kincaid threatened to go to the police in 1950, Kincaid wrote to tell his wife that he could not stand the shame. "I have done things," he wrote, "that I should not have done."[141] However, these once fairly common reports of personal failings leading to financial woes now surfaced infrequently at inquests. Good times were forgiving times.

Prosperity continued through the 1950s and 1960s. Short recessions punctuated these decades, but none initiated enduring pessimism and the National government's spending on infrastructure kept wages high and unemployment low.[142] Working conditions, judged by the inquests, seemed better; dismissal and harassment appeared rarely in testimony. The world-wide recession of the late 1950s momentarily and marginally increased the number of suicides with an economic motive. Among the 1958 and 1960 cases, witnesses and suicide notes mentioned a handful of large and small business failures. Stockbroker Jock Fraser wrote to his wife that "we are in a hopeless mess at the office and we can't carry on. The mess was due to shortages by Dad and Uncle Donald but we have had to take the blame."[143] On the day that Thomas Hyslop had planned to see a real estate agent to put his grocery store on the market, he took a fatal course instead. The suburban location had not been paying.[144] Financial stress intensified friction among business partners. A radio repairman told his partner that "he would be better on his own."[145] The operators of a small manufacturing concern decided "to wind up" their business because of the domestic troubles of one partner, and that individual felt let down at a vulnerable moment.[146] As in any period, a very few men with access to company funds committed fraud and could not face the shame of exposure. For years, Bill Robarts, who collected insurance premiums for Provident Life Assurance, had falsified his accounts.[147]

Farmers in the 1950s and 1960s continued to contend with physical and business cares. "Getting physically weak" and finding the "worry of running a farm too much for him," Donald Duguid drowned in a likely suicide.[148] As in earlier times, older farmers had problems adjusting. When he had to scale down, John Lloyd felt diminished.[149] Rural life was and remained a world apart; many farmers thrived on a pride in property. Elsewhere men and women who found themselves out of work arrived in that predicament due to particular circumstances rather than as cast-offs from a downturn or casualties of nature. Economic and work motives for suicide in the 1950s and 1960s originated in assorted troubles stamped with individual rather than labour-market or business-cycle hallmarks. People made poor business decisions, faced competition, collapsed from overwork, experienced setbacks amidst rising expectations, failed to reach high goals, and suffered disabling mishaps.[150] They succumbed to the debilities of alcoholism, which persisted as a source of material and mental misery.[151]

Male profligacy continued to bring financial suffering, although some reckless leisure-time pursuits, available in the livelier cities, deviated from the grooves of earlier times when workers simply sought escape at a tavern. Drugs now ruined a few men; the numbers of drug users among the suicides of the young would grow in the 1980s and 1990s. Ted Richmond was a 1960s harbinger. His employment as a waiter in night cafes brought him into contact with assorted temptations that undermined his family life. "He was associated with what could be called theatre society and cafe habitués, and was known to his intimates as a braggart. It is known that he associated with a suspected drug peddler." His circumstances were only partly new. He had also fallen behind on maintenance payments.[152] For decades, other men had done likewise.[153] Alcohol abuse has always interfered with earning a living. Labourer William Parsons slipped away to a hotel bar during his hours of employment. His boss found out and sacked him. Soon afterward, someone tampered with the brakes on company trucks. The police suspected

Parsons.[154] According to his wife, tailor Paul Hardy's excessive drinking destroyed his business. "For the past 18 months the deceased has been drinking fairly heavily and because of this he has failed to fulfill orders for suits and tailoring."[155] Gambling put men in financial difficulties; there was nothing new about living for the big win and running up debts.[156] However, the men involved were more likely than in prior years to have steady jobs, viable businesses, or pensions. Their dreams of escape were consumption-based, not survival-driven.

Pressure at work, labour scarcity, and perfectionism contributed to mental breakdowns. Overworked professionals included the doctor who "worried over his inability to treat his patients correctly."[157] Another doctor wrote that "my work has overwhelmed me. Ring my nurse and cancel patients."[158] In the wake of post-war medical advances, doctors were expected by patients to tackle a greater range of ailments more effectively; social security assured easier patient access to care. Other professionals and managers could not give up work, even when work undermined mental health. Like farmers, men who ran other types of enterprises and who needed to see progress were exhausted by their efforts. A dairy company manager, who shouldered more work than necessary because he was a perfectionist, was advised by a doctor to take early retirement. He refused and had a breakdown.[159] Particular occupations were stressful in ways other than fear of unemployment. Individuals in prosperous times worried less about a lack of work, but were burdened by workloads and unrealized goals. Addressing a perceived failure in his career, a company secretary wrote a terse note: "A loser quits."[160] A long-time employee with a large company applied for an executive position. His wife believed that this bid put him under strain and contributed to his heavy drinking.[161]

The foregoing episodes were rare, and inquests during the years of long prosperity portray good times even in the midst of the tragedies of suicide. Witnesses left us with remarkably few images of lean lonely men reflecting on empty lives as they lay sleepless in a boarding-house.

CONCLUDING OBSERVATIONS

By at least the early 1950s, general practitioners and psychiatrists mentioned that patients suffered from "reactive depression" on account of worries about work. Even when the term was not used, these close observers noted that material conditions and associated stress adversely impacted mental states. With the idea that this proposition should only be a starting point for discussion, we turned to case files for more illuminating details. We asked how precisely material circumstances affected suicide rates. Correlations of aggregate data are mute about the exact sources of hardships such as labour market practices, poor wages, and work hazards. With the advantage of case-based evidence, we identified four groups of economic determinants. First, the overall economic state affected people's circumstances. The Great Depression and the years of prosperity illustrate this proposition by way of a contrast between bad and good times. Aggregate data adequately demonstrates this one determinant, but there was more to economic life than the business cycle, and it is from this point forward that aggregate data is found inadequate.

Economic growth was a necessary condition for a better life, but not the only one. Thus, we encounter a second connection between economic life and suicides: the economy's structure. Asymmetries of power between employer and employee and an absence of support for people in need were important. An expanding economy that ground down labour and operated with substantial unemployment delivered casualties including suicides. Third, by their own actions individuals put themselves in a financial hole. Finally, there were always chance debilitating mishaps, prominent among them assorted natural events that kept farmers on edge.

It should be added that the misery of unemployment was not always about money. A few older farmers with property, who could have sold assets to cover their retirement years, felt a loss of purpose from surrendering their life's work. Some individuals who continued to work in hard times to make ends meet had to leave former trades and felt diminished by new menial tasks. Work assumed psychological importance for men raised with a work ethic. When William Moana retired in 1982, he told his daughter "that he was no longer any use to anyone and he might as well go out back and shoot himself."[162]

Economic and work-related motives for suicide were perhaps more significant than our cautious statistical estimates have allowed. At the beginning of this chapter, we reported that for the whole century, economic motives for suicides among working men accounted for roughly one in six (13.8 percent). We erred on the side of caution.

Were relationship problems, through legal costs and maintenance orders, a source of economic distress, or was a personal economic disaster the cause of misdirected anger and a related disintegration of relationships? Was mental illness a motive with isolated origins or, in many instances, did economic worry inflict mental harm? The evidence from people's lives makes us wary of bald assertions about an overwhelming connection between suicide and mental illness. Often an end state truly did disclose a mental illness broadly defined, but the pathways leading to a clinical condition merit attention if suicide is to be properly understood. One well-trodden pathway ran through the thickets of financial or work-related trouble. Thus, we return to another statistic mentioned at this chapter's beginning. Half of the men in the workforce who took their own lives had work or financial difficulties (50.9 percent).

There remains an immense unresolved problem. Why would suicide be adopted by a few men as a solution to their financial or work-related troubles? We suggest ideas in chapter eight where we consider how individuals assessed their future, reasoned or acted on impulse, designated their exit as revenge or sacrifice, integrated their belief in an afterlife with a fatal decision, looked for courage, and experienced prior physical pain.

In the next chapter, the cluster of motives is one that appears to be the least puzzling of all. Physical suffering is viscerally understood and makes self-euthanasia a plausible course, although we are going to show that as an escape from pain, suicide is a complicated subject. Due to the variety of medical conditions encountered and the involvement of popular fears, discerning a threshold for self-euthanasia is not straightforward. In the late twentieth century, the weighing of medical conditions, palliative options, and suicide became a matter of public debate when advocates of self-euthanasia grabbed media attention. Behind the occasional eruptions of public controversy and political debate in the late twentieth century, there was the reality of self-euthanasia evident in private decisions.

4

Life Diminished: Illness and Trauma, 1900–2000

From 1900 until about 1980, when the long prosperity ended, the proportion of individuals who committed suicide and for whom physical illness was the leading motive remained constant at about one in five. This ratio held true for women as well as men. The mean age for these women and men increased after World War II due to the medical revolution and the welfare state, which together made life more bearable for many in physical distress. The age of morbidity had begun to rise, and with it the mean age of the people who took their own lives on account of illnesses (Graph 4.1).

On a case-by-case examination we see the consequences of work hazards, recreational injuries, traffic accidents, the pleasurable excesses of smoking and drinking destroying vital organs, the advance of chronic diseases, and the inexorable debilities of aging. For some people, even the years of golden weather were leaden times, because illness or injury restricted their lives. Pain, impeded mobility, loss of employment, insomnia, and intense fear of an impending end affected mental outlooks. Insomnia plagued the acutely ill. "The pain is somting ofal," wrote Gordon Lee. "I cant sleep at night i will have to end my days theay cant do any more for me."[1] In his suicide note, Wallace Barnard mourned that "I just roll around in bed in agony most of the night."[2] Moods darkened when sufferers lay awake immersed in morbid thought night after night. Witnesses routinely remarked on "fits of depression" and "despondency." Mental instability frequently evolved in association with serious diseases or disabilities. Recurrent references to physical decline and depression connect ailments to reactive depression.

Across the century, several leading motives rose during economic downturns and fell in boom times; however, until the years of economic crises, illnesses held a stable position as a major reason for self-destruction. A smaller proportion of illness motives appeared in the years of economic crises, when more and more young people took their own lives. They rarely did so for reasons of physical decline. With the rates of youth suicide rising, the firm standing of physical illness as a major motive faded. In its many decades of prominence, the frequency of this common cluster of motives rose as the life-course advanced. It continued to do so late in the century when it was relatively less significant. With increasing age, anxieties shifted from sexual and domestic relations or financial and work troubles to illnesses and infirmities. When mortality figured in the thoughts of older people, fear of hospitals, suffering, and the indignities of incapacitation erupted (Table 4.1). Individuals' encounters with mortality were symptomatic of reflections that extend beyond the suicide cases. Self-destruction was an extreme response to pain or a failing body, but the statements of the people who chose suicide reveal universal ordeals. People everywhere have experienced fear, torment, and humiliating incapacity. Seldom can we "hear" their cries in the middle of the night. Now we can.

RATIONAL AND IRRATIONAL FEAR

The roles of physical illnesses in the suicides of mature men and women were usually straightforward and comprehensible. Many suffered dreadfully. One autopsy disclosed that "the right lung shows emphysema, the left lung is missing and is replaced by a large cavity containing brownish necrotic material. The prostate is slightly enlarged. Coronary arteries show sclerosis and calcification."[3] Rarely were circumstances so fully catalogued. On occasion men and women made their own erroneous analysis and assumed wrongly but stubbornly that a terminal illness tortured their body. Dread fuelled a morbid imagination. Fear of worse to come rather than fear of an imminent death figured unexpectedly in many instances of what at first looked like self-euthanasia. The deeply fearful insisted they were finished before they received a diagnosis. Pointing to blood in his phlegm, Charles McIntyre wept before a fellow labourer, "I am buggered any day."[4] Perhaps he was finished, but many were not. Year in, year out, individuals stubbornly assessed their own health and ignored doctors. Widowed farmer John Forsyth wrote in 1902 that "my health is done. I do not care what the Doctor says."[5] Decade after decade, similar attitudes cropped up to challenge a perfect separation of physical and mental illness.

An obsessive fear of cancer persisted throughout the century.[6] Auckland butcher John Walmsley missed work often in 1930 likely due to a gastric ulcer, but he feared cancer. If he had it, he told his wife, "he would go mad."[7] In 1944, labourer Cyril Harding "knew that he had Haemorrhoids but also harboured a fear that he had cancer."[8] Alfred Ashwood's doctor claimed that this patient "developed a fixed cancerophobia."[9] A case from a half-century later shows how persistent fear helps explain a puzzling phenomenon that could be dismissed as hypochondria. A fifty-year-old man, separated from his wife, had a history of abdominal pains; the autopsy discovered a huge duodenal ulcer. Two of his grandparents had died of cancer and he had watched a friend's painful demise.[10] Cancer inspired waking nightmares, because of widespread familiarity with its degradation and the fearful crudeness of treatments. For much of the century, medical intervention inspired fright, and not just about cancer treatment, although cancer was the predominant nightmare.

Until the 1920s, medical care likely killed more often than it cured. Folk memory of unsuccessful and excruciating medical intrusions persisted for generations. An ulcerated growth on her breast convinced Edna Bowers that she would become ill and helpless, a fate she rejected. "I suppose it is Cancer," she wrote.[11] When a close friend died from cancer, Bert Adams said "he would shoot himself if he ever got cancer." Forty years later he had cancer and ended his life.[12] The reasoning of suicidal individuals may seldom accord with our ideas, but that does not mean that they all acted wholly irrationally. They pre-empted private fear and pain. Out of respect to them, the burden falls on us to attempt to explain how they reasoned. In this quest, mental states cannot be set aside to favour material causes. Physical illness and mental distress mingled.

Boundaries between physical and mental were not always well demarcated. Leonard Best's wife explained the carryover from physical to mental distress when she testified that after removal of his kidney "he appears to have suffered mentally from the shock of the operation."[13] Another boundary problem appears with respect to alcoholism. In certain instances, the proximate reason for a suicide was incurable cirrhosis of the liver or advanced heart disease, but the underlying condition was excessive drink.[14] Vagueness obscures the exact medical condition in many more cases, although the evidence still conveys unbearable suffering. In his suicide note, Samuel Ricketts wrote, "I have been suffering a lot with that old pain, and its making it so hard to carry on, that I can't stick it any longer."[15] What old pain? In the early decades of the twentieth century, witnesses often testified vaguely that a deceased was "old and unwell." The social circumstances of these old and unwell men and women deserve attention, since many lacked the support of friends and relatives. Social isolation of the enfeebled added to the risk of suicide. Medical, social, and mental states were conjoined in people's lives. Attempts at an orderly analysis of motives and mental states, therefore, have to be disrupted by messy authentic details.

Unusual patterns of thought can point to overlooked truths. For most of the chapter, this proposition applies to individuals' assessments of their physical maladies and injuries plus their unwillingness to bear them. In certain instances, suicide seems an excessive reaction to the physical crisis. However, the decision deserves to be explained from the individual's standpoint and not from a pre-emptive suggestion of irrationality. An admittedly unique example can illustrate the idea that ailing but rational individuals could and did choose to die on their own terms. Shortly after his hundredth birthday, John Walton discharged himself from a hospital geriatric ward and took an overdose of a barbiturate. He was described as "a very independent man and disliked receiving help from others."[16]

In the late twentieth century, media attention to self-destruction was substantial. Controversy about euthanasia coincided with a surge of publicity about youth suicide during the 1980s and 1990s. Newspaper and television journalists, attentive to human interest stories, seized upon unnatural deaths. Moreover, in an increasingly secular society, dying was no longer seen on all occasions as God's will. Painful and terminal conditions could be managed by palliative care. For some non-conformists, the next step was to avoid this managed interlude and go directly to euthanasia. People did not have to accept their fate and suffer, nor did they need to endure an amateurish suicide.

EUTHANASIA REALITIES AND DILEMMAS

The range of medical conditions that led to suicide decisions throws up an issue to be confronted by New Zealand parliamentarians if they legalize medically assisted suicide. Bills were defeated in 1995 and 2003, and at the time of writing a new private member's bill has been drafted.[17] In any debate over principles and administrative details, proponents would have to consider carefully how far to push eligibility. Tightly controlled access would allow the terminally ill to seek assistance. Undiagnosed fears of a fatal illness or claims of being tired of life, circumstances occasionally found in the suicide files, would not qualify under this rule. Proponents of an absolute right to die could make an argument that such applications should be considered, but they would encounter ethical and practical objections to permitting assistance in these circumstances. Finding doctors willing to assist might be difficult. The diminished-quality-of-life appeal is a trickier subject. Realizing that this is contentious, individuals who were affected by an incurable paralysis or degenerative disease and who committed suicide in the late twentieth century were vocal in asserting their rights. Inquests showed that self-euthanasia formed a long-standing subset of suicides and that the more richly documented episodes at the end of the century overflowed with evidence of dilemmas and with statements about individual rights.

In New Zealand and other affluent countries, suicides by people with grave illnesses have been publicized in hotly contested debates over legalizing medically assisted suicide. Rehearsed before the courts, in political chambers, and in the media, the arguments for and against are well known. Serious controversy flared up intermittently once euthanasia societies began campaigning for the right to an assisted death, publishing advice books, and providing advance declaration forms instructing doctors not to administer life-sustaining treatment. In New Zealand these activities began with the formation of the Auckland Voluntary Euthanasia Society in 1978. Judging from inquests, this society and later branches possessed committed adherents in the 1980s and especially in the 1990s.

Firm advocates of legalizing access to medical assistance have insisted that individuals have rights, including the right to choose when and how to die. Adamant opponents refuted this rights position with an uncompromising stand of their own. Death ought to be left solely to God. On a secular plane, critics envisaged self-interested relatives encouraging someone's self-destruction, and pointed out that medical doctors are enjoined not to do harm. To obviate suffering, they recommended palliative care at a hospice, an innovation that began in the United Kingdom in the 1950s and spread to other countries including New Zealand.[18]

Can evidence from actual self-euthanasia actions contribute to the debate? It seems so, because well-documented cases late in the century show people with resolve, intelligence, and a sense of personal rights. They rejected drawn-out medication. Witnesses' depositions depict gentle deaths along with frightful ones that in their own way make an argument for assisted suicide. The plastic bags, plus handcuffs to forestall the reflex to rip the bag off, were not decent trappings for the death of a loved one, but were suggested as effective by euthanasia society publications.[19]

Suicides by the terminally ill have been evident for a long time. The inquest files for the twentieth century show that a few individuals every year exercised their free will while they still had the ability to do so; they had decided to end their lives on account of illnesses. A few also acted to end what they judged was a severely diminished quality of life.[20] These latter instances for which there was no likelihood of an imminent death have complicated euthanasia debates; however, they were not unusual. As a result of tobacco smoking, the country had substantial numbers of patients with emphysema or what became known in the 1990s as chronic obstructive pulmonary disease. Later in this chapter we present quite a few suicides that originated from an excruciating struggle to breathe. Paralyzed accident victims or individuals with a paralyzing disease brooded over their immobility, but also their loss of control over bodily functions. Brandon Dumain had transverse myelitis and was paralyzed from the waist. He could not pass urine for months, and could not work; his former girlfriend became simply his friend. She reported that "he talked only about the good times he would never have again."[21] In every year, moreover, there were suicides by older men and women who declared they were "tired of life." Ethical questions abound when these assorted non-terminal cases are encountered, but for the sake of working with a consistent idea of self-euthanasia, we applied a narrow guideline.

The designation of a death as self-euthanasia required a research judgement on each potential case, because officially a suicide is a suicide. A coroner explained the situation in 1998. In his opinion, the deceased in question did not have an unsound mind. "On the contrary," the coroner elaborated, "I believe he was of very sound mind but overwhelmed by the deterioration in his health. I am happy to describe it as a case of euthanasia but unfortunately for statistical purposes I must give it the label of suicide because that is the way it is legally classified."[22] When reading the case files it was necessary to be aware of this distinction between life's tragic realities and the legal definition. The latter affected statistics on suicide cited in government publications, which had no place for an important elaboration on some suicides as self-euthanasia.

Exercising an independent judgement that went beyond the coroners' formal findings, we found instances of self-euthanasia in every year of the century. Some seemed like self-euthanasia, but included people who were not terminally ill, although in their estimation they suffered serious life-diminishing conditions. It was decided that the only self-euthanasia cases to be marked in the data set would be those where the individual was conscious, rational, and experiencing an incurable illness that would result in death. For the first half of the century, when medical records were not regularly consulted or were vague, we estimated self-euthanasia cases at between three and five percent from year to year. In the second half of the century, when medical records were sufficiently routine and detailed to make a firm judgement, and when a few individuals used the term euthanasia, it appears that the number of self-euthanasia cases varied annually from five to eight percent of all suicides. Stated another way, self-euthanasia constituted a quarter to a third of all suicides where an illness or injury was deemed the primary motive.

In raw numbers, twenty-five to thirty individuals annually undertook self-euthanasia in the late twentieth century. As will be seen shortly, witnesses' references to self-euthanasia escalated sharply in these years due to advocacy by euthanasia societies. More cases could have been added if the standard had been relaxed to include people who evaluated their physical quality of life as severely diminished as a result of a degenerative disease, stroke, emphysema, or spinal accident. While these diminished-quality-of-life cases were excluded from our statistics on self-euthanasia in order to adhere to a narrow definition, they certainly figure in the discussion of ethical questions about legalized assisted suicide. If medical assistance for euthanasia had been available in New Zealand at the end of the century, probably more men and women would have opted for it than was the case, because the number of such deaths as a percentage of all deaths amounts to 1.0 percent for Belgium, 0.5 percent for Switzerland, and 0.2 percent for Oregon. All three have legalized assisted suicide.[23] The threat of prosecution in New Zealand precluded some individuals from going ahead, because without help, they worried about botching their end. A long-time sufferer of lung problems said he would shoot himself but feared being unsuccessful. He was not unique.[24]

Judging from the differences between the percentage of self-euthanasia cases in New Zealand and the percentage of instances in jurisdictions where it has been legalized, the threat of criminal charges against those who wanted to help probably stopped some acts of self-euthanasia. Patients asked doctors to finish them off painlessly, but the doctors declined, or so witnesses reported.[25] The law could have encouraged virtuous perjury. Self-euthanasia with a strict definition has occurred often enough to be a noticeable trend at inquests, plus there were an unknown number of failed attempts, as well as 'natural' deaths advanced by stepped-up medication. These realities of misfortune within the finiteness of life have long been with us. But something changed in the culture. Greater public awareness and insistence are novel developments captured in depositions for the 1980s and 1990s.

Fear of criminal prosecution has not deterred everyone from assisting. Although iron-clad evidence of an assisted suicide could not be found in the instances that we read, assistance was occasionally hinted at. The fact that there were such intimations is remarkable, because inquests occurred in a courtroom setting with police present. Thus from witnesses we learn that a young woman with multiple sclerosis nearing the end was informed about her sleeping medication. "She knew that she was dying." She also knew that the tablets that helped her sleep "would knock her out in a few minutes."[26]

Sympathetic helpers could act in a grey area between the levels of morphine needed to relieve pain and the amount for permanent sleep. The police investigated the deaths of individuals who may have had help, but they laid no charges. Testimony could be honest but abridged. Thus, in one instance, a wife "administered morphine to the deceased to alleviate his suffering." Cancer had spread through the lungs, the pancreas, the gallbladder, and the large intestine.[27] There were suspicions but no prosecution. Cecilia Harper planned her death using the book *The Final Step*; her family knew and determined to allow her to go ahead. No police prosecution was ever contemplated.[28] Auckland lawyer Michael Crew wanted his death to spark public debate. The quadriplegic "held a big farewell party; he told his mother he had found someone who would help him die."[29] The possibility of criminal action did not stop subtle collusion, and perhaps occasionally there was more going on *sub rosa*.

The debate over medically assisted suicide is long on argument and short on exposure to people who viscerally confronted the subject. Authenticity is what documents-based history can deliver. Witnesses brought to light doctors' dilemmas, the disparate sensitivities of medical practitioners, the judicious silences of family and friends who worried about the law but did what they could, and the determination of hard-luck sufferers. Insights into self-euthanasia can be arranged by placing protagonists into two camps. The medical establishment forms one. It includes doctors, nurses, and pharmaceutical companies; public hospital personnel are possibly in a more conflicted position, with costs to manage but ethics to follow. Doctors are bound by oath to do no harm; moreover, many doctors and drug companies are committed to treatment for the prolongation of life. They aspire to do it well. Doctors varied in their ability to appreciate the plight of patients. Some took talk of suicide as an unbalanced wilful threat, and could not fathom the action.[30] Others sensed the complete despair. In a consultation with the wife of a dying man, a doctor remarked that "the only way one could really guarantee against a suicidal attempt would be to incarcerate him in an institution for the sum total of his days. Even this course is no guarantee against suicide."[31] He comprehended his patient's state of mind. Not everyone did.

Many patients enrolled in the fight-to-live camp, but of course not the ones who died by suicide. Probably others endured the struggle right up to their natural end but did so reluctantly, inhibited by a fear of failing or by the encouragement of persuasive therapists. Time and again, doctors in this camp did not foresee the suicide; they thought that the patient was coping because they assumed patients shared their values in the battle to beat cancer, heart disease, or some other serious ailment. Medical teams were heroic and inventive. The living suffocation of emphysema, for example, called up radical measures, including single-lung transplants seen first in the early 1980s and double transplants in the late 1980s. All the same, individual campaigns could fail. A recipient of a double transplant in 1994 despaired when he developed bronchial fibrosis anew. He experienced extreme pain.[32] The suicide of an emphysema patient came as a complete surprise to a doctor who felt this elderly man was coping well, although in addition to breathing trouble he had hypertension, generalized joint and muscle pain, an aortic aneurism, and prostatic disease. Medication included Prednisone, Digoxin,

Allopurinol, Pulmicort, Combivent, Enalapril, and Amiodarone.[33] A multiple sclerosis sufferer was taking Baclofen, Tegretol, Prednisone, Premarin, and Amitriptyline.[34] Each prescription reminded of diminished capacity.

Only suffers knew what they endured, and some of what they ruefully tolerated was medical intervention. Martin Kuiper "was receiving cobalt treatment which seemed to cause him dreadful pain." He was using Indomethacin, Senokot, Ventolin, Dexamethasone, Dilantin, Quibron, and Solu-Medrol. He took up to fifty tablets a day.[35] Patients showed resolution or cunning when confronted by well-meaning life-savers going about their duties. A doctor believed that Paula Pasternak, a nurse and psychologist, was considered a risk to herself because she had expressed frustration and anger about being cheated of life by lymphoma. He dispatched the Rapid Response Team from Health Waikato to her hospice; she escorted the paramedics out stating that "she now intended to attend to her roses." They considered detaining her under the Mental Health Act, but concluded she was mentally sound.[36]

By the early 1980s, the other camp, the independent-minded patients' camp, consisted of people who were well-informed, feisty, and emphatic about the right to end their lives.[37] We have seen several already. During the previous three-quarters of the century, the men and women who exercised self-euthanasia went ahead without a proclamation. They said their private goodbyes, but neither connected their pending death to a cause nor proclaimed a right. Toward the end of the century, however, there was a pronounced assertiveness about death as a right.[38] "Let me die," wrote an elderly retired nurse; "it is my right."[39] The right to die entered the culture of the ailing and elderly, along with the recognition of the word "euthanasia" that the euthanasia society had advanced. It was symptomatic of this growing awareness that in 1982 an elderly man with liver cancer asked his daughter to spell euthanasia. She wrote it on a piece of paper.[40]

Awareness led to impatience with meddlers. "A wasted man" aged seventy-eight whose leap from a building had not accomplished a quick end was asked by a caregiver at Hawthorn Eden Rest Home, "Harry why did you want to do it?" "Fuck you I want to die."[41] Similarly, an independent man, an author suffering with emphysema, let loose a stream of criticism about laws forbidding assisted suicide. "It terrifies me to think," he stated in his final letter, "that compassionate doctors or relatives anxious to initiate peaceful sleep would be deterred by those self-centred busybodies who are today persuading Government to maintain laws making it a criminal offence."[42]

The eruption of forcefulness owed much to euthanasia societies. The first reference to one at an inquest came in 1986; however, later inquests disclosed longer connections between individuals and the societies. A husband at a 1988 inquest reported that his wife had been a member for five years; in 1998 an inquest discovered that a couple involve in a suicide pact had been members for fifteen years.[43] Members figured in a handful of euthanasia deaths in the 1990s.[44] Some close observers suspected that these organizations provided more than publications. At the end of a 1994 inquest, coroner R.G. McElrea wondered how far the society's United Kingdom office had aided a woman who had motor neuron disease. Had it supplied her with morphine? Someone had to have done so, he believed, because of stringent hospital controls. A police investigation concluded that while funds had been forwarded to England, it remained unclear who had supplied the morphine. Investigators were satisfied that "no other persons were responsible or offered material assistance."[45] The probe straddled a dilemma. It served as a warning, but also as a sign that zealous enforcement on this occasion was not in the public interest.

To bring order to our upcoming representation of physical-crisis suicides as profoundly individual acts, the sections of this chapter now will follow phases in the life-course. They examine the physical burdens afflicting people in their prime, their years of transition, and their senior years. To retain the idea of the uniqueness of each instance and to avoid allowing a conceptual scaffolding to create an impression of order, the chapter's watchwords are subjectivity and fluidity. With respect to the former, the words of suicide 'victim' Julia Bessant are enlightening. "I don't think anyone can understand what people go through that get cancer, unless they have had cancer themselves."[46] Her sentiments on a powerful subjective experience could apply to journeys through other serious illnesses and trauma. As for fluidity, the typical ailments associated with suicide changed as people aged. The life-course provides an orderly starting point, but it is indispensable to truth to consider medical problems in relation to other difficulties in people's lives, the unique course of an ailment, the subjectivity of the experience, and changing times. With reference to the latter, medicine scored triumphs at mid-century; some terrifying fears were largely defeated or their symptoms better

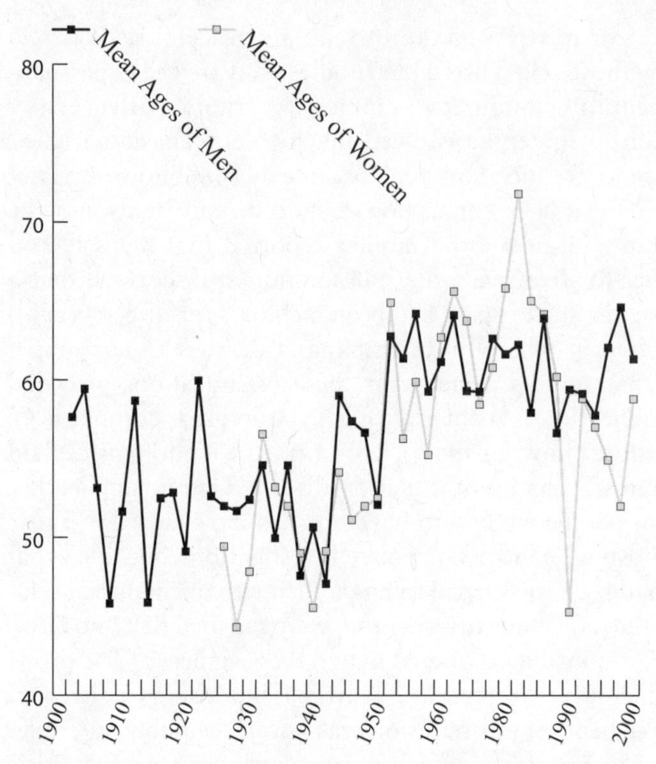

Graph 4.1
Mean ages of men and women whose motive was a physical ailment, 1900–98

managed. As well, social welfare alleviated anxieties arising from a loss of income due to injury or illness. To recognize how much better life had become for mature men and women by the 1950s, it is useful to remind ourselves of the medical burdens and fears of prior decades. It is helpful that family, friends, and doctors unburdened themselves and left intimate glimpses of fear and suffering.

In our opinion, the intimate accounts that follow advance the case for medically assisted suicide, while concurrently exposing the challenges of defining the terms of access. Not all sufferers faced imminent death. Does that matter?

SHATTERED IN THE PRIME OF LIFE

Seniors were over-represented among illness-related suicides; however, the number of individuals in the prime of life was large enough

Table 4.1
Distribution of physical illness cases by life-course phase, 1900–98

Life-course phase	N *with a leading physical illness motive*	*Overall n of suicides in the life-course phase*	*% of leading physical illness motives within life phase*
Pre-adolescent	3	77	3.9
Adolescent	34	615	5.1
Prime of life	634	5,908	9.5
Transitional years	364	2,023	16.4
Seniors	945	2,236	40.9
Unknown age	16	132	9.4
Total	1,996	11,000	20.0

to warrant an opening discussion of their trials (Table 4.2). More than proportions separated the life-course phases. The physical health crises that struck down men and women in their prime were distinct from the medical problems that afflicted older people. Individuals in their thirties and forties who took their own lives typically had the misfortune of a disabling accident or a medical problem with an early onset – tuberculosis, epilepsy, diabetes, and kidney diseases (Table 4.2). After World War II, several changes influenced this pattern. Workplace accidents that resulted in brain damage, the loss of a limb, or back pain were evident throughout the century; however, accidents outside the workplace that injured the spine or brain increased after mid-century. They originated in recreational activities or auto accidents.[47] Affluence introduced distinctive hazards. Simultaneously, a post-war upsurge in pharmaceutical developments reduced the medical motives for suicide among people in their prime. Tuberculosis had once caused immense suffering. Testimony at inquests bares the physical anguish and feelings of hopelessness, but morbidity and mortality due to "the white plague" began to recede after mid-century on account of new inexpensive and readily administered drugs.[48] From mid-century, diabetes and goitre were also subject to better treatment. Crippling disorders such as rheumatoid arthritis, stroke, multiple sclerosis, motor neuron disease, and head injuries remained. In one respect, the last did change over time; their origins shifted from work to leisure.

Work-related accidents for the first half of the century often involved men and animals. A horse threw Sidney White, who

Table 4.2
Ascending mean ages and life-course phases of individuals for whom a physical ailment was a primary motive for suicide, 1900–98

Group of ailments	*Mean age of men and women (life-course phase)*	*Standard deviation*	*N of cases*
Venereal diseases	33.8 (prime)	3.4	6
Non-work injury	37.0 (prime)	19.1	23
AIDS	42.0 (prime)	13.5	3
Epilepsy	42.6 (prime)	14.7	23
Tuberculosis	42.8 (prime)	13.4	37
Influenza	43.7 (prime)	15.9	68
Severe headaches or tinnitus	44.2 (prime)	13.5	41
Obesity	47.2 (prime)	21.9	9
Disabling work injury	47.5 (prime/transitional)	16.1	26
Head injury	48.3 (prime/transitional)	17.0	18
Lingering incurable ailments	49.6 (transitional)	18.0	76
Assorted ailments: liver, stomach ulcers, goitre, gall bladder, appendicitis, broken limbs, fevers	50.7 (transitional)	17.7	245
Kidney disease	51.1 (transitional)	16.8	28
Unspecified but failing health	51.4 (transitional)	16.6	178
Back pains	52.0 (transitional)	16.4	37
Diabetes	54.4 (transitional)	14.8	30
Breast cancer	55.0 (transitional)	11.8	7
Breathing ailments: emphysema, miner's phthisis, asthma	59.4 (transitional/senior)	17.1	159
Cancer diagnosed and type specified	60.2 (transitional/senior)	16.7	140
Cancer feared but not diagnosed	60.1 (transitional/senior)	14.2	71
Arthritis of various types	60.4 (transitional/senior)	16.8	72
Heart disease and related ailments	61.7 (transitional/senior)	15.4	222
Blind or becoming blind	62.3 (senior)	19.7	27
Stroke	65.1 (senior)	14.1	111
Prostate cancer	70.0 (senior)	12.3	38
Old and unwell	74.9 (senior)	11.7	157

sustained a head injury; the young man had persistent headaches and underwent a change in character. He was described as "eccentric" after the incident.[49] Adolf Bergen was twenty when he fell from a horse; during the two years between that incident and his death, he complained of severe headaches. After a fit, he confided to his friend James Harris, "Well, Jim, if I thought that my head was going to be bad again often like it was last week, I would sooner be dead."[50] Dizzy spells from a fall off a horse bothered James Kinnear to such a degree that he told his wife that "if he didn't get better he hoped he would die."[51] Young farmer Charles O'Neill had fallen from a horse and been unconscious for forty hours; in subsequent years he experienced severe headaches.[52] Farm and forestry work held other dangers for labourers. A piece of machinery at a saw mill struck William Bignal in the head. "He was never the same afterwards," his wife reported.[53] Family members and friends stressed that head injuries altered character and precipitated a history of headaches. Victims had likely suffered a severe concussion with long-term cerebral damage.

Injuries had multiple consequences, including pain and loss of work. Farmer Jacob Graham said that he had a "great pain in his back and sometimes thought it would drive him off his head."[54] Wharf labourer James Burnell, according to his aunt, "met with an accident six weeks ago and hurt his back and was unable to follow his occupation. He seemed depressed but endeavoured to bear up." He reported to the docks but could not work. He hanged himself the following day.[55] At forty-eight, John Walsh was perhaps no longer in his prime for a risky line of work. He had been in hospital three times on account of separate accidents while working on scaffolds. He could no longer work.[56] A father of a large family, James Scott, could not work on the railway due to a back injury. A friend testified that "his one anxiety was to get back to work."[57] Invisible back injuries, challenged by employers, had multiple consequences.

As an adjunct to pain and unemployment, there was despondency and references to depression. A connection between injury and mental state was noticed by those closest. Builder Francis Cameron "had a fall from a building and was unconscious for some hours. Since then deceased has not been well." His wife mentioned that he "was suffering from depression."[58] A neck injury prevented David Nelson from working as a forklift operator. "His depression occurred in that context," according to his wife.[59] These remarks by wives were unexceptional and contribute to the idea that episodes treated as mental illnesses could have material origins. That proposition is pursued in the next chapter.

Injuries instigated mental conditions, one of many complicating facts that call for subtlety and awareness of patients' histories on the part of those psychiatrists and psychologists who today link mental illness and suicide. It preyed on the minds of men that they could not provide for their families. Masculinity, built firmly on the idea of the breadwinner, had disturbing implications for disabled men. Frustration wrought changes in character that could compound troubles. Edward Ryan had been partly paralyzed by an accident to his back at work; his condition made him hostile and put him at odds with the law.[60] Work-related injuries that plunged families into destitution mostly appeared in the first three decades. In later times, social security assisted individuals with workplace injuries, but it alone could never fully compensate for a crippling injury, nor erase the low self-worth of working-age men.[61]

In the early decades of the century, witnesses seldom could specify medical problems with clinical precision; however, they described symptoms. They also recounted the collateral consequences of a chronic illness. Unemployment was a principal concern. Farmer Michael Conroy, who took his life in 1902, often told his wife Bessie that "he wished he could leave this world as life was a misery to him." A long illness had put him in hospital three times in four years. He could no longer work and that promoted despondency.[62] At the age of forty-five, Philip Barker had begun to lose his memory and was deemed "not fit to work." His wife said he "often spoke of committing suicide."[63] After a chronic disease hit younger men and women, they realized they would never get better and could not expect to live the life they wanted. Kidney diseases rendered patients pessimistic.[64] Thirty-year-old labourer Thomas Whitehouse knew he had poor prospects. A friend commented that Whitehouse's kidney trouble "preyed on his mind and he said he was useless."[65] By the early 1920s, medical descriptions at inquests had improved and some doctors connected physical ailments to depression.[66] At the 1924 inquest into the death of twenty-seven-year-old war veteran Clifford Lloyd, the doctor who conducted a post-mortem stated that "the heart was fatty, and the muscle friable. There was an extensive adhesion of the pericardium. The right lung contained a chronic abscess filled with thick pus. The state of the deceased's health would produce lowered vitality and depression."[67] Mary Evan's doctor believed that "the death of her relatives and kidney trouble was enough to cause depression."[68] A "leaking kidney" and a poor prognosis distressed Rex Beattie.[69]

Until the second half of the century, a diagnosis of tuberculosis imposed a life sentence of delicate health or early death. It demoralized people in their prime. It precipitated periods of depression even among patients supported by excellent professional care and a loving family.[70] Edith Stanley's doctor felt that her bereavement over her husband's death was made worse because she was "always rather delicate in consequence of tubercular disease."[71] Unemployed cook Ernest Beguely, at the age of thirty-six, told his wife after his release from a five-month stay in hospital that "life was not worth living."[72] At least two operations for tuberculosis left Arthur Tuke "very easily depressed and subject to fits of prolonged melancholia." According to his doctor, "he took a jaundiced view of everything on every occasion." A crisis developed when his latest surgical scar did not heal.[73] At forty-eight, shopkeeper William Ginsberg was prosperous and happily married, but no treatment in New Zealand or Australia could relieve his tuberculosis, and consequently he was in "a state of depression."[74] Mary Tahu, a twenty-year-old housemaid, endured the pain of tuberculosis in both lungs, but threatened to kill herself if sent to a hospital.[75] Long hospital stays contributed to the dread that overwhelmed many. Only in his early twenties when he entered hospital with pulmonary tuberculosis, Hugh Reddie was already labelled a hopeless case. His wife commented that "he had been very depressed and suffered a great deal."[76]

Depression understandably overwhelmed tuberculosis sufferers.[77] Thirty-nine-year-old labourer and war veteran William Wilkins occupied a tuberculosis shelter at Auckland Hospital. The police report on his death in 1924 noted that "he had been gradually dying of tuberculosis disease for two years."[78] Discharged from the hospital without hope of recovery, John Reid returned home, went into the kitchen, and sat with his wife crying for about half an hour before killing himself.[79] Suicides arising from fatalism about tuberculosis peaked in the 1940s and were rarely seen after the 1960s.[80] Before social security had become integrated into the country's fabric, men blended their identity with their capacity to work. Tuberculosis left many totally incapacitated or undertaking light work.[81] Thus this disease hit at several levels: men were in pain, lacked hope, forfeited income, and lost their sense of manhood. Farm labourer Thomas Parkinson, thirty-six and single, had required care and charitable support for two years prior to his death. His tuberculosis "was progressing" and he feared that the local charitable aid board would cut off assistance. He was in a panic and alone.[82] Tuberculosis made miner Denis Gavin an invalid at forty. He told his landlady that when his savings were finished "he would be finished as he would not accept charity."[83] A stoic pride in self-sufficiency and physical prowess exercised considerable influence among men, perhaps diminishing with the challenges of the Great Depression.

Some diseases were grotesquely frightening. Hydatid disease was one. Caused by the larval stages of tapeworm, it was a terrifying affliction known well through experience and legend in a rural society. Archibald Beaton ended his life in 1916 at the age of thirty, because hydatids had reached his lungs. He was "wasted to skin and bone."[84] Twenty-six-year-old gardener Thomas Hatherley had an operation in August 1923 for a tumour on the appendix; it was a hydatid cyst the size of a large orange. He made a recovery, but according to his doctor there may have been other cysts that accounted for his continuing pain.[85] Fear of this parasite persisted for decades.[86]

Terror of an internal growth materialized in many accounts of cancer. Not everyone waited for a diagnosis or treatment; some decided to forgo pain and a wasting death by choosing to die in their own time by their own means. A firm prognosis was one thing, unsubstantiated fear another. Fear was a common motive, although more so among seniors. Nevertheless, fear of cancer overwhelmed people in their prime too. Twenty-five-year-old Harry Dale had strained himself lifting a bag of chaff onto a dray. It appeared that he had pulled the muscles in his chest and had to abandon hard work. "He told his sister that he either had heart disease or cancer coming."[87] According to her doctor, forty-eight-year-old Hannah Seebeck "was afraid to face the results of the X-ray and thought she had cancer." Her fear was stoked, as it was for many, by firsthand familiarity with the disease's progression. "Her sister had been operated on for cancer and her mother had died for it," said her husband, "and she was obsessed with the idea that she had cancer."[88]

Unexpected observations such as the fear of cancer call for explanation, not dismissal as statistical outliers. This maxim also applies to the linkage of suicide and influenza. Influenza was mentioned often for people in their prime. Physicians also remarked that influenza increased the risk of suicide. "Influenza is a disease well known to cause sudden impulsive mental aberration."[89] Influenza was linked to depression, low spirits, nervous breakdowns, and unbalanced behaviour on account of fatigue. Wharf worker Harry Barlow explained how influenza undermined his will to live. He survived a self-inflicted pistol shot to the head long enough to say, "I got very weak from the influenza and I didn't think it worthwhile."

His suicide note simply read, "I am suffering terribly. I can hardly stand up."[90] A friend of labourer George Hill had seen him a week earlier. "He was then recovering from a severe attack of influenza. He was very much pulled down."[91] As late as 1922, the mother of a poor, unemployed, and melancholy farm labourer mentioned at his inquest that "he had influenza in the epidemic of 1918."[92]

Remarks about influenza and depression preceded the 1918 pandemic. In 1902, a farmer's wife stated that after the influenza her husband was not the same man.[93] Amelia Dunn testified that her husband had "a very bad case of influenza from which he never properly recovered. He complained of severe pains in the head. He thought he was going mad."[94] A witness at the inquest for a young engineer in 1910 reported that "for about five weeks prior to his disappearance he was ill with influenza which left him in an unusually depressed state."[95] Ruby Hunter said that her father "was taken ill with influenza which later developed into insanity."[96] Auckland physician Alfred Knight held influenza responsible after the death of a young man in 1902 without domestic or money problems. "Influenza is responsible for producing mental depression. There are recorded cases leading to suicide."[97] Other physicians also remarked on connections among influenza, depression, and suicide.[98]

A possible tie-in between influenza and mental illnesses prompted Sir William Osler to write in *The Principles and Practice of Medicine* (1912) that "almost every form of disease of the nervous system may follow influenza." Osler stressed that "the most important nervous sequelae are depression of spirits, melancholia, and in some cases dementia."[99] The medical profession in the early twentieth century had settled on the idea that influenza disturbed mental stability. During influenza outbreaks in 1926 and 1928, physicians continued to connect the flu with mental illness when they testified at suicide inquests. Influenza weakened men and women struggling with other debilities and worries. For decades, doctors related influenza to depression and suicide.[100] As late as 1986, a psychiatrist attributed a suicide to a brain infection associated with influenza, and in 1996 another referred to "post influenza depression."[101] At the end of the twentieth century, virologists suggested that reports of mental disorders from around the world during the 1918–19 pandemic were probably explained by the virus entering the central nervous system.[102]

The physiological and work-for-pay divisions between the sexes produced several gender-based health motives. Post-natal depression was a factor in some suicides. So too was the inability to give birth. Elsie Osborn at twenty-six wanted children and had been married for seven years; her hopes were dashed when she had a hysterectomy. She was described as "very depressed."[103] Breast cancer and cervical cancer were feared.[104] A lump frightened Ethel Bird, who wrote, "I know I am not getting any better. I suppose it is cancer and I would rather be dead than ill and helpless."[105] Esther Halverson "underwent an operation for bowel and womb trouble" and emerged "very depressed."[106] Not only did men have male diseases, but certain pursuits of manliness had terrible outcomes. Occasionally sport injuries left men with enduring problems. A cook and amateur boxer, Jock Gunn had lost a match in Australia in 1912; friends reported pains in his head and forgetfulness.[107] While boxing in 1916, George Richardson received a bad blow on the head which "left him with great pain and at intervals after that he suffered pain in the same place and at such times he seemed erratic and gradually got worse." Just before his death in 1928, his condition had become "very bad."[108] Air Force engineer Anthony Boult told a wartime friend that he had done a good deal of boxing and suffered a good deal from headaches. "He often asked me for Aspros."[109] In 1954, a doctor explained the likely source of Dan Morrow's excruciating headaches: "He had fought some strongly contested bouts in the boxing ring and it is possible that there was some residual damage to the cranial contents."[110]

The long prosperity witnessed the rise in sport, recreational, and motoring accidents that left individuals paralyzed or partly paralyzed. Some people with seizures, loss of limbs, brain damage, or paralysis could not endure what they saw as a diminished quality of life.[111] Epilepsy was mentioned occasionally.[112] Seizures may have led to imposed or self-imposed isolation, and thus limited exposure to education and other people.[113] Henry Angel lived at home and was subject to epileptic fits and was disabled. His father found his crutches lying on the river bank.[114] Minnie Arndt "became very depressed after suffering epileptic fits."[115] Accidents unrelated to work had a presence among the suicides of people in their prime. An auto accident, followed by months in a coma, deprived thirty-two-year-old John Andrews of the quality of life he had known. "He would shake with anger."[116] Pelvic injuries from an auto crash left George Milton with pain and declining mobility.[117] The most notable instance of suicide on account of paralysis concerned Michael Crew, a prominent lawyer who advocated euthanasia. We mentioned him in the earlier section on discourses about euthanasia, because he had arranged for assistance. While on vacation in Fiji in 1987, Crew had been pushed in fun into shallow water, shattered his vertebrae, and lost almost all use of his body. He was "very depressed and on several occasions had said 'I want to die.'"[118] In 1993, his death was featured in an episode of TVNZ Frontline that explored the case for euthanasia. Frontline's account of Crew's suicide also raised the contentious question of whether media coverage of suicide deterred or encouraged such deaths.

BAD FORTUNE AND ACCUMULATED RISK

Accidents to men in their transitional years undermined their ability to work with the result that they felt useless. Crushed between a car and a tram, fifty-four-year-old William Murdoch lost a leg. A friend testified that "he worried for some time about not being able to work" and was "in a state of great depression."[119] As workers aged, they succumbed to occupational diseases. Miners suffered from "miners' complaint," the lung ailment also known as phthisis.[120] Retired miner Joseph Williams realized he was dying and, according to his doctor, pleaded that "he was suffering such torture from his difficult breathing and sleeplessness that he thought I ought to give him a big enough dose of Morphia to enable him to die in comfort. I explained I could not administer a lethal dose, but would see that he had enough sedative to relieve his symptoms."[121]

There were scores of ailments with well-described consequences; together these assorted illnesses were a major presence at inquests, but there were not enough cases of each to merit separate designations. Examples will convey the diversity along with the themes of illness and pain, and illness triggering poverty and mental distress. Severe rheumatism kept sufferers from working or from merely moving about the home.[122] After an operation for appendicitis, farm labourer John Moyan could no longer do heavy work and according to his doctor "in consequence he was getting hard up."[123] Stomach ulcers sometimes prompted the cancer fear, but they were also intrinsically painful.[124] "I am so tired of this pain in my inside," wrote Thomas Browne.[125] Like ulcers, goitre was uncomfortable and on occasion initiated a cancer scare.[126] Ada Line had a swelling in the throat which her doctor insisted was a goitre but she would not have it. For several weeks she had pains and great difficulty in getting her breath.[127] Felix McGarry told his wife, "I cannot stand this any longer, the goitres are choking me."[128] We could cite many examples of specific illnesses and the ways in which they upended the routines of everyday life. John Coles' spinal meningitis required pain-relieving injections daily.[129] Hyperthyroidism and an associated heart condition kept widower Henry Harwood from his railway job.[130] The list of circumstances is long.

It is difficult to place diabetes in one phase of the life-course. In the form we know as Type 1, it could have an early onset with severe consequences before the widespread use of insulin. Twenty-six-year-old William McBeath suffered from diabetes and, in his brother's assessment, "had been depressed." His doctor described him as a severe diabetic and extremely ill-nourished. Illness deprived him of employment for three years.[131] Some individuals with Type 2 diabetes had physical problems or behaviour that intensified their diabetes. At fifty-four, Violet Grace had been quite ill with diabetes; it did not help that she was a very heavy woman.[132] "Advanced diabetes, a condition of which he was fully aware," did not bring Harry Burrows to a sensible course of action. "I've had enough of hospitals; I should rather take a dose of poison."[133] At sixty-one, Arthur Naylor's diabetes had become severe enough that his doctor warned of comas; illness led to twelve months' unemployment.[134] Diminished capacity accompanied cases of congenital ailments such as spina bifida, degenerative diseases such as Parkinson's Disease, motor neuron disease, and multiple sclerosis, and lingering disorders such as Crohn's Disease, cerebral palsy, systemic lupus erythematosis, and spondylosis of the cervical spine.[135]

Lung diseases with symptoms of near-suffocation comprised one of the more numerous sources of a diminished quality of life, lack of sleep, and illness-induced depression. Unable to sleep because "he could not lie down for difficulty in breathing," Peter Tindall was exhausted and depressed.[136] Harry Meadley had "bad turns" attributed to asthma and bronchitis. His wife remarked that "sometimes his health made him depressed."[137] Pensioner Richard Hopkins "seemed to have a dread of smothering because of his bronchial complaint."[138] Consider farmer William Hurst, who "through coughing during the night ... had not been sleeping too well of late."[139] Some years later, at the end of the century, Norman Tanner told his wife that "things are not right, harder to breath at night."[140] Later that same year, Morton Flannery complained to his wife about "the bad nights and the breathing."[141] Time and again, family and friends passed off emphysema as asthma or bronchitis.[142] By the 1980s, a new label – chronic obstructive airways disease – came into use.[143] Whatever the label, the symptoms of a lung disease amounted to unremitting torture; the shortness of breath kept men out of work and unable to sleep.[144] "Let me die," pleaded Ronald Anthony after stabbing himself in a lung.[145] Not once in the first half of the century did witnesses at a suicide inquest remark on a connection between heavy smoking and attendant lung disease, but rather they attributed racking coughs and shortness of breath to asthma and bronchitis. Casual remarks added details about chain smoking. "Life was a continuing problem" for Charlie Logan, who received an invalid's benefit and was "living on beer and cigarettes."[146]

By mid-century a greater recourse to autopsies cleared up diagnostic uncertainties.[147] Carbon-occluded lungs and nicotine-stained fingers were described in reports. An inquest from late in the century illustrates precisely what afflicted many individuals across the century and what witnesses were afraid to admit. The deceased had been "out of breath a lot," according to his wife. The autopsy revealed "severe upper zone emphysema and abundant carbon pigment deposition usually associated with cigarette smoking."[148] The lungs were "clouded with smoker soot"[149] or "there were heavy carbon deposits on the surfaces of the lungs."[150] Witnesses' statements earlier in the century failed to get to the root cause of lung troubles, but they did not mince words about the ultimate misery. Maori labourer Henare Kohu "felt as if he was choking when he was breathing."[151] Farm manager Edward Christensen made it clear that the months he spent in hospital brought no relief. He would not return "because he had enough torture the last time he was there."[152] Despair was common across the decades. "I am sick of it all," wrote Martin Bullen. "Don't open the garage door. Ring Constable Watson."[153]

IS IT WORTH GOING ON? OLD AND UNWELL

Heart disease, including high blood pressure, hypertension, arterial sclerosis, angina pectoris, and heart attacks, accounted for many medical-related suicides. Seniors were at risk, as were people in their transitional years. According to her doctor, Ethel Hood's high blood pressure subjected her to a bout of neurasthenia "of a rather marked type." He thought that her case could only get worse.[154] A heart condition could inflict pain, a diminished capacity for favoured routines, and unemployment. Owing to loss of time through illness, Alfred Prince lost his job as a city council labourer during the Great Depression. His son noted that this loss "appeared to worry him."[155] "My husband," reported Frederick Wallace's wife, "became very worried since he stopped working [on account of heart trouble] and considered he should be doing more."[156] Suffering from heart disease, Clifford Fuller "worried about his health, not being able to work, and bring money into the house."[157] Heart disease and an occipital haemorrhage forced fifty-seven-year-old Thomas Wilson to leave his job as a tram driver; he was described as depressed.[158]

Great physical distress was a consideration. James Butcher's doctor stated that this elderly man "was suffering from heart disease in a distressing form. For the past month he has had a very bad time. Injections of morphia had to be administered to him about every four hours."[159] Joshua Machlin's doctor treated him for angina pectoris. "My God, how can I bear this," Machlin wrote.[160] Fifty-nine-year-old Sigrid Collie's son described her as "very miserable on account of her ill health." An autopsy brought to light that "her lungs were oedematous and congested. The heart was enlarged and showed fatty infiltration."[161] In another instance, a post-mortem examination found coronary arteries that were "thin thready vessels."[162] The number of heart disease cases peaked at an estimated one hundred for the 1950s, but numerous instances surfaced in all subsequent decades.[163] Severe heart trouble prevented James Hunter from working his farm and he worried about that. At night when in pain, he would call out to his wife, "Shoot me, shoot me, Annie."[164] "Sorry Bonnie I couldn't last another day with 15 pills," wrote heart patient Gerald Blair.[165]

Congestive heart disease left patients struggling to breathe and unable to sleep. Andrew Thurston "had to sit up in bed gasping for breathe." His doctor could only palliate.[166] Among seniors, heart and lung diseases occasionally occurred together. Exertion was agonizing.[167] Pensioner William Whitehouse "suffered from his heart and breathing." He despaired of recovering and let friends know that he wanted to use a gun on himself on account of the pain.[168] Bad heart attacks kept Hugh Hambleton in bed and out of work; a blood clot was found on a lung. He was about to resume work but worried about his capacity for labour at a foundry.[169] The considerable physical distress in heart-lung conditions undermined sufferers' mental outlook.[170] Time and again, decade after decade, witnesses described individuals with heart and lung ailments as "depressed" or suffering from "fits of depression."[171]

To be destitute and in pain early in the century was a terrible double misfortune. Single and suffering from heart trouble and a lung ailment, seventy-four-year-old retired labourer Peter Maskrey had saved little. His physical decline bothered him and "he wished someone would give him chloroform so he could pass away gently." The absence of a spouse and children meant that he would soon have to rely on charity. He said that "he would rather throw himself in front of the Express than go into the Old Men's Home."[172] In another case, arrangements had been made by a hotel keeper to get an ailing old bachelor into the old men's home when he was discharged from the hospital, but he would not go there.[173] Elderly men had a pronounced distaste for these institutions, for not only were the facilities rule-bound and spartan, but along with a disability or illness, these places signified an end to active lives.

Urine retention among older men warned of a prostate condition.[174] The inevitable progression was well known throughout the century. Treatments, such as a tube up the urinary tract to relieve the bladder, were a painful source of humiliation and despair.[175] Widower Edward Tamplin had an operation for relief in 1919, but his son said that over the next three years his father was "a wreck." At times, "he said he wished that he would die as he was suffering from great pain."[176] Despite his broken English, a Finnish immigrant wanted friends and family to know what caused him to end his life. "I left this note," he wrote. "I gott stoppis in mia vater. I can not do anni mor vork I am finnis I am gon Mom."[177] The doctor for sixty-eight-year-old farmer Henry Bilborough was in no doubt why he shot himself: "he was suffering from cancer of the prostate, which was incurable, and would cause him to suffer a lot of pain."[178] Ralph Barton had prostate obstruction "for which he had a further minor operation to insert a tube into the bladder." Depressed and worried about his wife caring for him, "he said that he would be better dead."[179] Prostate cancer as a motive for suicide remained throughout the century, although it featured less prominently after the 1950s. It could not be cured, but its progression could sometimes be controlled and discomfort alleviated, although intervention was not always successful. A few men simply felt that prostate trouble marked the end of their time. "I have been getting very thin and making my water is getting me worried," wrote a seventy-two-year-old retired labourer in 1972. "I know I am too old now for Hospital for the rest of my life."[180] Other men were in far worse shape. In 1980, cancer spread from Jack Cole's prostate through lymph nodes into his liver, to the genitalia, and the lower limbs; it produced malignant nodules on the skin of the groin and perineum.[181]

Whether imagined or real, cancer upset seniors. Reclusive old George Watson had a bladder infection; his niece testified that "he thought he had cancer."[182] A doctor attending seventy-nine-year-old Josiah Elphinstone told a coroner that "he had a suspicion he had cancer of the stomach."[183] Not long before his death, William Power complained of stomach troubles and remarked that he was afraid of cancer.[184] Mama Punaki, aged sixty-five, did have cancer of the stomach. "She was in very considerable pain throughout and was mentally depressed."[185] More than fear led John Miller, a farm labourer with incurable cancer and pain, to commit suicide.[186] Cancer of the face upset sixty-one-year-old William Winsfield. He had suffered from a growth which broke out periodically, but only recently had a doctor informed him it was cancer.[187] Tobacco precipitated many miseries, perhaps most often emphysema. Other tobacco-related health crises included cancer of the mouth, lip, jaw, tongue, and lungs.[188] The pain of a terminal lung tumour caused fifty-nine-year-old Ian Bourke to refer to a bullet as his lead painkiller.[189] James Carter, sixty-five, suffered from cancer of the tongue and jaw; he declined an operation.[190] Surgery for George McGregor's cancer of the tongue failed to cure him and he could endure no more treatments.[191] Sixty-year-old Patrick Herald likewise had an operation for cancer of the mouth, but feared a recurrence and another operation.[192] At the age of seventy, John Peter wrote in his diary that his condition, unspecified but likely cancer, made living an ordeal. Additionally, as was often the case with suicides by very ill people, he believed his exit would lift a burden from those he loved:

> Well this may be my last day. I have reached that stage of health when life to me is not worth living. I am too weak that I can't hardly walk. And the pain in my side is unbearable, and I know there is no cure, and I don't see why I should linger. I'm only a trouble to myself, and will be to others. I wish all my friends long life and free from pain and worry. Good-bye.[193]

Strokes and cerebral haemorrhages were motives for suicide among the elderly and for a few unfortunate younger people. Dean Smith was in his prime when a haemorrhage deprived him of short-term memory and most of his vision. His mother said that "when he went to do something that required sight he said he'd rather be dead than alive."[194] Paralysis could take away any joy for living, especially if the victim had been independent and active, as Emily Brown had been until a stroke. She then needed constant assistance and nursing.[195] Some stroke victims may have thought of themselves as a burden, but usually it was not a presumed burden but the loss of quality of life that tipped the balance. Ship modeller Tony Campbell could no longer engage in his beloved hobby.[196] At the age of eighty-six, Charles Duncan lived alone even after a stroke, but he confessed to his doctor that partial paralysis sapped his will to live.[197] Those around elderly Piripi Waipapa noticed that after a paralytic stroke he was not his usual self. "You could see the decline." One witness added that "he did not eat his food too well."[198] Strokes could have another effect leading to a rational suicide decision. When an eighty-year-old husband saw his wife immobilized and suffering indignities, the experience inspired a determination to remain in control. Michael Bowden resolved that he "didn't want to be in the same situation." He made it clear to his son that "after his dealings with mum he would consider taking his own life."[199]

Prior to the provision of social security medical benefits, an illness that required hospitalization put impoverished older men and women in the position of appealing for charity.[200] Victims of strokes were in difficult circumstances unless family members or charitable groups were available and willing to tend to them. Charles McDevitt, at eighty-six and without family, had a stroke that impaired his mind; sisters at a convent looked after him.[201] William Powell was fortunate too, because his wife looked after him when a stroke left him with memory loss.[202] Assistance was not always available. Even when it was provided, the elderly were prone to feel that they had become a burden. Widower John Ryder was partly paralyzed from a stroke, had symptoms of senile decay, and had come down with pleurisy. His son moved in for a few days until the old man could be moved to Mrs King's Nursing House in Christchurch, where he rebelled and had to be removed. Discomfort, a feeling of rejection, and a belief that he had become a burden led to his hanging himself.[203]

A few older men were still working at the time of their stroke and afterward had to retire.[204] Up to the age of seventy-three, pattern-maker William Coats continued to work until a paralytic stroke left him immobile. He tried to walk again but fell. His daughter commented that "at times he was despondent."[205] Some who had been deemed old and unwell acted on a mix of connected motives that included poverty, the absence of family, and the necessity of giving up work. Strokes also brought on additional physical complications. Inactive limbs became painfully ulcerated.[206] John Day's doctor described the effects on a stroke on the elderly man. "He could only swallow with difficulty. His drinks came back through his nose. He ran a risk daily of choking or getting septic pneumonia."[207]

For some people, aging brought worries about a loss of memory and sight.[208] These were predominantly but not exclusively frailties of the aged. Tram driver Ernest Wood, for example, was in his fifties when he went to see an optician and returned fearing a loss of sight.[209] Frank Kelleway was forty-eight when his memory loss became acute. His condition made him "quite depressed." He was to have seen a specialist but instead committed suicide.[210] More typical were individuals over sixty. Thomas Christiansen, a sixty-nine-year-old widower, knew he was losing his memory; his son heard him complain that "he was not altogether master of his mind."[211] Residing in Jubilee House, a private nursing home, on a ward with twelve other senile dementia patients, eighty-four-year-old Charlotte Clark insisted to a nurse that she was going to see her Jim. That was the name of her deceased husband.[212] Described as an old man, Daniel Kelly had become "childish of late." He told friends that he would "rather be dead."[213] Family members described James Reese as "childish through old age and he occasionally had fits of depression."[214] Mary Huntington explained that her late father "had been in the habit of wandering away."[215] Admitting that she had been failing fast for six years, Dorothy Butler wrote in her suicide note that "I cannot think out things like I used to."[216] Blindness depressed seventy-seven-year-old James Richardson.[217] Eighty-one-year-old Swiss immigrant George Jacklin worried about his failing sight, because he enjoyed reading.[218] Doubtless the many indignities endured by the elderly and the physical agonies experienced by other adults made their exits understandable.

When each ailment case is closely reviewed, it is possible to see a boundary between the conditions of men and women with a seriously diminished quality of life and individuals with a terminal illness. In the former instances, it is impossible to move from a position of sympathy and understanding to one of moral approval. The preservation of life takes precedence because to condone a pre-emptive death is to jeopardize the defenceless by shifting society's moral compass in a direction that could lead to unscrupulous parties spurring on someone's death for purposes of gain. Can even the plight of the terminally ill be transferred into a recommendation for assisted suicide? That was a question posed in the media and among politicians several times late in the century.

WAR TRAUMA AND THE TRAUMA OF WAR

In recent years in the United States, publicity about a high suicide rate among combat personnel returned from Iraq or Afghanistan has drawn press attention to war's physical and mental trauma. Reports on trauma convey graphic yet ambiguous stories that disclose discord over war's medical legacies. Abundant reports on suicides have official sanction and reveal that the military acknowledges a problem; it honours its soldiers and wants citizens to be understanding and helpful. Stories of mental trauma nevertheless leave an impression of scarred lives that can subvert a war effort. To offset some of the news surrounding physical trauma there have also been optimistic reports on combat medicine, physical rehabilitation, and advances in prosthesis engineering. Discussion in public about the current or future mental state of maimed soldiers is a missing page in these nearly celebratory accounts. "Look, these men are walking." Serious discussion about suicides among returned soldiers has opened and includes attention to unemployment; however, tales of medical progress do not project forward with plausible conjectures on post-rehabilitation work possibilities and mental states. The New Zealand case files indicate that wars have a lingering impact.

Combat medicine has undoubtedly progressed. Wounded soldiers from the armies of affluent and technically advanced countries have experienced historically high injury survival rates. The consequences of combat do not end with successful surgery and physical rehabilitation. The impact of maiming and amputations must be tracked over the long term and results publicized. Combat medicine's wonders ultimately need to be put in perspective by analysis covering the life-course of returned personnel. The lessons of World War I and World

War II may not be wholly applicable to current and future circumstances on account of improved combat medicine and rehabilitation practices, but case files of suicides by combatants from these wars suggest that physical and mental trauma have had devastating consequences. States engaging in wars must anticipate the multiple costs of rehabilitation, including the challenge of making soldiers emotionally whole when physically they are not. World War I was especially horrific for New Zealand troopers. The following account examines war injuries and how men felt about them. In a bridge to the next chapter on mental illness, the discussion turns briefly to mental trauma.

Two questions must be asked in any study of war trauma and soldier suicides. Are suicide rates for soldiers and returned soldiers any greater than the rates for men of the same age who did not see combat? If there is a difference, can the suicide case files of soldiers and returned soldiers suggest why? It is not easy to calculate rates for soldiers and returned soldiers for New Zealand. Only the suicides of men on New Zealand soil can be discovered, because the coroners' authority did not extend to overseas troops. Even in New Zealand, during World War I the army tried to put a lid on the topic of soldier suicides in military camps at home. Thus, case files capture only the suicides of men outside military jurisdiction. Another challenge comes from the shortcomings of population data and data on veterans.

To calculate a suicide rate for returned servicemen, we identified from our data only those men who committed suicide and had been overseas. That number (multiplied by 100,000 since rates are expressed in terms of 100,000 individuals) was divided by an estimate of surviving returned servicemen. To find that number, a variety of unpublished government reports on war pensions were located.[219] These reports calculated an annual figure of surviving war veterans from World War I and World War II by subtracting those who died each year. The 1939–40 report remarked that the life expectancy of the veterans appeared to have been ten years less than for men in the general population in 1935–36 and three years less in 1939–40.[220] Despite efforts by government and employers to reintegrate veterans into civilian society, the lives of many former servicemen were apparently unhealthier and unhappier than the lives of civilians in the same age cohort.

To show that difference between returned servicemen and civilians, estimates on the suicide rates of men who were of the same ages as the men who went overseas are required for comparison. During the war, the ages of service were set at a minimum of twenty and a maximum of forty-four. To estimate the number of men in that cohort in each of the sample years, the census age distribution data for 1921, 1926, and 1936 were used. The data for the missing years (1922, 1924, 1928, and 1930) were estimated by linear interpolation. As the cohort aged, the numbers of men in it were reduced accordingly to estimate the actual number of civilian men who survived in the cohort in each sample year. The essential data and results of the calculations appear in Table 4.4. Over the years, the suicide rate of the men who were in the same age cohort as returned servicemen increased because the cohort aged and, as we noted in chapter one, rates in this era increased with aging.

The rough but reasonable method of calculating a comparison shows a unmistakable pattern. Immediately after World War I, returned soldiers had a significantly higher suicide rate than their civilian counterparts. A comparable set of calculations was undertaken for World War II (Table 4.5). Once more the suicide rates of returned soldiers greatly exceeded the rates of civilians of the same age cohort. A comparison of marital status, class background, and current employment further indicates that the returned soldiers and the civilians were essentially identical. Combat alone differentiated them. Returned soldiers showed no preference for firearms; they selected methods of self-destruction common to all men at the time.

Taking into consideration all returned soldier–suicides from both wars, a number of facts stand forth. For the whole century, the five hundred and thirty-three returned soldier–suicides found in sample years account for one in fifteen male suicides (6.9 percent). An undeterminable number of these individuals might have taken their own lives even without the intrusion of war, because on close inspection the conduct and suicide motives of some returned soldiers were not absolutely attributable to war. A few men had alcohol abuse problems before their military service. Sydney Eaton's wife remarked with candour that her husband "was gassed in the war and his nerves had never recovered and his tendency to drink grew worse."[221] From time to time, witnesses claimed that trauma led to later alcohol abuse or elevated a predisposition. Friends of Mike Gillman claimed that "he did not drink as much before he went to the war as since he has come back."[222] It was difficult too for doctors to separate the morbidity caused by a non-war-related heart condition or to distinguish pulmonary tuberculosis from damage caused by a gas attack.[223] After his return from the front, Angus Watkins could do very little work because he was incapacitated from a gas attack. He had been occupying one of the tuberculosis shelters attached to the Auckland Hospital. The police report claimed that he was dying of tuberculosis.[224] Occasionally, a witness dropped a hint about war injuries but did not elaborate. A decade after the armistice, Jack Moore's wife said only that "he suffered from war wounds."[225]

Despite the existence of indeterminate or incomplete cases, there are sufficient applicable instances to show that war increased profound unhappiness. A decade after a conflict ended, its influence on suicide is uncertain. War trauma was an apparent but not a dominant presence among male suicides. Witnesses in over half of the cases of returned soldier–suicides (59.0 percent; n = 312) made no remarks at all about war injuries or shell shock. Men were described simply as returned soldiers; witnesses could not add more or chose not to. The absence of details means that physical and mental war trauma were under-described, although witnesses did think that the war was a significant enough factor in the suicide to deserve mention. In other instances, witnesses readily recounted in detail the type of war-related pain. It should be added that the majority of cases involving physical trauma were associated with World War I. That war's horrors marked more men physically and emotionally than World War II.

When witnesses supplied rich information, they frequently intimated that physical injuries had been an ongoing burden, possibly more numerically significant than so-called shell shock cases. Hesitation in claiming the outright primacy of physical injury comes from the fact that so many cases that identify a man as a returned soldier are silent about trauma. Among the well-documented instances, however, the sequence of cases is notable: wounded (15.0 percent; n = 82); shell-shocked according to witnesses (10.8 percent; n = 59); gassed (9.3 percent; n = 51); prisoner of war (6.6 percent; n = 36). Suicides among returned soldiers have multiple origins connected to their war experiences. For some, the trauma was primarily emotional strain; for some, it was irreversible physical damage. Details depict injuries intruding on men's lives and undermining their mental health. The inquest files disclose how a few men felt about their loss of a limb, their succession of operations, and their gas-scarred lungs.

One of the first instances of suicide connected with a severe and permanent injury reveals a man aware of his fate and then encountering a military system that had yet to accept responsibility for what industrial-scale warfare was doing to men. Wounded in the head at Messines in 1916, Fred Sheriff was sent home on a hospital ship in July 1916. His injuries and his reaction to them persuaded the army to consider him insane; it sent him back to New Zealand without notifying his family. The intent was to provide him with the best medical care while at the same time keeping him out of the public eye. He railed against his fate. On board the hospital ship, he was "put in irons or in a cell." On landing in New Zealand, he was whisked away to a hospital and held as an insane patient "under control" for three months, without formal hearing as required by law. More will be said about these illegal practices in the next chapter. Discharged from the army in October 1917, Sheriff was labelled "a head case."[226] Other so-called head cases appeared in the suicide case files during and after the war. The men complained of head pains from their wounds, difficulty adjusting, and an inability to work steadily. Friends and family remarked on mood changes.[227] Some witnesses advanced the unverifiable suggestion that temper tantrums were a result of head wounds.[228]

Military and civilian doctors innovated and worked diligently to reconstruct men. Expressions such as "severely wounded" and "many operations" appeared in case files. These phrases described Thomas Hanley. To rebuild a badly fractured thigh, "part of another man's bone had been graphed." His father told the coroner that his son "had recently complained a great deal as the result of his injuries and said that life was a torture to him."[229] Much the same history burdened Sydney Kidd. Wounded at the Battle of the Somme, he would later speak to a friend about the awfulness of that experience and "to his injuries received there and to his treatment in hospital later and to the pain he suffered." Another friend stated that "his war experiences used to bother him and he used to suffer from the effects of his wounds."[230] Reconstructive surgery continued for years. In 1924, a returned soldier told his brother "that he would sooner do away with himself than undergo another operation."[231] In many cases of severe wounds, the men could not return to their former lines of work, which for most had involved physical labour.[232] Francis McGregor suffered mental trauma, but the main reason why he could not work was his "crippled arm."[233] William Wallace's shrapnel wound made his arm useless and painful. "He has done very little work since his return," testified an acquaintance. Another witness stated that "he told me he still felt the effects of the war."[234]

How could war injuries not have been felt? How could the injured have avoided reflecting on the quality of life lost, particularly in a culture of work and recreation that accented physical prowess? Not all despondent wounded men who took their own lives were disabled; some were able-bodied but in agony. The abundance of shrapnel wounds in World War I meant that surgeons were removing metal shards years after the war. Doctors could not always extract shell fragments and the pain revived the horrors.[235] The father of a farmer who shot himself in 1930 reported that pieces of a shell could not be extracted and that these contributed to his son's nightmares. He woke up terrified; "it was pitiful to see Howard in the state he was in as he appeared to be going over his war experiences all over again. His bed was wet with perspiration."[236] Shrapnel disfigured men. A shell wound to the face discomfited Vincent Stewart.[237]

The number of definite war-related suicides declined by the late 1920s; war-related motives for suicide now vied in witnesses' narratives with the more commonplace ones such as lack of work and marital discord.[238] Still, a few men had endured war injuries for years only to collapse in despair after long suffering. Archibald MacKay had been disabled with a bullet in the spine. "As a rule he suffered intense pain. The bullet had never been extracted." Unable to endure more agony, he ended his life in his bedroom in 1928.[239] A young veteran's mother reported in the same year that her son "for some years had been in bad health the result of being gassed in the war and a wound in his chest."[240] Suicides attributable to war trauma still appeared in the 1940s and in ever smaller numbers into the 1950s.[241] Badly wounded at the Somme where he lost a lung, farmer William Lewis "had to exercise great care with regard to his general health and recently became very ill and depressed on account of this." He shot his son, wife, and himself in 1952.[242] Herbert Perry endured one of the longest periods of suffering where war trauma was a leading motive for suicide. "From his return from overseas in 1919 in a state of collapse, deceased had a history of bad health. He spent a good deal of his time in hospital, the latest of which was two years ago when he underwent a severe operation. He complained about pains in the head and stomach for years." He ended his life in 1954.[243]

Gas attacks were unique to World War I and men who survived them had recurrent medical problems. Incapacitated veterans survived on a pension. Invalided out of the army in 1917, Archibald Gilmour been gassed. To his family he seemed "since his return to have melancholy fits and to be strange in his ways, and mentally depressed."[244] Farmer Alfred Hawkes knew that his lungs had been permanently damaged; recurrent illnesses convinced him not only that his condition was incurable but that he would always be subject to painful attacks.[245] According to his family, Michael Mansfield had returned from the war in a serious condition and "suffered with his lungs."[246] Russell Winters had been gassed. A neighbour testified that "since his return from the war he has not done much work. He was addicted to drink and appeared to me to be sometimes queer in the head."[247] Since he had enlisted when he was eighteen, it was unlikely that alcoholism was a pre-war condition. Among some older men, however, alcohol abuse was a likely precondition.[248]

In addition to injuries, the war subjected men to illnesses that they otherwise might have escaped; most plainly they would have avoided malaria had they not served in Egypt and Palestine. As a witness explained about his brother, "he got over the fever and returned to the front on light duty. This would be about the end of war. He has suffered from the after effects of the fever. At different times he had complained to me of pains in his head as after effects of the fever."[249] Medical conditions contracted on account of military service persisted in peacetime or recurred. Witnesses linked them to suicides. Meningitis from army camps and pneumonia from the trenches affected the health of men after demobilization.[250] Venereal diseases were another category of possible war-related ailments.[251]

When war trauma was a physical injury, a relationship between suicides and war could be strong and visible. But it also could be confused with troubles that preceded or followed the war. Pension boards were alert to these possibilities when they laboured to minimize the government's obligations; by 1936 about a fifth of veterans still qualified (15,474 pensions; 73,707 survivors).[252] Mental trauma was particularly difficult to affirm or dismiss. Occasionally, men were known by friends and family to have suffered real physical harm and their odd conduct was put down to a combination of war-related physical and mental distress. Witnesses testified that men had been gassed and suffered from shell shock, or had been wounded and had shell shock.[253] Mental trauma could have multiple roots: injuries; injuries and illness; injuries and terrifying experiences; experiences and fatigue; grieving; and on and on. Mental trauma varied in severity.

Junior medical officers at the front adopted 'shell shock' as a catch-all term for a host of mental conditions including exhaustion, breakdowns, depression, and psychoses. They determined on the spot that an individual's mental state made it pointless to send him immediately back into combat. The worst cases were returned to New Zealand and the medical corps made local hospital arrangements commensurate with the presumed degree of severity. Processing and treatment became more sophisticated as the war lengthened, but the term "shell shock" spread from 1916 forward. Returned soldiers and the public quickly adopted this blanket term. Its widespread use meant that coroners only needed to hear it mentioned by a witness in order to find grounds for a finding of suicide while mentally unbalanced. Thus, not every case of war trauma was well described.

The relationship of physical injuries to suicidal despair could be palpable on account of vivid testimony, or it could be as vague as a brief remark that the individual was a returned man, as if that were enough to explain his action. A similar range of evidence is apparent for shell shock cases. Some amounted to a psychosis but were covered by the courtesy of a shell shock or nervous breakdown designation.[254] Labourer Arthur Donald, according to his employer, had had a breakdown and "was labouring under a delusion and he passed a remark that he was going to be executed that morning."[255] Another returned soldier "said the Germans were after him."[256] A soldier who survived Gallipoli and several battles in France returned home before war's end on account of a mental collapse culminating in aphasia that lasted three months. His mother and brother travelled to see him at a psychiatric facility in New Zealand where, with speech regained, he recounted his ordeals. His brother recalled that "in relating his experiences at the front, he would break out in tears, thoroughly breakdown."[257] A quiet man aged forty-four, George Madden, was described by a close friend "as an old soldier." He had been invalided home sometime before 1918 and became more silent than ever; he stayed in his boarding-house room; a doctor provided an unspecified treatment for shell shock. To his landlady, he confided that "he would sooner have come back with a limb off than be in the state of mind he was in."[258] Men sent home in a fragile state collapsed when they heard of the combat death of a mate. At home, a few men who saw unspeakable things treated life recklessly or became habitual gamblers.[259] Men chain-smoked to relieve their anxiety and spoke of their state of depression.[260] After the Armistice, World War I went on killing.

World War II claimed its victims of trauma too. Due to the greater visibility and shocking quality of wounds from the previous war, descriptions of wounds from World War II seem comparatively scarce. As had been the case with quite a few suicides of World War I veterans, witnesses assumed that the investigating constable and coroner would be familiar with the individual and required no further information than that the man had "suffered a certain amount of shock during the time he was at war."[261] In file after file, a key witness mentioned a war disability pension but not the nature of the claim.[262] Occasionally, witnesses added a little more. It was said of farmer Norman Simms that he had "received injuries."[263] Detailed accounts were seldom provided and even the better descriptions were terse. A head wound at Monte Cassino left John Strathmore blind in one eye, and that is all we learn.[264] Service in the South Pacific left Henry Stephenson ill with a respiratory problem for a year on his return. His wife remarked that "after my husband's service in the Islands I noticed a big change in him in that his nervous and physical energies were depleted."[265] Arthur Taylor's injuries qualified him for a pension, but he was unable to work and this condition, according to his wife, made him depressed and irritable.[266]

Unlucky men in World War I were killed, wounded, or gassed. Only two prisoners of war from that conflict turned up among suicides. The German advances of World War II rounded up numerous prisoners. Their camp experiences, especially toward the end of the war, were wretched. Some were in captivity for over four years.[267] In explaining her husband's mental state, one woman told the coroner that "during the last war, my husband was a prisoner of war in Germany from 1941 to 1944 and on his return to New Zealand was not in good health. His nervous condition was bad and during the last month up until the 4th May had been very bad."[268] Carpenter Denis Symington never settled down or recovered his health after his imprisonment and forced labour in a German-run mine.[269] Mental trauma was not mentioned often in the case files of veterans of World War II, but when instances were discussed during the war by patriotic organizations and the government, they were known as "psychosis cases," not as shell shock.[270]

Table 4.3
Average age of death of civilians and soldiers in same cohort (20 to 44 during the war): Annual report of the New Zealand Expeditionary Force, Statistics for 1939–40

Year	*Civilians*	*Soldiers*
1935–36	62.5	51.9
1936–37	58.0	54.0
1937–38	60.0	54.7
1938–39	50.0 (?)	53.3
1939–40	57.6	54.6

Source: Archives New Zealand, SS7 W2756, Box 17, Accounts, Miscellaneous Publicity and Returns – Returned Servicemen – Miscellaneous Statistics, Annual Returns on Pensions, 1936–56, Annual Report of the New Zealand Expeditionary Force, Statistics for 1939–40.

Suicide scholars have identified wartime as a period of low suicide rates, allegedly because a society on a war footing demands an engagement with common purposeful tasks in an atmosphere of patriotism. Potentially alienated or isolated people became integrated into society and too busy to worry about petty troubles. This superficial guess promoted first by Émile Durkheim persists in recent literature. Simple suppositions derived from guesswork theories are unworthy of trust. A factually based explanation indicates, first, that a good portion of a high-risk population is out of the country. At home, there was close to full employment. Moreover, the claim about war's integrative service leaves an impression that war distracts people from trivial worries. Thomas Joiner in 2005 cited a study from 1933 to the effect that war prevents people from "brooding over individual troubles and disappointments."[271] On the contrary, case files show vividly how war exacerbated troubles and disappointment (Graph 4.2). During both world wars, people worried about running farms and businesses short-handed and families brooded about the hazards to "their boys" overseas. Bereavement suicides captured awful "disappointment."[272] When Matilda Clements received the news that her youngest son had been killed, she had a breakdown and had to be attended to by a doctor.[273] When labourer George Ready spoke about his son "he would sob and cry like a child."[274] In another of the bereavement suicides, a witness testified that "the deceased had two brothers killed in the war. He used to grieve about them. Whenever their names were mentioned in the house he would always get up and walk out. The deceased killed himself with a rifle that belonged to one of his dead brothers."[275]

Table 4.4
Estimated suicide rate for returned World War I soldiers relative to civilian males in the same age cohort, selected post-war years

Year	*Approx. n of surviving returned servicemen*	*Min. n of suicides by returned servicemen*	*Approx. rate of suicide of returned servicemen per 100,000*	*Approx. n of all men in age cohort of servicemen*	*Est. of men in cohort who never served*	*Suicides of men in service age cohort who never served*	*Approx. rate of suicide of men in service age cohort who never served*
1920	79,500	32	40.0	471,100	391,600	34	8.7
1922	79,100	21	26.5	461,685	382,585	44	11.5
1924	78,700	23	29.0	452,260	373,560	52	14.0
1926	78,300	15	19.2	442,835	364,535	57	15.6
1928	77,900	21	27.6	417,561	339,661	61	18.0
1930	77,400	22	30.0	392,287	314,887	72	22.9

Table 4.5
Estimated suicide rate for returned World War II soldiers relative to civilian males in the same age cohort, selected post-war years

Year	*Approx. n of surviving returned servicemen*	*Min. n of suicides by returned servicemen*	*Approx. rate of suicide of returned servicemen per 100,000*	*Approx. n of all men in age cohort of servicemen*	*Est. of men in cohort who never served*	*Suicides of men in service age cohort who never served*	*Approx. rate of suicide of men in service age cohort who never served*
1946	145,000	21	14.5	660,500	515,500	35	6.7
1948	140,440	38	27.1	660,000	519,560	41	7.9
1950	137, 700	29	21.1	611,000	473,300	56	11.8

Table 4.6
War experiences among male suicides

Type of war experience	*Boer War*	*World War I*	*World War II*	*Korea or Vietnam*
Served; no additional information	7 (1.3%)	177 (33.2%)	107 (20.1%)	21 (3.9%)
Wounded or serious illness	–	52 (9.8%)	46 (8.6%)	–
Gassed	–	31 (5.8%)	–	–
Shell shock; nervous breakdown	–	71 (13.3%)	4 (0.8%)	–
Prisoner of war	–	2 (0.4%)	15 (2.8%)	–
Total	7	333	172	21

Civilians in World War II suffered as they had in the previous war, worrying about sons in the army. The shortage of labour made farmers anxious about crops, the wool clip, and ultimately debts. In some of these instances, it is impossible to hold the war entirely responsible, because there were pre- and post-war troubles. However, evidence in several cases made the war the obvious cause. In 1946, farmer Thomas Shaw testified that his wife was "not in good health and was suffering from a nervous breakdown caused through the death of her son on active service."[276] Awful wartime tragedies afflicted people for years until they had a breakdown. At the time of their fatal decision, they may have been mentally ill, but that label evades life's heartbreaking misfortunes. In 1956 Helen De Jonge took her own life, after years of bearing nervous trouble as a result of her husband having been tortured and murdered by the Japanese during the occupation of the Dutch East Indies (Indonesia). In the words of her sister, she "had been had been very concerned of his death and had never really recovered from his death. About six months ago it was noticed that she was beginning to show signs of being depressed and she used to talk of his death."[277]

The shift in subject from war trauma experienced by soldiers to the trauma of war affecting civilians heralds the end of a topic and the beginning of another, because the pain experienced by civilians was mental anguish, a distinct form of torment. From physical ailments, discussion must shortly turn to mental illnesses in general. Before making that transition, a summary of findings from this chapter is in order.

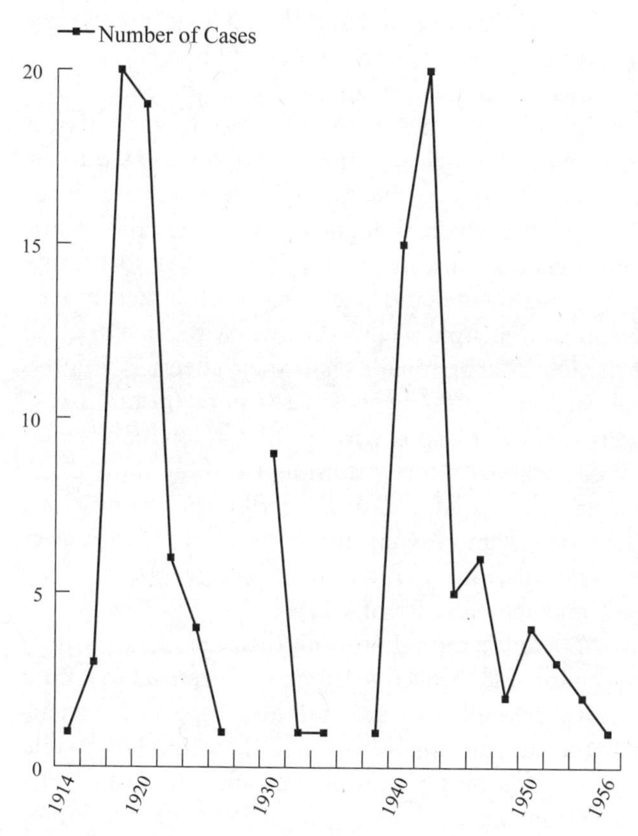

Graph 4.2
Number of suicides of civilians potentially affected by war, 1900–60

CONCLUDING OBSERVATIONS

Fields of study that cater to a human yearning for simplicity and solutions have their work cut out for them when dealing with suicide, because these expectations for tidiness are overthrown by nonconformity, unexpected mental processes and fears, and the intrusion of momentous historical events. The latter can never be predicted. Despite the likelihood of complications, we had expected that diseases and injuries would turn out to be comprehensible motives for suicide because a healthy body has long been integrated with notions of a full life. Self-euthanasia seemed the most understandable of all motives for suicide even if it is immensely upsetting. However, things proved not so simple. For one thing, the number of self-euthanasia cases was small. Furthermore, on a number of occasions, individuals perceived they had a terminal illness when they did not.

Individuals' knowledge about their medical conditions, possibilities for treatment, and prospects for recovery has been imperfect and in some cases clouded by their nightmares. We think it would be wrong to consider these people as mentally ill; there were explanations for how a number of them thought the way they did. There were lags between a generation's memories of a relative's suffering through ineffectual treatments and the arrival of better practices. Morbidly pessimistic people weighed down with illnesses and injuries were at greater risk of suicide than their cheerier counterparts; however, pessimism should be considered in relation to background. There were and are reasons why specific individuals feared pain and protracted incapacitation. Additionally, some individuals simply could not get over the idea that serious injuries from work, war, or play had robbed them of what they believed was a complete life. Their prior lives and values coloured their perceptions. They brooded about a diminished quality of life.

The complexity of people's thoughts about their health is a principal finding of this chapter. It showed up in people's refusal to secure a diagnosis or follow a course of treatment. It also appeared in a pattern of denial by witnesses and suicide victims who seemed incapable of accepting the role of smoking in causing chronic lung disorders.

There are observations about war trauma that connect to larger themes. Apart from the pain of war wounds, there was an embedded cultural aspect to injuries. If bodies were maimed, men's expectations for a normal life as marked out by culture were also curtailed. This point offers a clue to a better understanding of suicide, because it is the idea of a diminished life defined in many ways that turns up often in the records, including some cases discussed in the following chapter on mental illnesses. They have not only been intrinsically hard to bear but, in the minds of the men and women who endured them, they diminished the capacity for a full life, due in part to the persistent stigma. In relation to particular times and places, this idea of a diminished life was more than a misplaced perception. Social practices and conventional values did not accommodate people who seemed disabled or different, and they recognized their marginalized status.

5

Mental Illnesses: Representation and Therapy, 1900–2000

Social historians of medicine insist on including patients. Regrettably, the annals of psychiatry provide few accounts for mental health patients. Freud urged uninhibited talk, but his published cases comprise a short list.[1] More patients are encountered in Dale Peterson's anthology *A Mad People's History of Madness* and Roy Porter's path-breaking *A Social History of Madness*.[2] Both advocated a patient's perspective and assumed a sceptical attitude toward the medical profession. Porter declined to identify syndromes from autobiographies, because he considered the individuals unique and their thoughts worthy of review principally as commentaries on the age when they were written. Moreover, he distrusted diagnoses; all were flawed by their attachment to far-fetched rationalizing schemes. He acknowledged that the patients whose lives he recounted were "a hopelessly unrepresentative minority."[3] Since the 1980s, more and more former patients have published reminiscences about institutionalized psychiatric care; a few have published memoirs recounting their struggles to achieve mental health.[4]

Historians have opened asylum records to reach the patients. Files on admissions, disciplinary action, and censorship have exposed routines of control but also the involvement of family members in committing or taking an interest in relatives.[5] Porter and the asylums' historians established a standard for investigation.[6] This chapter follows their critical leads, but can add unique narratives, because coroners, when considering physical evidence that pointed to the possibility of a suicide, next had to make inquiries into the deceased's state of mind.[7] The abundant evidence from these inquiries discloses diversity, evolution, guesswork, pretention, and chaos in mental health care as it was actually practiced. There is plenty to criticize, but most of the nearly one thousand doctors whom we encountered treating mental illness were not self-assured fantasists. They included a significant number of unassuming individuals who examined or cared for patients in homes, private practices, clinics, public and private psychiatric hospitals, and general hospitals. Many were compassionate but overworked. To their credit, some were deeply interested in the personal histories of patients.[8] Variety, confusion, and humane concern have largely remained out of sight. They appear here through openings provided by inquests. Professional thinking about mental illness has been complicated, evolving, personalized, and uncertain. Intellectual histories of mental illness have exposed this confusion, but the public faces of psychiatry and psychology have projected undue confidence, because clinicians and therapists have worried about losing public faith or patients' trust.[9] There is also a public expectation that experts should radiate confidence, and so they have.[10]

DISCOURSES ON DEPRESSION AS MENTAL ILLNESS

Mental illness occupied legions of doctors outside psychiatric hospitals. Asylum historians had merely scratched the surface. Doctors outside the institutions treated individuals who presented a wide range of symptoms of confusion. Some of the considerable diversity, it must be admitted, originated in medical imperialism. Psychiatrists and later psychologists annexed a variety of conduct into mental health. They drew depression, substance abuse, and so-called personality disorders into their practices. Notions that addictions are matters of health and the mind originated in the reasonable idea that an abuse of intoxicants caused neural damage that could induce psychoses. Alcohol was entangled in representations of mental illnesses throughout the entire century. Expansion of mental illnesses did not stop with the plausible inclusion of addictions. By the late 1960s, a few psychiatrists treated men for homosexual tendencies.[11] Official reports beginning in the mid-1960s cited a host of vague 'disorders' such as personality disorder, emotional instability, passive dependence, aggressiveness, and asocial personality.[12] In these years, wrote Edward Shorter, personality disorders became "a whole sandbox for empire building."[13] Parasuicide joined other disorders.

In the 1990s, a burst of media attention about suicide prompted psychiatrists and now psychologists to promote their utility, which they did by declaring a firm and overwhelming connection between self-destruction and mental illness. That claim raises questions about medical doctors and psychologists "pathologizing" the troubles, sorrows, and suffering arising from everyday living. Assertions that most suicides were committed by people with mental illnesses were weakly supported, and certainly not backed by studies of numerous completed suicides. We found that in most years of the century, between twenty-five and forty percent of individuals who took their own lives had some form of mental health motive (Table 1.3). The percentages would have been higher if alcohol and drug addiction had been added to mental illness rather than considered separately as we have done.

The breakdown of motives into categories that subtract from the mental illness count is a step that promotes transparency, perhaps at the expense of a few psychiatrists and psychologists who pronounced on the subject of suicide and mental illness during a panic about youth suicide in the late 1980s and early 1990s. The emphasis which clinicians and affiliated researchers placed on mental disorders and suicide is rife with curious features. The case files are packed with evidence about the enduring stigma of mental illness and its demoralizing impact on individuals. Self-awareness of the conventional shame of mental illness could have precipitated a few suicides. In a final note to his wife, a businessman wrote, "it is this or Porirua [psychiatric hospital]."[14] Stigma is a persistent theme. Clinicians recognized this prejudice and combatted it. Could they not then have realized that their public claims about a link between mental illness and suicide injected a troubling message into a culture that still stigmatized mental illness? Mental illness was certainly prominent, but the concept needs to be probed, broken down, and studied in relation to the stresses of the times. In chapter seven, much will be said about the rashness of youth, unprecedented economic and cultural upheavals, and claims about mental illness and suicide (Graph 5.1).

To demonstrate transparency, we should explain again the quality of our records, but this time highlight the medical testimony. A few files from early in the century contained a deposition or letter from a doctor that detailed symptoms, diagnosis, and treatment. In many instances, there were only several sentences. By mid-century, medical

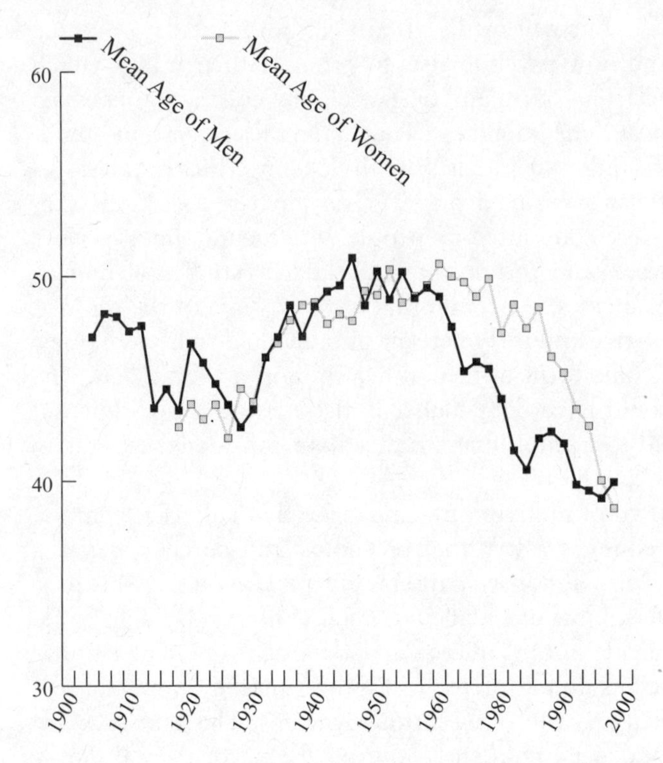

Graph 5.1
Mean ages of men and women with a mental illness motive: Three-year moving average

reports were common and extensive. Late in the century, doctors came under intense questioning and scrutiny at inquests; therefore, by the 1980s, files routinely contained remarkably detailed information. At least twenty percent of the individuals who committed suicide in the last two decades of the century received specialized psychiatric treatment (Table 5.1). Approximately 800 files from 1980 to 1998 contain the doctors' notes or reports summarizing the deceased's medical and related history. While there was a greater volume of evidence on the diagnosis and treatment for each case during the last decades of the century, the proportion of mental illness–related suicides had not increased remarkably from early decades (Table 5.1). Most mental illnesses mentioned at inquests in the late twentieth century were labelled either depression or schizophrenia (Table 5.2). In prosperous countries with passable health statistics, these two widely used categories accounted for most psychiatric

Table 5.1
References to depression at suicide inquests, 1900–2000

Usage of the word "depression" and related words and phrases	1900–50	1980–2000
Depressed appearance according to witnesses	24.5 % (n = 1,032)	32.0% (n = 2,333)
Mental depression as a motive for suicide attributed by witnesses	11.3% (n = 478)	12.4% (n = 961)
Medical treatment for mental depression evident in file	9.5% (n = 401)	8.5% (n = 652)

Table 5.2
Motives for suicide: Broad categories of mental illness, 1900–2000

Broad category of mental illness	N *of suicides*	*% of mental illness suicide cases*	*% of all suicide cases*
Depression, melancholia, nerves	2,048	64.1	17.8
Unspecified mental illnesses	429	13.4	3.7
Schizophrenia	311	9.7	2.7
Various others (anxiety, neurosis)	159	5.0	1.4
Bi-polar, manic-depressive disorder	109	3.4	0.9
Paranoia	73	2.3	0.6
Paranoid schizophrenia	60	1.9	0.5
Multiple personality disorder	4	0.1	0.0
Total	3,193	100.0	27.6

hospital admissions, with depression leading schizophrenia by roughly five to one.[15] Public discussion, diagnosis, and treatment of illnesses covered by these two labels occupy the bulk of this chapter.

At the beginning of the twentieth century, specialists in nervous disorders, influenced by German psychiatry, elevated depression to the status of a disease. By the 1920s, psychiatrists were splitting depression and labelling the sub-types. Many accepted the idea that there was endogenous depression, which was considered unprovoked and affected the body's entire vital feelings; there was also reactive depression, allegedly caused by external difficulties that promoted deep sadness.[16] How far did these developments, based on the analyses of discipline-founding psychiatrists in Europe, reach? New Zealand case files reveal that the intellectual formulations of psychiatry quickly filtered down to general medical practices. Non-medical witnesses, meanwhile, used the term depression alone, although their explanations confirm the usefulness of the expression "reactive depression."

Beginning in 1900, witnesses at inquests mentioned depression, and disclosed an interest in its association with various sources of stress. Complicating this picture of a public recognition of depression as an illness, the word "depression" had multiple applications. Sometimes it merely summarized a short-term emotional state, and in these instances it is hard to separate reactive depression from sadness. At the age of seventy-one in 1906, Patrick McCall had to work as "he was a labourer not a pensioner." His wife reported that he was weak and had had no income for a fortnight. "He was very much depressed."[17] In the same year, an elderly widower was described as having had "fits of depression for many years."[18] "My husband," testified another wife in a contemporaneous case, "had suffered from depression for a good while."[19] Duration suggested an order of complaint separate from sadness on account of an immediate crisis. When doctors and lay people tried to distinguish depression from sadness, they frequently mentioned the period of suffering, but an enduring stigma associated with mental illness further complicates a retrospective sorting of cases into endogenous depression, reactive depression, and sadness.

At century's end, after years of public education about mental illness, witnesses still avoided a mental health connection if possible. They emphasized 'normal depression' – sadness or possibly reactive depression – to avoid shame. Marie Taylor's mother testified that her daughter was separated, had financial troubles, and suffered from Crohn's Disease. "She also at times became depressed but her depression was as suffered by any normal person."[20] Depression caused by material distress was normal. By inference, depression without apparent cause was not considered to be normal. Throughout the century, when family members or doctors attempted to assign depression either to a medical condition or to a mere emotional state, they were struggling to avoid statements or actions that would invoke the stigma of mental illness. To help achieve a separation between the medical and the emotional, doctors and lay witnesses referenced traumatic events, symptoms, and the duration of the suffering. Although they modified the term, depression remained the hard pivot amidst adjectives.

Grassroots confusion about depression was always apparent, although only in the late twentieth century did media reports begin to question whether it was an illness. Critics then claimed that psychiatrists and pharmaceutical companies had transformed the ubiquitous – "normal" – emotional state of sadness into a medical diagnosis.[21] Sceptics queried whether any so-called mental illnesses – not just depression – were illnesses.[22] A few writers romanticized mental illnesses as creative and liberating, and denounced treatments as oppression.[23] This position had supporters in New Zealand in the 1970s.[24]

A prolific critic with an international following, Thomas Szasz, denied that any mental illnesses had an objective reality, because they had no physical substrata.[25] People suffered torment, but to Szasz the mind was not a physical organ and thus, for example, depression did not require medical intervention. The problem with this position was that, although the mind was not an organ, an organ created it. A cautious observer, Laura Hirshbein, proposed that while depression was an illness, it had been over-diagnosed in the United States on account of a fixation on happiness and trends in American psychiatry. In pursuit of scientific rationality during the 1950s and 1960s, American psychiatry started to downplay personal histories in favour of supposedly more detached scientific assessments leading to drug therapy.[26] Depression thus acquired standing as a widespread disease concurrent with the introduction of medication for mental illnesses generally.

By turning away from an older practice of learning about a patient's family and life circumstances and toward a reliance on psychological tests that American psychiatrists promoted as objective, the profession there fashioned a problem that doctors could credit themselves with solving through tests and medication.[27] This account of American psychiatry establishes a benchmark for considering where New Zealand psychiatrists stood in the final decades of the twentieth century. Hirschbein contends that in the 1970s, American psychiatrists were not especially interested in how or why patients developed symptoms, "so long as researchers could all agree on the significance of those symptoms."[28] New Zealand's specialists retained a psychodynamic approach and continued to compile information about the patient's family history, economic setbacks, substance abuse, and relationship troubles. In its brief to a 1972 Hospital Commission, the Medical Association of New Zealand concluded "that the two most important things an individual could do to insure mental health is to choose his parents (from the point of view of genetics) and ensure that he is a wanted child."[29] In but one example of a psychiatrist's attention to background, notes prepared for an inquest several years later stated that "the depression was caused by a series of personal circumstances, particularly in regard to the farm."[30] As we have seen in chapter four, New Zealand's country life was fraught with stress. As well, doctors frequently reported universal background troubles: a disturbed upbringing, an alcoholic parent, early school-leaving, and years of heavy drinking.[31]

The American approach had adherents at the University of Auckland. In the early 1980s, a university-based initiative to advance the biochemical treatment of schizophrenia proposed that patients' records be maintained on a computer so that psychiatrists might ask common questions, keep track of undesirable treatments and side effects, check congruence of diagnosis and medication, and ultimately develop a computer decision tree to expedite psychiatric work. The advocates noted that psychiatrists averaged fifty minutes a week with patients. That was too long. Critics of computer-assisted decision-making insisted that mental illnesses defied patterns and the time spent with each patient was warranted.[32] During the 1980s and 1990s, New Zealand psychiatry was criss-crossed with professional divisions, but seldom did controversy or doubt emerge in public. Confidence, even assertiveness, prevailed when mental illness and suicide came up for public discussion. Otherwise what would patients think?

American psychiatrists, meanwhile, responded to Szasz by building a case for depression as a disease that originated in trauma and heredity, caused abundant suffering, and contributed to suicides. They reported a cluster of syndromes: deep lingering sadness, loss of appetite, difficulty sleeping, and trouble concentrating. Psychiatrist Peter Kramer listed these symptoms and added that depression progressed as a disease with remissions and recurrences. To help his argument along, Kramer cited historical acceptance of the term.[33] His enlistment of history does not advance his case, because an acceptance of a term does not mean lexical precision. In New Zealand, the label was mentioned by doctors and the public before World War I, but what it meant was truly murky, perhaps slightly clearer when supported with adjectives, and somewhat clearer still when symptoms were detailed

The chief obstacle to considering depression as an illness was the apparent absence of a somatic feature. The public craved physical evidence and family members and doctors even 'discovered it,' because it lifted the stigma of mental illness. A family doctor in 1906 found "evidence of organic disease of the nervous system having set in. He was in a condition tending to insanity and I told him he needed three months absolute rest."[34] In 1918, the family of a man with neurasthenia wanted a post-mortem examination of his brain in the hope of finding an abnormality, thereby proving "that deceased was unacquainted with the nature and quality of the act that ended his life."[35] He was considered free of responsibility, a victim of a disorder, and clear of the stigmatizing designation of insanity. Seventy years later, a solicitor argued on behalf a man's surviving family that "I have heard of others having had this same type of 'flu' that carried such a depression."[36] In some cases, syphilis was blamed. It was preferable to attribute depression to a physical condition, or to invoke the fiction of going to a clinic for treatment of a physical ailment.[37] If a somatic feature was not available, there was another way to dampen the distress created by a suggestion of depression as a mental illness. Throughout the century, individuals would be diagnosed as severely and persistently depressed, yet not "certifiable."[38]

Psychiatrists recognized that in the absence of markers, the designation of depression as an illness was mistrusted. Years before any evidence of a neurological connection, psychiatrists assured patients that their suffering originated in a disease. One reason for doing so was to convince them that they were not suffering from a fault of character. In her 1986 report to a coroner regarding the suicide of a depressed young woman, a New Zealand psychiatrist insisted that her depression had "a biological basis" and was "a biological illness." She admitted to taking this stance because she wanted the patient to stop feeling unworthy and responsible.[39] Assertions that suicide has a strong connection with depression, and that depression is an illness, might have worked to diminish the individual's responsibility. That would have served the purposes of some socially nervous family members, as well as doctors who were expanding the domain of mental illness. However, a few individuals who committed suicide knew of this inclination to reduce their rationality and they objected. They wanted their act understood as a reasonable decision; they wanted their troubles known. "I am in my right mind."[40] "I am making a rational decision."[41] Doctors and family members shied away from representing depression as insanity. Meanwhile, as the critical participants describing their own illness, patients emphatically rejected the idea that they were acting irrationally.

The missing somatic factor was filled in late in the twentieth century by a plausible theory of neural effects that could lead to depression.[42] During most of the century, no evidence supported a biomedical connection; however, in a few instances there were references to high blood pressure. Interactions between poor physical health and mental illness were surely common two-way situations. Without exact somatic features to point to, lay witnesses muddled along with the term "depression," but importantly they often situated its origins amidst life's stressful events. Doctors did the same.

It is important to emphasize at this point that depression was not invented by psychiatry and pharmacology in recent times. On that point critics were wrong. Their claims of over-diagnosis are another matter; depression could not be readily separated from individuals' life experiences. Had stresses inflicted neural harm, or were they short-term and immediate causes for deep sadness? For at least a century, depression straddled socio-cultural troubles and medical agony. The people directly affected and their families sought immediate aid and not distant social reform or the uncertain results of family counselling. Exigency brought in the doctors.

In the pre-barbiturate years, from 1900 to 1950, witnesses at almost a quarter of suicide inquests (24.5 percent) described the deceased in terms that suggest what became known in later years as clinical depression. While this is a significant proportion, some people mentioned depression in the same breath as serious concrete crises. In many instances, a doctor had been called in to prescribe a sedative, and it was difficult to determine if a symptom such as loss of sleep expressed depression or resulted from immediate stress. The patient was unemployed, had sold the farm and felt useless, had marital or romantic troubles, suffered from a debilitating illness, or had experienced a recent death in the family. Additionally, there were historically unique sources of stress. The loss of a son in war was a terrible shock; the great influenza epidemic laid people low.

When witnesses went beyond recounting how life's crises had disturbed the suicide victim and added remarks about mental depression, their statements show a lay form of "diagnostic creep." It had started with the earliest reports. Families wanted help with deeply upset loved ones. To whom could they turn but a family doctor? The impetus for a medical treatment of depression came from families. Appearances were not enough to convince us that a quarter of all suicides from 1900 to 1950 arose from depression as mental illness. There were other factors, conditions that simply would have depressed anyone. For their own reasons, family members accepted a doctor's expression and incorporated it into their conversations. To doctors and family members early in the century, depression was not insanity. However, it intimated that the balance of the mind had been upset sufficiently to explain the act of suicide and suggest that it was abnormal. Therefore, the word "depression" served the cultural function of explaining a suicide as irrational without suggesting madness.

Sometimes suicide seems to have been precipitated directly by great existential distress. Even so, we did not dismiss the idea of depression as an illness, although the term's perpetual imprecision made it susceptible to over-diagnosis. In each file, we looked for more than witnesses' descriptions of someone appearing depressed. During the first half of the century, witnesses in over one in ten cases of suicide (11.4 percent) specifically attributed self-destruction to a motive associated with depression, nerves, nervous breakdown, or neurasthenia (Table 5.1). As part of this early evidence that depression, as an illness, had been a motive for suicide, there were indications that general practitioners really did see something disturbing, something more than sadness or mourning. In some cases, their familiarity with the individuals enabled them to detect a change in character. They continued to have difficulties finding the right words, or at any rate being consistent in how they used "depression," "melancholia," and "neurasthenia." Before World War I, they resorted to linked terms to emphasize more than a temporary upset; they positioned depression in association with neurasthenia and melancholia. These latter two terms were fading from use by the 1920s, but they had been drawn into older descriptions to bolster the idea of mental distress greater than common sadness. In her doctor's estimation, Elizabeth McKay, who took her life in 1900, "was suffering from melancholia and was subject to fits of depression." Another general practitioner stated in 1914 that his late patient "was suffering from marked melancholia and depression."[43]

More helpfully, doctors and lay witnesses occasionally mentioned symptoms. When a patient cried, stayed in bed, and refused to eat, his doctor remarked that "he was suffering from neurasthenia. Neurasthenia has the effect of depression."[44] In late 1912, one of two doctors who had been seeing Frederick Farquhar testified that he "suffered from sleeplessness and fits of depression. I came to the conclusion that he was suffering from neurasthenia."[45] Harold Morgan's doctor stated in 1918 that his patient was depressed and in an advanced stage of neurasthenia "bordering on melancholia with marked suicidal tendencies."[46] Depression's symptoms were richly, movingly, described by lay people. Relatives and friends emphasized an individual's insomnia; they reported how the deceased found small problems insuperable, appeared detached, and fretted about trifles. The duration of misery indicated something beyond unhappiness. In 1906, Elizabeth Mills mentioned at an inquest that "my husband had suffered from depression for a good while."[47] Popular sensitivity to mental illness was notable even in remote rural areas. Farmer Paul Carter's oldest son visited him in 1918 and thought he was in good physical health but "suffering from nervous or mental depression." "A suggestive therapist" from town had been treating him for neurasthenia and migraine.[48] If depression has been medicalized, then that process began early in the century and resulted from an interaction of doctors, patients, and family members.

Post-partum depression was a well-known and distinctive form of depression. Its symptoms were described in language comparable to that used about mental depression generally.[49] Marie Redman's doctor reported that "she was in a depressive condition and she felt too miserable to do anything."[50] If witnesses were reporting diligently and consistently on suicide and post-partum depression throughout the century (a bold assumption), then something notable was happening in New Zealand that should be observed and studied further. The incidents of suicide attributed to post-partum depression were rare, and most occurred before World War I. It is possible that the country's unique Plunket Society, established in 1907 and thriving by 1914, had a role. It was organized to support recent mothers and ensure that their babies had good care and a nutritious diet. Its supervisory activities may incidentally have reduced post-partum anxiety.

In whatever circumstances it originated, depression was regarded as distinct from insanity. In 1906, private hospital owner Evelyn Lucas offered the opinion that a patient who had suffered for eighteen months "with his head" was "a little depressed but not insane."[51] Lay people also made this distinction. Boarding-house keeper Gina Martin described a resident's mental state to a coroner in 1912: "I do not consider that he was insane but severely depressed."[52] In 1920, Elizabeth Watkins had been told by her doctor that her husband "suffered from nerves and was mentally depressed, particularly depressed." After her husband's suicide, she reported that "I have always kept a guard over him as the doctor informed me to do."[53] In this case and others, a doctor recognized danger but recoiled from committal.

Doctors preferred home care for depression. In the opinion of his doctor, veteran Palmer Hatley, described in 1940 as "shell-shocked and nervy," was "actually never insane at any time."[54] A morose unsmiling farmer was described as very depressed and diagnosed in 1942 with involutional melancholia. His doctor felt "he was not certifiably insane, but would have become so, had he lived, within the next year."[55] In his 1918 suicide note, David Webber intimated that his depression could lead to insanity. "I am terribly depressed. I sleep worse each night. I fear that madness is not far off and I decline to inflict an imbecile husband and father on my wife and child."[56] Patients could be depressed but in touch with reality, asserting sanity, taking responsibility for actions, and writing lucid final letters. "No doctor in my position," said a family practitioner about his patient in 1906, "could conscientiously commit him to an Asylum, though he was near the border line."[57]

For decades before the introduction of anti-depressants, instances of mental depression were handled as more than a deeply emotional state yet less than insanity. Roughly one in ten suicides (9.5 per cent) from 1900 to 1950 had been treated by a doctor for what contemporary witnesses called melancholia, nerves, or far more often depression (Table 5.1). If they wanted to underscore that the individual's state was exceedingly miserable, they did not escalate to a designation of insanity, but applied expressions such as "great depression," "extreme depression," "depressive condition," "nervous depression," "mental depression," and "severe mental depression."[58] Doctors and lay witnesses described individuals being uninterested in things going on around them, being too miserable to do anything, staying in bed, avoiding people, crying fitfully, and having extraordinary trouble sleeping for days on end. A patient described in 1906 as suffering from "mental depression" told his doctor that "he didn't feel ill, but he seemed to have some mental worry." He could not face work.[59] Similar immobility was mentioned by witnesses throughout the century.

Early-twentieth-century doctors and nurses believed that unhappiness or sadness could be shaken off, but observed that depression was tenacious. Patients expressed this idea too. Jessie Thomas told her doctor in 1904 that "she could not shake off her depression" and that was why she could not eat or take an interest in things.[60] Treated as a neurasthenic, George Brock told his wife that "he suffered every minute of his life."[61] Repeated visits from his doctor in 1912 could not help Andrew Thompson, who told his son "he would like to die on account of his depression."[62] An afflicted shopkeeper could not open his store; a teacher could not enter a classroom. Sufferers found it difficult to eat or socialize.[63] "Oh God," wrote Arthur Graham in 1920, "my brain is a whirl. No sleep for ten nights. It is awful. My nerves are shattered and done. Feel I am going mad."[64] Going mad, but not mad! That distinction was always important.

AN ERA OF KINDNESS THERAPY

To treat suffering, doctors conversed with patients; they prescribed separately or in combinations sleeping draughts, holidays or even more work, a change of air, fresh air, and cold baths. A prominent businessman "suffering from neurasthenia" was advised in 1918 to "change his occupation and go to the country."[65] A woman in 1940 was described as "in a depressed state, but actually mentally deranged." Her family physician and her husband advised that she should go for a holiday.[66] A rest for the more affluent at a spa or the seaside remained a leading treatment for depression until the favourable publicity for electro-convulsive shock as a cure swept all before it in the late 1940s.[67] The patient-centred approach, appearing in the files for the first thirty or more years of the century, likely reflected the influence of Adolf Meyer, a contemporary of Freud who had more impact on individual lives. Meyer recommended collecting diverse biographical information about a patient and then recommending a suitable mode of occupational therapy to restore the individual to a balanced life (Figure 5.4).[68] His individualized system of analysis and treatment meshed with the established family practitioner arrangement.

Throughout the first half of the century, family practitioners commonly recommended a suicide watch for individuals with depression.[69] Some doctors tried to reassure patients that they were not insane, while others warned them to pull themselves together or face committal. In a rare instance, a depressed patient was subjected to restraint at a hospital. Doctors committed James Power to a "mental hospital" in 1902 due to "acute melancholia and mental depression" so debilitating that he frequently had to be fed by force. In this case, the patient may have experienced a form of schizophrenia that presented similarities with depression, for schizophrenia flattened moods and reduced enjoyment.

The general therapeutic approach for depression is well summarized by a doctor who in 1920 advised "rest and care."[70] Beyond kindness prescriptions, doctors groped in the dark. In 1910, a doctor detailed this course of treatment for a man suffering "from marked depression of spirits": the patient was to walk every morning for two to three miles, have lunch, take a hot bath, have a cold douche along the spine, undergo a vigorous rub-down, walk five miles, rest for a half hour, have dinner, rest for a half hour, walk about two miles, take a hot bath, and retire to bed. The doctor also prescribed a purgative of calomel, quinine, and tonics.[71] There were also short-lived modern faddish cures. A neurasthenic patient entered a private hospital voluntarily in 1916 to receive a treatment by electric bulbs and massage.[72] For the first half of the century, the only chemical treatment was a sedative – typically chloral hydrate – to deal with insomnia.[73]

Doctors early in the century preferred that patients stayed in their homes. In a statement for a 1900 inquest into the suicide of a melancholic young farmer, the lad's doctor mentioned specifically that the symptoms did not require confinement.[74] Two doctors treated Agnes Crombie for melancholia in 1902, but "did not consider her a fit subject for the Asylum."[75] Robert Coxon was described by his wife as "very depressed. It was really a nervous breakdown." His doctor treated him in spring 1912 for melancholy "but he was not bad enough to certify him as a lunatic."[76] Often general practitioners cautioned family members to keep a close watch on the patient because they felt depression carried a risk of suicide.[77] Delicate calculations followed from this belief, because doctors feared that if a patient seemed suicidal then committal or close supervision by a nurse or family member could make that person feel greater helplessness, shame, and anxiety. To suggest a psychiatric hospital was almost certain to precipitate a crisis. "I feel depressed," wrote Ada Glaspell in 1920, "and feel I would rather face death than Seacliffe."[78] This challenge of managing a patient to minimize self-harm without deepening a mental crisis persisted throughout the century. When hospitalization was felt necessary, great effort was made to reassure the patient about the quality of care. Later in the century, former patients were even asked to mediate with testimonials.[79]

SHELL SHOCK AND MODEST NEW DIRECTIONS

World War I precipitated mental health problems that called for additional nuanced reactions. Public awareness of traumatized soldiers from World War I helped somewhat in legitimizing mental illness. The return of shell-shocked soldiers forced the government to intervene in mental health more than it would have liked. Public demand for treatment of war trauma promoted the training of specialists during and immediately after the war. Within the history of psychiatry, researchers have identified war neurosis as significant in the history of medico-psychological thought.[80] Whereas general practitioners had recognized and treated mental depression before the war, open discussion was modest. War trauma opened a more substantial exploration into neurotic or functional disorders and highlighted the need for psychotherapeutic out-patient, as well as in-patient, treatments.[81]

Soldiers' and veterans' associations in a number of countries lobbied to blunt the stigmatization of mental illness for men returning from the battlefield. The Federation of New Zealand Patriotic War Relief Societies lobbied in mid-1917 for special treatment for "light mental disorders or neurasthenia and shell shock," suggesting that these men "require more care and attention than they can expect to receive in a boarding house." "Is it right that these men should be discharged to roam aimlessly? Surely they are the care of the State."[82] The associations did not want men trundled off to "mental hospitals."[83] They would have preferred that shell-shocked men be "placed in homes where they could receive special attention, and their lives be made bright as possible."[84] An officer responsible for contacting next-of-kin complained in December 1917 that the terse designation "mental" that he put into telegraphs gave no sense of prospects for recovery. "Omitting deaths, these messages probably cause more distress to the next of kin than any other."[85] Families and friends did not seek a general reorganization of mental health services, just special treatment and thereby a validation of sanity for their boys.[86] Shell shock or neurasthenia labels satisfied community emotional needs even if, in particular cases, they fulfilled no medical purpose.[87] Shell shock posed diagnostic challenges similar to those of depression.

Wartime and post-war governments also heard from public health administrators and army medical officers. Junior and senior medical personnel clashed over explanations for neurological problems and the degree of the army's responsibility for the mental health of returned soldiers. During the war, the medical services collected more and more information about mental illness as the war progressed, and briefed the Minister of Defence. But the goal was to get men back in action.[88] In practice, there was a softer side to the diagnosis and treatment of war trauma. By at least August 1917, the medical service had in place a special neurological section at Number 1 New Zealand General Hospital, Brockenhurst. "The urgent demand for expert advice and special treatment for the wide group of functional disorders, eg. neurasthenia, shell shock, etc." was met here. Captain Marshall MacDonald, who had had experience with neurological cases in France early in the war and had returned to New Zealand, was sent to England to supervise the unit.[89] The inclusion of neurasthenia – classified as a non-somatic illness associated with depression – for treatment at Brockenhurst is important, because it implies that some army doctors had accepted emotional trauma as a legitimate source of mental incapacity. Moreover, a new space (figuratively and concretely) outside the home was about to be created for the treatment of depression.

At home, military and civilian authorities misled the public about how profoundly the conflict affected some soldiers' mental health. Press censorship was imposed on soldier suicides. The Director of Military Hospitals cautioned his superiors that it was unwise to commit soldiers to "mental hospitals," a step which required a hearing in open court. "The public would no doubt much resent any soldier with mental symptoms being committed to the ordinary Mental Hospitals if such could be avoided."[90] If returned soldiers were committed to mental hospitals, "a great howl will be raised."[91] The immediate remedy was to place mentally ill soldiers in a mental hospital under remand for observation without a formal committal in court.[92] Less violent cases could be placed in cottage annexes on the grounds of mental hospitals.

Larger psychiatric hospitals in New Zealand since 1900 kept pace with the latest innovations and provided annexes or cottages for light or improving cases. Mental health experts laboured to classify patients; improving ones progressed to these on-site facilities and then on to parole or experimental leaves. By 1914, New Zealand's psychiatric hospitals practised arranging patients in eight classes, each with special staff and facilities. The civilian mental health authorities quickly discovered that with respect to some soldiers, they had bitten off more than they could chew. The director of one hospital reported: "We have come to the crossroads as to the destiny of neuropath troopers who cannot be managed in outside quarters."[93] "Regarding the prospects of recovery," he wrote to the Director of Army Hospitals, "I am sorry to say that there is going to be a larger proportion of hopeless chronics than we hoped."[94] War experience reinforced the pre-established classification and separation of patients.

Significantly for the development of mental health and especially for the treatment of depression, the army decided to manage selected war trauma cases on its own. Partly for show, it transformed a mountain spa into a psychotherapy institute. By late 1916 the army was sending some functional mental illness cases to Queen Mary Hospital at Hanmer Springs (Figure 5.1) even as it sent other men, with more severe problems, without committal papers to existing "mental hospitals." Isolation played a role in the selection of Hanmer, because the army worried about disorderly conduct by returned men, and refused to place them in private convalescent homes where their presence could demoralize the war effort.[95] By 1918, the army streamed men into, through, within, and among institutions. The army by now called presumed light cases of shell shock or neurasthenia 'borderland cases.' Exceptionally light cases proceeded directly from hospital ships and demobilization camps to Hanmer. Patients at district psychiatric hospitals also went to Hanmer if they showed progress. For serious alcoholics, the army arranged for committals by family members or the men themselves to the Salvation Army's inebriates camp on Rotoroa Island at Auckland, a quasi-public facility that continued to provide "drying out" programs for the rest of the twentieth century.[96] New Zealand had a mental health network, a tiered system of public, charitable, and private institutions, and a managing bureaucracy.

After World War I, attitudes changed. New debates arose. Field control over the number of traumatized soldiers ceased, replaced by looser evaluation processes at home and a greater willingness to accept the legitimacy of neurasthenia as a service illness. The military dam controlling the flow of shell-shock and neurasthenia cases home was about to burst with mass demobilization. Senior army officers knew this, and realized too that it would be difficult to deny demobilized soldiers medical help for trauma if and when requested.

In planning for demobilization, the army prepared for a deluge of shell-shock cases and hoped to avoid committing many men to mental hospitals, because patriotic and returned soldiers' associations kept attacking the mixing of shell-shock cases with "the worst lunatics."[97]

There were going to be thousands of discharged men in uniform milling about the country for a while, and the army was under no illusions about the mental state of some. Senior officers sought to minimize government involvement in committals by convincing returned soldiers to go voluntarily to a hospital, or to have a relative initiate a committal.[98] From early 1916 until at least 1922, a number of traumatized returned soldiers stood before magistrates, facing committals. With or without court appearances, it is likely that mental illness of all classes led to the institutional confinement of 1,500 returned soldiers, or about 1.5 percent of the army.[99] How many traumatized men suffered without encountering a police magistrate for committal to a mental hospital or for conviction as drunk and disorderly? We can never know.

At a conference in Wellington on 18–21 March 1919, the army decided to concentrate shell-shock and neurasthenia rehabilitation efforts at Hanmer. Thanks to the medical service's demobilization anxieties, a modest revolution occurred in the treatment of mental illness. At war's start, the standard approach for helping treatable patients consisted of encouraging words, sunshine, music, walks, gardening, vocational instruction in carpentry and mat-making, and activities generally calculated to keep men busy. By late 1918, the medical service edged beyond these practices; it accepted the legitimacy of more recent ideas from European military psychiatry to the extent of sponsoring the training of personnel in neurology and psychotherapy in London and bringing them home to treat returned soldiers. The Minister of Defence was briefed in November 1918 on "the neuroses of war."[100] In February 1919 the army decided that two or more medical officers should stay in London for training in "psychotherapy for treating functional nerve cases."[101] The DGMS, Brigadier-General D.J. McGavin, minuted this cable: "I consider this is a [useful] suggestion and that two medical officers should be trained in psychotherapy on modern lines – a science which has developed much during the war."[102]

New practices made their way to New Zealand by way of army-sponsored initiatives, but at Hanmer the old gentle therapies were going strong in 1919 and much longer. Men there were exposed to "bracing climate, the quiet games and baths, and last, but not the least, work."[103] Hanmer remained a distinct treatment centre into the 1920s and beyond; it was soon made available to members of the public with light mental ailments. Beginning in January 1921, Hanmer started to accept "civilians suffering from neurasthenia, psychasthenia, etc." Civilian health authorities notified doctors throughout the country that they could now recommend patients for specialist treatment by applying though Medical Health Officers situated in cities and major towns.[104] Hanmer's superintendent thought that women were "the biggest field" for expansion.[105] Women were "pathologized."

Hanmer became a busy post-war centre for the treatment of depression in women and men, but if more severe symptoms or disorderly conduct surfaced, family members were notified "to come and take the patient home."[106] The hospital continued to specialize in allegedly moderate or functional mental illnesses for decades.[107] It simultaneously branched out into treating alcoholism and drug abuse. During and immediately after World War II it returned to its military rehabilitation role (Figure 5.2).[108] Subsequently, it once more treated light mental illness until 1965; in the mid-1950s, mental health officials advertised its spa-like facilities to combat public fear of psychiatric hospitals (Figure 5.3). From 1965 until its closure in 2003, it focused exclusively on alcoholism and drug abuse. In the even-numbered years from 1924 to 1998, thirty-eight individuals who had received treatment at Hanmer committed suicide; most had suffered from mental illness, although eleven had been in an alcohol or drug addiction program.

THE ERAS OF SHOCK AND PHARMACEUTICAL TREATMENTS

Terms such as "depression" and "depressed," "mental depression" and "mentally depressed," were used regularly before World War I. Wartime developments affected public consciousness and psychiatry was no longer confined to the country's mental hospitals. Freudian psychiatry even made a tiny appearance in the extraordinary case of Edna Gillespie, who went to the former shell-shock treatment centre at Hanmer for nerves. The twenty-four-year-old had had formal training for self-analysis. "Her mind had been disturbed," claimed her disapproving doctor, "by analyzing herself by the methods of psychoanalysis for which she had been taught some years previously." His remedy was a sleeping draught.[109] Gillespie is the exception that demonstrates that Freudian psychoanalysis had little influence on mental health in New Zealand. Her doctor projected the commonplace quest for physical or chemical intervention, although his was an old remedy. When new therapies appeared in the late 1930s, they were not Freudian.

In the 1920s and 1930s, doctors continued to describe their patients as having suffered from depression, but they increasingly added modifiers. To deal with his "mental depression," John Hardy had gone to Hanmer mental hospital for four months in 1927.[110] The expression "mental depression" was an attempt at clarity that owed something to the war's legitimization of the idea that not all mental illnesses displayed disabling symptoms. In the 1920s, a few coroners attempted to distinguish between temporary states of sadness-depression, mental depression, and even deep mental depression. A New Plymouth coroner in 1928 found that a returned soldier with a medical history of shell shock had taken his life "while in a mentally depressed state."[111] In the same year, a Christchurch coroner found that a civic employee had committed suicide "while in a state of mental depression."[112]

Mental depression had entered official discourse. An expansion of diagnostic terms and the existence of the special hospital at Hanmer allowed patients to continue to shake off the label "insane." General practitioners and specialists preferred words that seemed to refine diagnosis and avoided mentioning insanity, at least when the patient was alive. In 1930, labourer Hamish McDonald was admitted to Hanmer "suffering from Anxiety Neurosis and borderline Psychosis." After his suicide, a Hanmer specialist read McDonald's letters and revised his assessment: "He was insane."[113] As they had before the war, witnesses in the 1920s and 1930s connected depression to stressors such as ill health, finances, marital strife, menopause, and grieving over a death. The nebulousness of labels such as "depression" and "depressed" was not cleared up with the routine appearance of the modestly more descriptive term "mental depression." Coroners by 1930 may have too freely invoked it, because it provided a compassionate finding that comforted a grieving family. Mental depression did not have the hard edge of a finding of insanity, but sustained the important notion that the deceased had not acted freely.

According to Warwick Brunton, who studied the practices at New Zealand's psychiatric hospitals before World War II, the country emphasized institutional care, but this included unlocked wards and parole.[114] However, treatment was not static. During the 1930s and 1940s, treatment of depression began to include aggressive therapies. Insulin coma therapy arrived first, although it was used almost exclusively for schizophrenia. Developed in Austria in 1935, a typical six-to-eight-week course of treatment consisted of daily comas induced by insulin injections. The Department of Health's psychiatric hospital at Seacliff introduced the therapy to New Zealand in June 1938. Wartime nursing shortages interrupted its application, but Seacliff resumed it in 1948. By that year, electro-convulsive treatment (ECT), which came to New Zealand first in 1943, was commonly used to treat depression.[115] Seacliff became the country's main centre for ECT, but later it was practiced in other psychiatric hospitals (Figure 5.7).[116]

The suicide case files show a post-war surge in ECT at private facilities. From the late 1940s to the end of the century, general practitioners up and down the country could refer patients with depression to the isolated government facility at Seacliff or to inconspicuous private clinics and small private hospitals in larger cities. Most small private facilities cared for elderly dementia patients; a rare one handled ECT.[117] Psychiatrists at Auckland's Bexley Clinic assessed referrals and recommended that individuals with acute cases of depression attend the Selwyn Hospital. If the number of suicides by patients is any indication, the doctors and nurses engaged at these places were exceedingly busy treating depression. In the even years from 1960 to the end of the century, thirty-one patients who had been examined by doctors at the Bexley Clinic died by their own hands. Fifty-four patients who had been treated at the Selwyn Hospital committed suicide in the sample years extending from 1945, when the Selwyn commenced ECT treatments, to 2000. Suicides of patients and former patients peaked in the late 1960s and early 1970s, decades which marked the high point of ECT treatment. Registered as a private post-operative hospital, the Selwyn was described by government inspectors as "really a psychiatric hospital" for patients who could pay.[118] Despite the hospital's concentration on acute psychiatric cases, management as late as 1960 wanted it considered "surgical" because this designation avoided the stigma of mental illness.[119]

Aggressive therapies were controversial. Like many countries, New Zealand by the early 1970s had an anti-psychiatry organization, the Campaign against Psychiatric Atrocities, which targeted ECT for its ostensible brutality and claimed memory loss.[120] Applications of ECT may have declined, but they continued for the rest of the century.[121] Patients were not uniformly critical, although most inquest files involved patients who were at least fearful of it, which may have inhibited effective treatment.[122] The Selwyn Hospital's interest in disguising its true nature made sense in relation to prevailing attitudes. The husband of a patient remarked that shock treatment for her nervous breakdown in 1957 had "seemed to cure her of her mental problems, but she did not like it and was always worried that if she had any further problems, she would again be given shock treatments."[123]

After mid-century, mental health specialists introduced the term "depressive psychosis," which joined "mental depression" as yet another way to designate a suspected ailment as opposed to unhappiness.[124] "Neurotic depression" appeared too, but rarely.[125] Beginning in the 1950s, evidence on the mental state of the deceased increasingly came from mental health specialists and less and less from general practitioners.[126] With the rise of specialists, more elaborate labels came into use. A medical officer at Seacliff Hospital described William Herd in 1954 as "suffering from depressive psychosis. He had lost confidence in himself, was listless, apathetic, and sleeping poorly."[127] Technical expressions contributed to a growing effort by professionals to separate themselves from concerned family members; however, the symptoms described by general practitioners, psychiatrists, lay witnesses, and the patients themselves resembled those from prior decades (Table 5.2). Early inquests provided lists of symptoms consistent with later reports like the following ones. A young mother in 1964 "worried about everything in general" and felt low self-esteem.[128] Roberta Black "would worry about little things, she would get very quiet and just start looking into space."[129] In 1976, Julia McDougall felt she could not go on, because "no matter what I do or say my mind won't let me accept my faith in myself. It is just too big for me."[130] Another patient in the same year was described as unable to sleep, tired, gloomy, and excessively reserved.[131] In 2000, a young woman had "low mood, decreased energy, poor sleep, poor appetite, poor concentration and motivation."[132] It was all familiar, authentic, and hazy.

During the first half of the century, general practitioners routinely treated depression with reassuring words and a sedative, primarily chloral hydrate. Chemical intervention changed radically after World War II; thereafter the introductions of new medication were relatively frequent. In 1948, barbiturates appeared in the records. By 1960, psychiatrists were prescribing anti-depressant drugs such as Chlorpromazine, Amitriptyline, and Librium. The first of the tricyclic anti-depressants was introduced in 1959.[133] Since some drugs required 10–14 days to take effect, it was pointed out to a patient that "she would need all her courage as she was very severely depressed indeed."[134] Doctors were now seeking cures, not mere short-term relief.

The unrealistic optimism attending ECT or pharmaceuticals in the 1960s was exposed when patients with depressive psychosis did not respond.[135] A doctor at Porirua Psychiatric Hospital commented about a patient that "despite all forms of treatment his mental state failed to make any significant improvement."[136] The mental state seemed to let the drug down. If heavy drinking accompanied ECT or "high doses of anti-depressants," doctors explained that patients could not shake their melancholy.[137] One of the most widely used tranquilizers, Valium, was praised in 1980 for "unmasking depressions."[138] However, in that same year psychiatrists and family doctors recognized that patients could became drug-dependent.[139] Specialists and general practitioners in the pharmaceutical age succumbed to pulses of hopeful enthusiasm and disappointment. Failure, harm, and limits to knowledge were not willingly shared with the public. Inquests and associated media attention provided a modicum of exposure.

In the 1980s and 1990s, the volume of evidence on mental illness at inquests soared. Witnesses described more than a third of the people who committed suicide (34.2 percent) as depressed. Witnesses at almost one in five suicide inquests (19.8 percent) cited depression as the paramount motive for the act, but that was roughly the percentage for the whole century (Table 5.2). Witnesses spoke more about an individual's demeanour; however, the presence of depression as a general motive for suicide was fairly consistent throughout the century. There was further continuity. As in prior periods, various stresses were mentioned as contributing to depression. Individuals were deeply affected by a failed relationship, unemployment, pressure at work, an impossible workload, poor health, a serious auto accident, the death of a loved one, or a miscarriage. By the 1960s, exam pressure joined the list.[140] Psychiatrists now remarked on "psycho-social stressors" and the interaction of social and psychiatric difficulties.

There was a new medical trend. The entanglement of mental illness with other troubles was now represented as more complex, because it was alleged by mental health professionals that mental illnesses could precipitate a sequence of economic and social troubles, not just the other way around. Denis Herd had his first psychiatric crisis in 1968. According to a consulting psychiatrist, spending money made Denis feel better. By the early 1980s he had encountered financial difficulties, and faced fraud and "drink driving" charges; his mother died; his wife left him, and he moved into boarding-houses. He was then diagnosed with "a major depressive disorder" and considered bi-polar as well.[141] Cases such as this raised the prospect that mental illnesses might lead to material difficulties as well as the other way around. Psychiatrists had long accepted that stress had a hand in precipitating depression, but in the late twentieth century they and psychologists were alert to instances that inverted this causal sequence. This switch elevated their professional significance or, to be less suspicious, it made use of their training. As we will show in chapter six, this inversion of causality was prominent in mental health circles when the youth suicide panic erupted in the late 1980s.

Presenting the circumstances as either mental illness causing material hardship or vice versa seems profoundly unhelpful. Individuals had their own histories in which the combinations of stresses and predispositions were unique. One line of insight does not preclude the other, although a fusion leaves proportions up in the air, and especially so because our case-based understanding of suicide accents individuality and changes over time. Fortunately, too, a doctrinaire inversion of causality was not the sole professional position. During the economically stressful late 1980s, the national organization representing psychotherapists and counsellors warned the government of "the rising number of clients our members are seeing whose difficulties are related more to the stress of economic and social change than underlying personality problems."[142] Concurrently, the Mental Health Foundation of New Zealand regarded the stress and frustration of unemployment as mental health issues.[143]

In late-twentieth-century New Zealand, many witnesses emphasized that a depressed individual was more than unhappy or sad.

They read the face, noticed the perpetual down-turned look of misery, or interpreted conduct to conclude that the deceased was "deeply depressed," "depressed for many years," "depressed and withdrawn," "depressed and feared he could not cope," "had low self-esteem and was depressed," was "depressed because she could not handle life's problems," was "anxious and depressed," had "periods of severe depression" or "increasingly severe depression," was "depressed and hysterical," or showed "depressed and abnormal behaviour." As in prior decades, an occasional suicide note presented a devastating self-assessment. Marie Scott was in a private psychiatric hospital in 1990 being treated for depression when she wrote to her family: "you are all so wonderful and I am not anymore."[144] In his mid-thirties when he died, Stephen Ashely had written, "my depression has destroyed my life and I can't fight it any longer and I know that I always will be [depressed]."[145]

Police officers and coroners in the late twentieth century requested and received more information than in earlier years. Details surfaced regularly about the duration of anguish. The length of suffering suggested a condition more grave than transient unhappiness. "For many years, the deceased had bouts of depression"; the deceased had a "longstanding chronical depressive illness"; the deceased had "suffered from depression for five or six years"; "Lydia has had a history of mental depression over the last eight years"; a son "suffered from depression for fifteen years."[146] A husband noted in 1980 that his wife had suffered depression for thirty years; a wife stated in 1989 that her husband had been depressed for twenty-eight years and "treated almost permanently for the last twenty years."[147]

The vocabulary associated with depression widened by the mid-twentieth century to include exogenous depression precipitated by an external crisis, endogenous depression or depression that originated without a stressor but had a genetic basis, and dysthymic or mild depression. First proposed in 1934 by Aubrey Lewis at London's Maudsley Hospital, the concept of endogenous depression appears rarely in files until the early 1980s.[148] By the late 1960s, American psychiatrists had started to question "the endogenous-reactive split." [149] Some New Zealand doctors, accepting these terms late, retained the distinction. Through to the end of the century New Zealand psychiatrists also continued to mention dysthymic disorder. Treated in 1981 for alcohol abuse at a cottage facility on the grounds of a psychiatric hospital, Richard Warren was diagnosed with a personality disorder and dysthymia. A hospital psychiatrist wrote that "his episodes were usually in response to social circumstances and generally felt not to be associated with a major psychiatric disorder."[150]

Depression continued to be situated as an illness but not madness, not insanity. There were gradations; background events were considered important enough to be recorded at length in patients' files. Doctors in clinical dealings were slow to pick up and then slow to discard intellectual trends from the two major sources of ideas from the English-speaking world, the United Kingdom and the United States. Whether this uneven adoption of trends was generational we cannot tell, but confusion as well as compassion are apparent in medical reports.

At century's end, depression was represented as a group of illnesses: endogenous depression described a suspected genetically based depression; reactive depression could be trauma-induced or adversity-based. Doctors helpfully identified adversity in many instances. Bert McBeath, who committed suicide in 1986, "was suffering from reactive depression and stress mainly connected with the death of his wife."[151] A psychiatrist reported that Douglas Heathcote "suffered a major depressive episode in the context of bankruptcy which he had experienced with a huge and bitter sense of disappointment."[152] James McLeod "had a history of depression due to relationship problems."[153] Elderly Nora Prescott "suffered severe depression secondary to her on-going medical illnesses [at least five]."[154] Genetic predisposition could only be assumed on the basis of family history, as it was with Keith Moffatt. His mother's depression suggested "genetic loading," although a psychiatrist observed "significant vocational stress [business troubles]."[155] In 2000, a director of regional mental health services questioned his profession's tendency to connect suicide and depression. After reviewing of a suicide case, he discounted a major depressive episode but pointed to "life experiences and personality."

> The threat of suicide is often not related to a biological illness but rather to one's life experiences and attitudes, something that I have difficulty getting used to ... I don't know why this is but I do think that particularly among young males, our society in New Zealand has forgotten the "shame" of suicide and its effects on families in general. It is considered an "option" here.[156]

The fact of the matter was that talk of depression was in the air. Witnesses' references to depression, for example, increased after the introduction of anti-depressants, and the shroud of professional jargon was commonplace and increased clinical space. When there was no firm evidence of depression, there could be dysthymia, which a doctor at an inquest in 2000 described "as a sub-clinical version of depression. In lay terms it could be seen as a precursor."[157] Another patient in the same year "never showed a major depression but often indicated symptoms that were consistent with anhedonia (lack of enjoyment in his life)."[158] Improving patients were "euthymic" (in good spirits).[159] If patients had side effects from switching medications, they expressed "a discontinuation syndrome." While psychiatrists coined new terms that occluded everyday comprehension, there was growing public recourse to the word "depression" (Table 5.2). Yet, despite discussion of depression in the culture at large, inquests fail to show an enormous leap in rate of treatment of depression. Fewer than one in ten suicides in the 1980s and 1990s (8.5 percent) had been treated at some time for depression, a figure similar to that between 1900 and 1950 (Table 5.1). Witnesses were more inclined to assign a motive of depression for suicides among women than men, but many men appeared depressed and sought medical attention (Table 5.3).

There was greater open talk about depression at century's end, but not necessarily an upsurge in medical involvement, because in our review of case files it was apparent that depression had been treated often in earlier decades, although in those times medical intervention was free from specialized language and involved family members. The coining of new terms captured psychiatry's emphasis on treatment to the neglect of care. With respect to this change, mental health professionals executed an even more spectacular move than a linguistic turn. Over the century, treatment altered astonishingly. The solitary general practitioners of old, equipped with compassion and chloral hydrate, had been replaced by teams of psychiatrists who tried one drug after another, adjusting dosages along the way. In the late 1990s, for example, a young teenage girl with a "major depressive disorder" was prescribed successively Prozac, Aropax, Thioridazine, and Risperidone.[160] The very concept of "teenage depression" was novel.[161] By the late 1990s, pharmaceutical developments and new trademark designations appeared with such rapidity that our

Table 5.3
Attributes of depression taken from inquests, 1900–2000

Years	*Labels*	*Symptoms*	*Remarks and associations*	*Common treatments*	*Stressors*
1900–20	Depressed, depressed in spirits, very depressed, deeply depressed, nervous depression	No attraction to former interests, prolonged sadness, insomnia, unaccountable feelings of loss	Mentioned with nerves, neurasthenia, nervous breakdown	Rest, work, fresh air, vacation, sedative	Romantic upset, death of someone close, loss of work, alcohol abuse, prolonged illness
1920–50	Mentally depressed	Similar	Mentioned in connection with shell shock	Same as above plus insulin shock, electro-convulsive shock	Same as above plus shell shock or war trauma from WWI and WWII
1980–2000	Depressive psychosis, endogenous depression, reactive depression	Similar		Electro-convulsive shock treatment into the 1990s; anti-depressants	Romantic upset, death of someone close, loss of work, substance abuse, prolonged illness, long-term welfare support

Table 5.4
Gender distribution of depression cases, 1900–98

Attributes of depression	*Men 1900–50*	*Women 1900–50*	*Men 1980–98*	*Women 1980–98*
Appeared depressed	70.1% (*n* = 723)	29.9% (*n* = 309)	70.9% (*n* = 1,104)	29.1% (*n* = 453)
Depression as motive for suicide	58.2% (*n* = 278)	41.8% (*n* = 199)	61.1% (*n* = 552)	38.9% (*n* = 351)
Treated for depression	65.1% (*n* = 261)	35.1% (*n* = 140)	64.7% (*n* = 315)	35.3% (*n* = 171)
Total suicide cases	79.1% (*n* = 3,337)	20.8% (*n* = 883)	78.6% (*n* = 3,508)	19.1% (*n* = 1,039)

list of medications taken in fatal overdoses became outdated from one study year to the next.

IDENTIFYING AND EXPLAINING SCHIZOPHRENIA

As an illness, depression was difficult to isolate, but another leading mental illness associated with suicides had more vivid symptoms. In the throes of an extreme episode of schizophrenia, individuals could experience hallucinations. Voices rather than visions predominated. Voices alone were not the cause for concern; the upsets for the individual and those in close association occurred when the voices gave instructions or criticized. If schizophrenia was fairly easy to identify, its causes were unclear. However, in a few well-documented instances, they appeared to stem from brain damage attending substance abuse. Alcohol seems implicated.

Around World War I, there was an abrupt decline in reports of alcohol-induced hallucinations, because heavy drinking of distilled spirits fell off during the war, never to recover fully. Before the war, the case files offered abundant descriptions of erratic conduct, usually explained by witnesses as the result of outrageous alcohol abuse. Hallucinations described in those years were numerous; some were perhaps labelled alcohol-related when they could have been designated schizophrenia, and vice versa. One instance from among many can illustrate the problem of establishing a causal sequence based on evidence from the early twentieth century. In 1924, labourer Patrick Duff – “a hard working man who gets on periodic drinking bouts” – had a persistent delusion that detectives were after him.[162] Many decades later, there were an astonishing number of cases where hallucinations arose from "drug and alcohol induced psychosis." To provide but one of many illustrative cases, in 2000, a twenty-five-year-old Māori suffering from "drug induced psychosis" responded to "hearing voices, at times nice ones and at times negative voices."[163]

In the late twentieth century, multiple examinations by specialists rather than general practitioners led to wider use of the term "schizophrenia," although medical records reveal doctors puzzling over the concurrent or interacting syndromes of alcoholism, drug abuse, and schizophrenia.[164] The records overflow with details that show professional assessments that located the source of mental disturbance in life events, with occasional references to a family history of mental illness that might indicate genetic predisposition.[165] What stands out is the frequency of details about stressful life circumstances.

In one doctor's estimation, made in 1970, Felicity Trenton "resembles the picture of a chronically institutionalized schizophrenic, despite her lack of hospitalization." It was concluded that she had "chronic brain syndrome from years of heavy alcohol intake."[166] Clinical records from 1972 described Martha Maxwell as an alcoholic schizophrenic.[167] Time and again a medical report remarked that schizophrenia was present in conjunction with "alcoholism and combined drug dependence"[168] or that schizophrenia had been "complicated by alcohol and drug abuse."[169] Quests to locate a precipitating cause, while occasionally acknowledging a possible hereditary predisposition, repeatedly mentioned drug and alcohol abuse. It was not unusual to see a statement that "drug and alcohol abuse predated the development of psychotic illness."[170]

By the 1980s, cannabis was often blamed for schizophrenia, and in chapter seven we show how it contributed to youth suicide. Other experiences surfaced as risk factors for schizophrenia; these included violent alcoholic fathers and war trauma. The deceased, concluded one medical report, "is one of the long term tragedies of war." He had suffered from "battle fatigue which had developed into chronic schizophrenia."[171] However, it is substance abuse that stands out in case after case, as it does on so many other fronts. Loss of employment, squandered money, petty crimes, shattered domestic relations, deteriorating health, road accidents, foetal alcohol syndrome, and mental illness made substance abuse the century's most stealthily destructive force in peacetime affluent societies.[172]

A calculation of alcohol-related harm found that in the late 1980s two-thirds of domestic disputes, driving accidents, and drownings in New Zealand were alcohol-related.[173] Delirium tremens of earlier times and some schizophrenia cases of the later decades were likely associated with neural harm due to excessive drinking.

Delusions were pronounced among individuals with schizophrenia. As befitted a century of technical innovation and later space travel, individuals described intrusions in terms of science. The voices of God, the Queen of Heaven, angels, and Satan were still heard as they had been for centuries.[174] However, in earlier centuries no one felt controlled, as they did early in the twentieth century, by giant batteries or electrical fields, or as they did later in the century by household plumbing, radios, cameras, televisions, or aliens.[175] Fearing that a company did the bidding of a representative of Martians bent on world domination, a young man in 1979 set fire to the company's building.[176] Drug and alcohol abuse complicated the case of an individual who believed "people from outer space were after him," but he was likely suffering from schizophrenia.[177] Patients were at risk of self-harm, because some heard voices that undermined self-esteem, expressed "nasty thoughts," and sometimes ordered that they kill themselves.[178] On occasion, a patient believed that the voices had to be killed.[179] Alcohol and drug abuse made diagnosis and treatment difficult.

Voices dictating harmful commands contributed to the shocking fact that patients with schizophrenia were over-represented among people who committed suicide by jumping from high places. From 1980 to 1998, roughly one in eight individuals with schizophrenia (13.0 percent; n = 33) jumped from buildings, bridges, and cliffs; only one in forty (2.5 percent; n = 105) other suicides were committed this way. A clinical psychologist reported in 1997 that Lee Mah had made many plans for suicide; all involved jumping from heights or in front of a vehicle. For most of the century, the beliefs that individuals with schizophrenia were more inclined to harm other persons or to damage property kept sufferers in cycles of committal, trial release, committal, trial release, and so on. Release from psychiatric hospitals had long been allowed, because there were periods of remission. Concurrently, there were characterizations of patients – characterizations of a combined medical and cultural formulation – that sustained hospitalization as a legitimate measure. At least as late as the 1960s, doctors described individuals with schizo-

Table 5.5
Anti-depressants and psychotropic drugs used in suicides

Name	*Year*	*Date of*	*Treats*	*Problems*
Acepromazine	1950	Development	Psychoses	Cardiac risk
Chlorpromazine	1950	Development	Psychoses	Akathisia, tardive dyskinesia
Perphenazine	1954	Released	Schizophrenia, bi-polar disorder	Akathisia, tardive dyskinesia
Thorazine (Chlorpromazine)	1954	Released	Psychoses	Akathisia, tardive dyskinesia
Clomipramine	1960–70	Released	Anxiety, depression	Dizziness, nightmares
Desipramine	1960–70	Released	Depression	Cardiac arrhythmia
Oxazepam	1960–70	Development	Anxiety	Dizziness, amnesia
Thioridazine	1962	Released in USA	Schizophrenia	Akathisia, tardive dyskinesia
Mianserin	1966	Development	Depression	Dizziness
Haloperidol	1967	Released in USA	Schizophrenia	Tardive dyskinesia
Amoxapine	1970–80	Released	Bi-polar disorder	Tardive dyskinesia
Prothiaden	1971	Patent	Depression	Drowsiness
Moclobemide	1977	Clinical Trials	Depression	Anxiety, blurred vision
Maprotiline	1980	Development	Depression	Dizziness, hypomania
Fluoxetine	1987–88	Development	Depression	Nausea, anxiety
Paroxetine	1992	Released	Depression	Nausea, anxiety
Dothiepin			Depression	Drowsiness
Nortriptyline			Depression	Suicide ideation

phrenia as “disabled persons”[180] or even “psychiatric cripples.”[181] Yet many decades before the medical profession’s embrace of deinstitutionalization in the late 1960s and early 1970s, psychiatric hospitals practiced trial releases, paroles, and day passes in recognition of the idea that sufferers were patients and not inmates, and that they experienced remissions and recurrences.

Hallucinations were prominent and memorable for witnesses, but psychiatrists generally grouped symptoms around the idea that an individual’s perceptions of the world were diverted from a conventional course.[182] It is helpful when considering the range of symptoms to keep in mind that schizophrenia was once called dementia praecox or premature dementia. That term kept cognitive disintegration in the foreground.[183] On occasion, however, a psychiatrist assigned the label when symptoms were described as “negative.” That is, they did not involve hallucinations. These individuals experienced flat and dulled responses, and a lack of interest in their former delights.[184] The symptoms led to compound diagnoses that linked schizophrenia with depression (Table 5.6). Thus doctors mentioned schizoaffective disorder with marked depression, schizophrenia with depressive episodes, schizophrenia with severe depressive episodes, and psychotic depression with schizophrenia. Psychiatrists proposed that schizophrenia had stages. "The major paranoid schizophrenia symptoms," wrote a psychiatrist in 1988, "have lifted and secondary ones of lassitude have developed."[185] Depression, he further suggested, was likely in long-term schizophrenia patients.[186] In 2000, a twenty-year sufferer was described by the doctor reviewing his file in terms that capture the essentials of hundreds of similar cases. His illness "was characterized by long periods of being fairly well interspersed with periods of unstable mood, intrusive thoughts, and lack of motivation."[187]

These complications remind us of individual manifestations and of a tension in psychiatry between check-list clinicians and those who extracted and assessed personal histories.[188] Personal histories, including medical events, disclose the multiple troubles of lived experience. It is difficult to imagine enduring James Gilbert's predicaments. He first presented symptoms of a psychiatric illness in 1957; he received electro-convulsive shock treatment in 1967; he entered hospital in 1968 and was diagnosed as manic-depressive; subsequently he was diagnosed with schizophrenia. He had to care for an invalid mother and a mentally ill son.[189]

DYING WITH RIGHTS PRESERVED

Significantly, the suicide inquest files in 1980s and 1990s contained a disproportionate number of schizophrenia cases compared to the 1930s and 1940s. Under-counting during earlier decades due to poorly described cases is a strong possibility, but a contributing explanation is the rushed de-institutionalization of the 1980s and the resulting gaps in psychiatric care.[190] The quantitative evidence is suggestive rather than conclusive; however, it is joined by the testimony of witnesses. Substance abuse with psychotic episodes is another possibility for a likely increase in suicides.

Waves of new pharmaceuticals during the late twentieth century brought hope to individuals with a complex illness, but medication introduced problems too. Side effects ranged from the annoying to the life-threatening; effective dosages and drug interactions were

Table 5.6
Deaths by suicide of individuals likely experiencing schizophrenia, 1900–98

Decade	*Est. n of schizophrenia cases*	*Est. n of schizophrenia suicides per 100,000 people*	*Remarks*
1900s	32	7.1	Designation based largely on symptoms which could be confused with delirium tremens
1910s	30	5.5	
1920s	35	5.5	Some cases possibly due to extreme instances of war trauma
1930s	15	2.0	No evident explanation for decline; possibly a high point for the committals for schizophrenia and close observation
1940s	17	2.0	Possible war service of some sufferers and institutionalization of many others
1980s	135	7.7	Closer attention to diagnosis; de-institutionalization; gaps in replacement system; retrenchment; drug and substance abuse with psychotic episodes
1990s	110	6.0	Mental health system works to reduce gaps in care left by de-institutionalization

imperfectly understood. Refinements to dosages, frank discussions about risks and benefits, studies on the relative merits of placebos and specific medications, and removals from treatment programs of some drugs, were measures that denoted greater caution. Initial enthusiasm and optimism faded with experience. Patients living outside hospitals went off medication for assorted reasons: side effects; periods of improvement; a conviction that problems were not medical; a feeling that the medication provided no help.

Leonard Carruther's life had gone badly. His daughter died in a motor accident and that precipitated a breakdown that hospitalized him for a month in 1969. Operations put him in hospital again in the 1970s. He stopped working and his wife resumed teaching. Around that time, he noted that the television sent him personal messages. To alleviate his insomnia, a doctor prescribed Mogadon and Valium; to manage his complex psychotic experiences, he was put on tricyclic anti-depressants together with the anti-psychotic drug Thioridazine.

He complained that the medication made him heady without relieving his psychotic experiences.[191] In another instance, an out-patient showed a friend his unused medication and complained that they "clouded his mind and he could not clear his mind."[192] Another patient stopped taking his medication as it made him feel "too jittery."[193] A manic-depressive clerk, a patient at psychiatric hospitals on about twenty occasions and undergoing treatment with Thyroxine, Haloperidol (Chlorpromazine), and Lithium Carbonate at an out-patient centre, experienced "involuntary tongue movement caused by long-term medication."[194] This side effect was widely observed for Chlorpromazine, an extremely heavily used drug from the early 1950s to the late 1960s.

The era of psychotropic drugs began in affluent countries in 1954 when Chlorpromazine (also known by the brand names of Thorazine in the United States and Largactil in England, Australia, and Canada) was licensed for use in the United States. Consumption soared around the world and the drug contributed to a universal decline in long-term hospital committals as well as promoting public acceptance of mental illnesses as 'diseases.'[195] Seacliff Mental Hospital received a small amount in 1954. It went next to other government psychiatric hospitals.[196] Word of wonderful results spread in a matter of months. Within a year of the Seacliff pilot study, S.W.P. Mirams, director of the country's Mental Health Division, Department of Health, reported that "these tablets are used extensively and with considerable benefit." The Department of Health established a national distribution system based at Seacliff. In 1957 private practitioners were allowed to prescribe it; in 1961 its cost to patients was covered by New Zealand Social Security.[197] Year after year, state purchases rose. To cut costs, supplies were purchased from companies in Canada and Italy that infringed on patent holders. New Zealand's consumption peaked during the twelve months ending 31 August 1967, when there had been 5,527,470 doses prescribed or 143.2 kilos.[198]

By now, side effects were known, and Mirams reflected on the hasty decade-long binge. "One might well argue," he wrote in a 1968 government memo, "that the use of psychotropic drugs would tend to be higher where there is a deficiency of psychiatric sophistication." He went on to say that "I know that it [Chlorpromazine] was used wastefully by doctors without psychiatric experience in many situations in the days when I did clinical work."[199] Despite its drawbacks and the fact that it had been superseded by later drugs, it was still widely used in the late 1960s and continued to be prescribed for the rest of the century.[200]

Patients' criticisms of medication clashed with doctors' self-assured enthusiasm. In 1980, a psychiatrist informed a coroner that a deceased patient who had been treated with the high-potency drug Pimozide "seemed better in terms of his schizophrenia, but to himself he probably didn't feel any better at all. He told me that anyway."[201] Patients who avoided medication were deemed "most uncooperative" or "insufficiently motivated."[202] From 1970 forward, when cost-cutting and a liberal-spirited retreat from committals allowed more patients greater freedom, the latter were expected to live under a regime of self-discipline, clinic appointments, and medication. It is possible to comprehend patients' defiance as an assertion of dignity and a rejection of chemical control, but occasionally non-cooperation truly proved disastrous. Patients relapsed into chronic schizophrenic states.[203] Psychiatrists implored patients to persist with the course of medication even if symptoms lifted. That was challenging.

Prescribing a psychotropic drug was not an exact science; cases were distinctive and New Zealand's mental health department encouraged its hospitals to experiment with new drugs once overseas clinical trials had been completed.[204] Medical professionals admitted that schizophrenia and other psychoses remained mysterious; doctors struggled to put their assessments into words. They could not always be certain about a diagnosis of schizophrenia, but they prescribed for it nonetheless, because the benefits of the latest psychotropic drugs seemed dazzling. In 1982 a young man with mood swings and fantasies was prescribed Navane and Cogentin. The attending psychiatrist "was suspicious that he saw early signs of schizophrenia."[205] Another young man in the same year was prescribed a course of ECT treatment after a psychiatric assessment described him as "a person with an underlying difficulty in the schizoid personality–schizophrenia areas as illustrated by impaired reality testing involving a fantasised relationship over a period of six years without an adequate basis in reality." In short, he had long been obsessed with a woman. A diagnosis of schizophrenia followed that jargon-riddled observation; subsequently, he was treated with Doxepin, Nitrazepam, Largactil, and Haloperidol. He declined ECT.[206] In another instance, the medical history of a middle-aged alcoholic mentioned a breakdown, paranoia, depression, anxiety attacks, and finally schizophrenia.[207] Trial-and-error diagnoses accompanied trial-and-error prescriptions and fiddling with dosages. Some patients, such as Robert Clark, contributed to experimentation; he "said he would like to try newer agents when his medications next needed to be changed. He also said he was well aware of the early signs of breakdown."[208]

About ten percent of suicides in New Zealand from 1980 to 1998 were committed by individuals under treatment for schizophrenia. We cannot say what the risk of suicide was for individuals with schizophrenia. There are too many variables; however, enormous complexity never stopped doctors from offering untenably precise risk assessments with overtones of unwarranted confidence. A medical officer at a regional hospital in 1980 stated that "suicidal tendencies are present in about 20% of all schizophrenics."[209] A dozen years later a psychiatrist informed a coroner that "suicide is a 10% risk in people with this disorder [schizophrenia]."[210] In 1988, another psychiatrist estimated that ten to fifteen percent of people with "major affective disorders ... do in fact commit suicide despite their therapist's best endeavours."[211]

These statements conceded that the healing arts could not always be effective. The statements demonstrated too that doctors lacked solid information when speaking publicly about mental illness and suicide. The base number of people with schizophrenia was a matter of guesswork, because of the slipperiness of diagnosis and the likelihood of undiagnosed cases. These unknowns were not taken into account. Estimates on risk left important questions unasked. Was the risk of suicide by people with schizophrenia a recent development? Should the percentages be understood in connection with a recent trend in de-institutionalization, or were they universal claims? Had de-institutionalization been bungled? A review of the literature on schizophrenia and suicide, published by the American Psychiatric Press in 1990, concluded that "suicidal behavior among schizophrenic patients occurs mainly among outpatients."[212] The authors did not explicitly suggest the possibility that de-institutionalization had a role. In their estimation, it was the aetiology of depression that required study.

Along with the desire to improve the lives of individuals, other considerations fuelled the introduction of anti-depressants and psychotropic drugs. Medication promised a way to treat patients outside psychiatric hospitals. For a century, confinement for psychoses had terrified the mentally ill. Had patients' fears and the attendant suicides of some of them been the only factors working against the hospitals, these institutions with their sprawling campuses and diversified facilities might have continued to flourish. During the 1950s across the affluent Western world, these hospitals had expanded as never before. Patients came and left; healing transpired; care accompanied treatment; abuses occurred; people entered never to leave. Practices and outcomes were mixed. The asylum had become the psychiatric hospital and its services had evolved substantially by the 1960s, just at the moment when critics began to warn of a ward culture of patients' dependence.[213]

In New Zealand, the novels and autobiography of Janet Frame contained emotive testimony about her terrifying ordeals with ECT and the stigma of being "sent down the line," meaning sent by train down the line to Seacliff. Internationally, *One Flew over the Cuckoo's Nest* made an assiduous but caricatured case against the hospitals and their treatments. An added push came from governments seeking to offload the costs of mental health, which were unrecoverable from many patients. Patients who could pay for psychotherapy or electro-convulsive shock treatment checked into private hospitals, where intervention included solicitous nurses. When radical treatments failed in private or public hospitals, they left profoundly disabled individuals "quite unable to live outside a hospital." The stigma and fear of psychiatric hospitals never abated. There were tragic instances that supported fear of a long unsuccessful courses of treatment.[214] One woman with bi-polar disorder spent almost twenty years in hospitals, beginning with a period in the 1950s in the private hospital Ashburn Hall where she had two leucotomy operations and 1,300 electro-convulsive shock treatments.[215]

Private hospitals and nursing homes had a presence in mental health care. They were well-patronized, but difficult patients were handed over to public institutions that generally employed male nurses.[216] There was an exception to this pattern. The leading private psychiatric hospital, Ashburn Hall in Dunedin, founded in 1889, attended to the full range of mental illnesses and had close relations with the University of Otago medical school and government institutions. Described by a coroner in 1999 as a hospital that "specialises in the treatment of highly intelligent people," it largely served middle-class patients who could pay for close attention, although it tried to accommodate all classes.[217] Public institutions were large, visible, a terror in popular lore, and they detained involuntary patients; consequently, they received the brunt of the anti-authoritarian criticism in the late 1960s and through the 1970s. There was principled support for patients' rights among mental health professionals and, judging from revisions to the Mental Health Act, sympathy from legislators. In 1969 a revised Mental Health Act shifted control of most psychiatric hospitals to local hospital boards effective in 1972.[218] In 2000, a new Act called for the least restrictive treatment environment possible, although that had long been a guiding philosophy among many psychiatrists.[219]

Community hospitals in the 1970s were ill-prepared for the influx of a new category of patients whom they were obliged to handle with light restrictions. Additionally, psychiatrists who were ashamed of their profession's previous enthusiasms and who now loathed detention erred on the side of 'freedom' if they did not see for themselves an indication of imminent harm. What if others such as family members had seen it? What did imminent mean? In 1978, a newly founded Schizophrenia Fellowship articulated a scathing assessment of a 'liberal' innovation. "It seems to be a matter of pride and satisfaction to the authorities that there are fewer people in mental hospitals but sadly, for some, hospital remains the only place where there is company and structured living. I wonder how much study has been put into what sort of conditions so many discharged 'cured' patients live under, especially where there is no family. Some find company at pubs with all the risks that involves."[220]

Supporting evidence for the criticism surfaced at inquests. Out of good intentions, doctors in 1980 sent a young man home from a psychiatric hospital, because they had been treating him for depression which they thought could be managed at home. According to his outraged father, "they thought that it would be better for him to get out of the hospital and on with his own life."[221] It was indicative of a new spirit in psychiatry that the doctors believed that he might become habituated to institutional life.

The medical profession had once been proud of the country's psychiatric hospitals and throughout the 1950s supported their expansion to alleviate overcrowding; in the 1970s some, but not all, psychiatrists found them debilitating and custodial care harmful.[222] Anti-authoritarianism swept the ranks of younger psychiatrists. The convergence of de-institutionalization, a retrenchment in expenditures, and pharmacological innovations proceeded in haste. Terrible consequences of the rush surfaced in suicide tragedies. Hasty discharges were sometimes failed gambles. They occurred at community hospitals which, as part of a new and allegedly kinder health care system, were to offer a local face to mental health care. Financial restraint created pressure for discharges. Staff looked for malingerers. A forty-year-old man who entered a local hospital as a voluntary patient – "very depressed and talking of suicide" – was discharged after a month and sent home with a three-month supply of Navane and Cogentin. Judged a chronic pot smoker and an excessive drinker, he was not the type wanted as a long-term patient.[223]

Some patients were held back. On account of "a long history of neurotic hypochondriasis but now presenting with endogenous depression," Cynthia Maynard was not discharged. "We were reluctant to discharge Cynthia directly to her own home because of her history of deterioration there and her need for support well beyond that which her daughter could reasonably be expected to provide."[224] Judgements such as this one ran against the grain during the era of de-institutionalization; the annual statistics on admissions and releases point to the use of hospitals as short-term care facilities in mental health cases. Medical personnel exercised considerable discretion and the determining factors were not always strictly medical.

As mental hospitals shut down or closed wings, the number of designated psychiatric wards at regional hospitals increased, as did out-patient clinics. Wards and clinics implemented group therapy, but psychiatry's newfound enthusiasm for freedom meant that patients were not required to attend.[225] Larger centres had licensed boarding-houses and halfway houses with varying levels of care.[226] Epsom Lodge in Auckland, for example, maintained an orderly and accepted many former residents of Carrington Psychiatric Hospital.[227] Files portray a system scrambling ceaselessly to adapt. As part of this effort during the 1990s, regional mental health services endeavoured to provide Māori health and social workers when individuals identified as Māori. In contrast to mainstream psychiatry, these specialists welcomed and promoted complete family involvement.[228]

From 1900 into the 1970s, the mental health archipelago consisted of spacious facilities on ample grounds; thereafter it lost a few grand establishments and acquired more small ones. More institutions reported to the department than before. There were eleven psychiatric units in general hospitals in 1974 and seventeen in 1988.

More individuals were counted in annual reports as admissions to hospitals and clinics because, with looser checkout provisions, there were greater numbers of multiple re-admissions as if through a revolving door.[229] While the mental health system in the 1980s and 1990s projected an air of comprehensive care with reduced coercion, it had flaws that frustrated coroners and that were repeatedly identified at suicide inquests.

Revised mental health acts made it difficult to commit individuals, but numerous patients experienced episodes that required assessment, and some were subsequently committed or subject to mandatory treatment orders. Psychiatrists worked to place as many patients as possible as soon as possible into communities, recurrently over objections from family and friends. By the 1980s, doctors worried about patients becoming dependent on an institution, but dependence on medication was a rising problem. In accord with the guiding new philosophy, professional networks developed to cater to mental health. Putting mental health into the community contributed to an awareness of services, and that helped establish an "advanced psychiatric society."[230] Family practitioners, psychiatrists, psychoanalysts, clinical psychologists, psychotherapists, marriage and family counsellors, psychiatric nurses, district nurses, occupational therapists, and community social service workers sought to assist people by building trust; new therapeutic tactics meant respecting the narratives, culture, privacy, and liberty of patients.[231] Mandated privacy plus the trust-building overtures of the mental health professionals narrowed the space for family involvement, most certainly so when patients rejected family participation or denied what family members said about their conduct.

In principle, building trust had merit.[232] When patients in psychiatric hospitals labelled nurses "screws" and "Gestapo," therapeutic relationships were impeded and a fresh system promised something better.[233] In practice, problems arose with trust-building through privacy when medical personnel marginalized family members. Inquests exposed bitter tensions between doctors on one side and, on the other, several interest groups and family members. Doctors asserted that they served the patient. If family members alerted a medical team to a patient's failure to take medication, to increased frequency of hallucinations, or to suicide threats, the medical professionals would ponder how, in their professional estimation, the patient had presented when last examined and on that basis claim superior knowledge of the patient. These assertions infuriated family members.[234]

Friends and family could not challenge professional judgement on the doctors' turf. Psychiatrists alleged that invoking mandatory treatment or heeding a family member might erode the patient's trust in the clinical team. The Schizophrenia Fellowship in 1979 took a contrary position: "It was felt that the law under the current Mental Health Act is designed to protect the patient to a point where it may no longer be protecting him at all."[235] In later years, branches of this association protested the closing of psychiatric hospitals, "the policy of 'everybody out.'"[236] Overall, mental health interest groups pointed out that the revolution in psychiatric care and treatment required more planning, better community-based services, and action to remedy "a very grim situation of accommodation for ex-psychiatric people."[237]

It was not only interested organizations that disparaged the poor execution of de-institutionalization. In the presence of a non-medical coroner, family members gained confidence. Loved ones closest to patients who took their own lives had a place to express their outrage, and medical professionals had an opportunity to learn how they had failed. The family of one young man thought that medical staff negligence bordered on the criminal. "We did as much as humanly possible to care for, love, and support him through his illness. I wonder," asked his sister, "can any of the health professionals say the same?"[238] Family members pleaded for medical personnel not to hide "under the well used cloak of 'the privacy act and client confidentiality'" and not to presume that they knew a patient better than family members.[239] These reactions erupted into a chorus of discontent during the 1990s and beyond.[240]

Coroners chimed in with suggestions that medical personnel pay attention to family members. "If there is a comprehensive review of problems in the Mental Health area I can only hope," stated one coroner in 2000, "that the position of the parent or caregiver is given adequate emphasis."[241] Regional health services employed lawyers to block the release of critical findings and to challenge allegations of neglect from close relatives.

A few patients severed ties with their family and medical team. Patients left incomplete medical dossiers strewn around the country. Medical reports trailed off with remarks such as the following: "we accepted him back as a day patient, but have no record that he attended at all";[242] "we had no further contact with the patient after that visit";[243] "after this she failed to keep her next appointment with me";[244] "she had not been attending follow-up appointments";[245] "he defaulted on his medications [major psychotropic drugs] and appointments and within a month or two was returned in a distressed state of mind";[246] "between episodes it was difficult to keep him engaged with psychiatric services";[247] Winston "moved out of our catchment area."[248] Letting patients determine their life-course led to sporadic care and greater opportunity for self-harm.[249] The medical profession was not united behind decentralization. A few specialists recognized patients' proclivity for avoiding appointments. A psychiatrist at a public hospital reported that Wilhelmina Grootman was "fit for release and intends to continue her vagrant way … The probability of an eventual successful suicide attempt is fairly high."[250]

In the past, doctors worried about unsettling depression patients with talk of institutionalization. In the 1980s, a comparable worry overtook psychiatrists working with individuals diagnosed with schizophrenia. Once committal ceased being the norm, recourse to compulsion reinforced a patient's pre-existing despair. Sensing this possibility and embracing a new ethos that distanced themselves from the old therapies of lobotomy and ECT, psychiatrists promoted freedom as the default measure. Insisting on the principle that a curtailment of liberty was an absolute last resort, medical personnel attempted to manage patients by means other than coercion and restraint. They wanted their liberal credentials and professional authority at the same time. An honest yet facetious compromise was reached by a doctor who stated, with respect to a psychotic patient who killed his wife, that "in retrospect we would have liked to have put him in cotton wool." The patient "didn't accept the need for counselling."[251]

Mimicking neo-liberal economic currents of the day, some medical staff encouraged patients in the 1980s to sign contracts to stop drinking, enter drug rehabilitation programs, or abandon ideas of suicide. Patients became clients who entered into contracts. Business language provoked debates among doctors, nurses, and administrators about the infiltration of commerce into the healing arts. The paternalism and patriarchy of old had been displaced by contractual relationships, and even more so by patient independence. Many patients in the 1980s and 1990s lived in residences with other patients, drew medical beneficiary payments, and partook of so-called recreational drugs or explored the mind-altering experiences of prescription medications. This novel way of life put patients in hazardous surroundings. As well, freedom of movement exposed gaps in the new mental health system.[252]

The well-being of patients who were not under supervision in an institution but suffered a psychotic episode depended on their getting treatment at a nearby hospital, sometimes after hours. On occasion, the patient's frustration at waiting for help led to a hasty departure from a hospital, a deepening psychotic episode, and ultimately self-harm. Staff inattention and absences were greatest after financial cutbacks that hit hospitals in the mid-1980s; coroners at the time worried about the well-being of unsupervised patients, under-staffing, and the failure of hospitals to furnish patient files to other hospitals.[253] In 1992, a psychiatric out-patient required urgent care only to be turned away from the community hospital because its psychiatric ward was full.[254] Shifting the burden of care quickly onto regional hospitals adversely affected some patients, but caregivers tried their utmost to help patients.

Psychologists backed up psychiatric services with counselling. Home-visiting psychiatric nurses provided supervision and medication, although supervision on a weekly or fortnightly basis hardly measured up to that in a hospital. Some patients, well-known as suicidal, received well-meaning but scanty attention.[255] Tragedies in psychiatric care continued into the twenty-first century; some suicides were the result of stretched resources and staff fatigue; some occurred due to an absolute insistence on patients' rights that discounted the words of family members and erred on the side of freedom at the expense of security against self-harm.[256]

By the mid-1990s, gaps and lapses in care had been repeatedly exposed at inquests. Consequently, hospitals required that individuals with psychotic symptoms were never to be left alone when they arrived. The challenge of scarce resources was met by implementing team approaches whereby one or more specialists conducted preliminary examinations at a hospital, made a diagnosis, and initiated a course of treatment pursued by whomever was available. Case notes might later be discussed by the hospital's psychiatric staff members. Following a suicide in 1988, the psychiatric staff at a regional hospital formed multi-disciplinary teams to review weekly all patients who failed to respond to therapy.[257] Psychiatric nurses at out-patient clinics administered prescribed injections, although this was often disrupted by a patient's moves.[258] District nurses could do the same in rural areas. A division of labour involving fewer doctors' hours but more duties for nurses and psychologists aimed at controlling costs; however, the legal requirement to observe patients' rights and simultaneously to protect them against themselves by unremitting vigilance drained staff stamina. The old psychiatric hospital system had been capital-intensive; the new patient-centred regime was labour-intensive in a disjointed way. In 2000, Murray Delany told a psychiatrist that along with frequent hospitalizations, the doctor was "the fourteenth or fifteenth psychiatrist he has seen" in thirty years.[259]

Pharmaceuticals in the new regime had two unfortunate features. In the first place, there were problems with the drugs *per se*. The side effects of some psychotropic drugs were dreadful, and understandably some patients abandoned medication. Chlorpromazine ceased being a leading culprit for side effects by the mid-1970s. There were problems, however, with its successors continuing to the end of the century and presumably beyond.[260] Shane Wanless told his father in 1996 that "he hated taking the drugs (Halopendol [sic] and Procyclidine)." "The Halopendol [sic] was knocking him around too much" and an experimental drug "did not seem to have any effect."[261] The powerful anti-psychotics Phenothiazine and Fluphenazine, given to people with schizophrenia who had poor compliance with medication and suffered frequent relapses, could cause facial grimaces or Parkinson's-like tremors, as Chlopromazine had done.[262] Brain damage was permanent. In the suicide inquests of the 1980s and 1990s, there are references to patients refusing to take medication as it clouded their minds.

The second unwelcome consequence was a proliferation of medication through the slackness of a few doctors and pharmacists, and fraudulent conduct by individuals who milked the health system.[263] A subculture of popping anti-depressants and psychotropic drugs fostered supply chains that originated with naïve doctors or with thefts from pharmacies.[264] Tripping out on medication joined conventional substance abuse, which, by the late 1990s, included using alcohol and heroin, smoking cannabis, sniffing solvents, and injecting methadone (Graph 1.8). Some medical professionals insisted that these abuses contributed to psychoses. Over the century, the agents for self-inflicted neural harm had expanded from alcohol and heroin to diverse substances, natural and synthetic.

CONCLUDING OBSERVATIONS

The mental health system of the early twentieth century shared attributes with other strands of modern state-building. In New Zealand, the government extended its departments into communities. An upsurge in state paternalism in the late 1800s and early 1900s had included schools, the national railway with housing estates, the telegraph and telephone systems, and hospitals and asylums. Among the latter were several immense establishments that assembled individuals with diverse illnesses and disabilities in places whose names became synonymous with lost hope. To citizens at large and even to many patients, the structures, grounds, and peripheral locales identified occupants as distinctive. In truth, by World War I the country's asylums were not monolithic but were instead composite places.[265] Patients were classified and assigned to diverse buildings and granted variable freedoms depending on their ailments and the presumed likelihood of their recovery. But named institutions seemingly homogenized individuals, as did the legal process for committal. Residents were deemed mad and the buildings made that madness real to friends, relatives, and the patients themselves. In the late twentieth century, a series of mutually reinforcing cultural and political changes overthrew mental hospitals and forced painful adjustments. A retrenching state sought to divest itself of several creations of its former pride. Mental hospitals were the first to be affected, in part because certain treatments were regarded as barbaric and because committal wounded dignity. The transformation left victims in its wake, because accidental gaps, liberal practices, and government retrenchment contributed to suicides.

An accent on patients' personal freedom created medical conundrums which were resolved to a degree by efforts to build self-discipline within individual patients by reminding them of appointments and getting them to sign contracts. The facility-based management of mental illness was replaced from the early 1970s into the new millennium by efforts at individualization assisted by medication. Evidence of the organization of self-disciplined individuals in the field of mental health did not stop with patients. The old order with its imposing hospitals behind fences protected doctors; the demise of the hospital estates exposed doctors, now situated in local hospitals, to critical scrutiny, especially when patients took their own lives in public places and when family members were in contact with these patients. The mental hospital had contained patients, managed family access, and shielded doctors. For self-protection, psychiatrists and other medical professionals during the liberal transformation disciplined themselves by holding debriefings after suicides, by participating in conferences and seminars, and by listening to advice from lawyers.[266]

In 1900 and for many decades afterward, outdoor recreation, work, and rest were thought to be restorative; body and brain were connected. By 2000, the idea of targeting a cerebral function with a chemical to alter mood or behaviour had been established for decades and it helped alter perceptions of the human condition in affluent countries. In the world of work, physical outdoor labour declined precipitously after 1950, and so too did therapy that valued outdoor activity as restorative. The mentally ill could subsequently resort to the chemical manipulation of mood and behaviour by legal means; additionally, young adults accessed therapeutic and recreational drugs illegally. In some instances, this experimentation with mood change precipitated psychotic episodes. In 1900, citizens' rights were few and protected if necessary by legal process; patients' rights once in an asylum were quite narrower. In 1900, family members and general practitioners were the parties who dealt first with individuals experiencing a mental illness. Family involvement at the end of the century remained spirited and positive in many instances, but families had less authority and influence. During much of the century, a doctor's authority was rarely questioned; however, by 1980, possibly earlier, irate family members aided by lawyers and alternative-medicine advocates turned up the heat and never relented.[267]

Both therapeutic and recreational drugs proliferated and at times interacted catastrophically in the last quarter of the century. Psychiatrists believed that recreational drugs compounded or even precipitated mental illnesses; the expression 'drug induced psychosis' appeared over and over again at inquests. "This man," reported a psychiatrist at Waikato Hospital in 1980, "has had a number of admissions to hospital with a severe psychotic illness which I consider was triggered off by illicit drug use."[268] The remark, with slight variations, was common.[269] A tattoo across the chest of an addict who committed suicide in 1996 spelled a coda for the end of the century: "Powered by Drugs."[270]

Finally, the de-institutionalization of mental health and the enabling pharmacological revolution revivified an Enlightenment-era ambition to restore people to mental health. In the last two decades of the century, the coroners' painstaking investigations into the suicides of men and women under treatment attempted to restore progress. Mistakes had been made, lives could have been saved, and corrections to medical practices should follow. Family members, most medical professionals, and coroners conducting inquests may have differed over what had led to a suicide, but they spoke in common terms about learning from a tragedy. At these intense moments when trust in medical care was fragile, medical professionals could have admitted their limitations as healers and reduced their responsibility. Or they could have defended medical science, which would have exposed personal liability as imperfect operators in a good system. In order to retain the trust of patients, doctors adapted a pair of arguments that enabled them to walk a fine line between these two damaging positions. First, they were not responsible when things went wrong, because the deceased patient had been wayward or was a member of a sub-population at high risk; second, the current system was basically fine but strapped for resources. Admissions about under-funding were awkward, however, for they risked undermining public trust.

Budget cutbacks accelerated de-institutionalization and curtailed district nursing operations.[271] During the ensuing years, efforts to bridge gaps in the mental health care system, the necessity of retaining legal counsel, and the funding of suicide prevention initiatives cut into the cost savings of reorganization. It is likely that the quality of life for many patients with mental illnesses had improved as a result of the great transformations at the end of the century, because the new mental health attitude shed the custodial or even the lingering penal attributes of the asylum. The word 'asylum,' as one student of New Zealand psychiatry remarked, evoked largely negative images, but "for some people it still meant 'refuge' and 'sanctuary'" (Figures 5.8 and 5.9).[272] That had been the case in 1998 for Tony Elliott, "who was upset that he had been released [from 'the Psych Unit'] and he didn't feel well enough."[273]

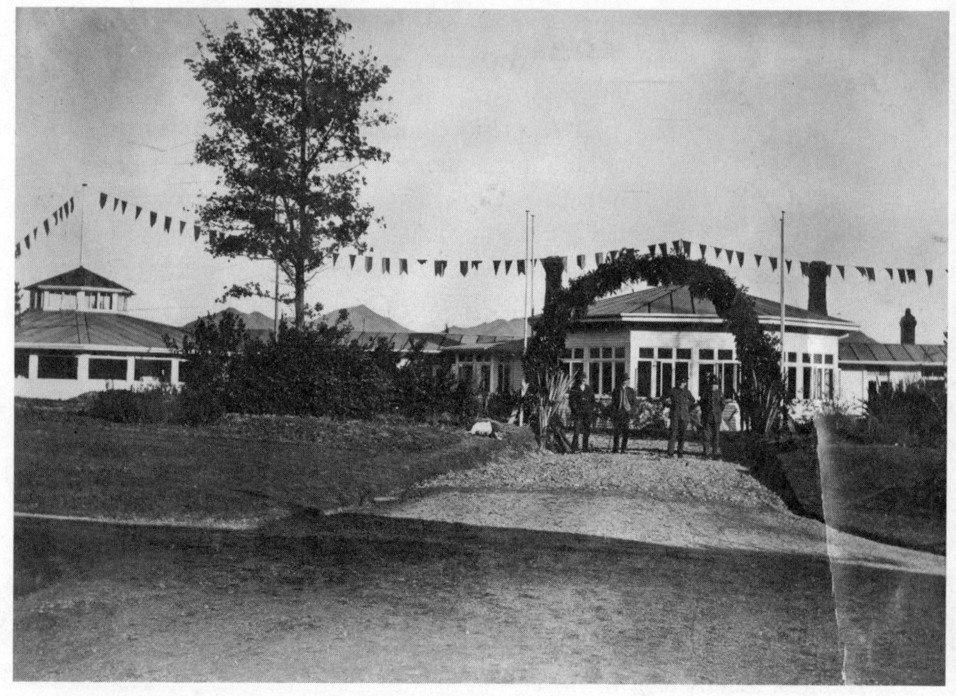

Figure 5.1
Opening day for the Queen Mary Hospital for convalescent soldiers with "shell shock," 3 July 1916. Between the two world wars and after World War II, the hospital treated light disorders. It was closed in 2003 and parts of the complex have been restored as a historic site. Courtesy of the Hurunui District Libraries. The web page for the library system maintains photographs on the hospital's history. See http://ketehurunui.peoplesnetworknz.info/en/queen_mary_hospital_hanmer_springs/all/images/. Accessed 18 February 2013.

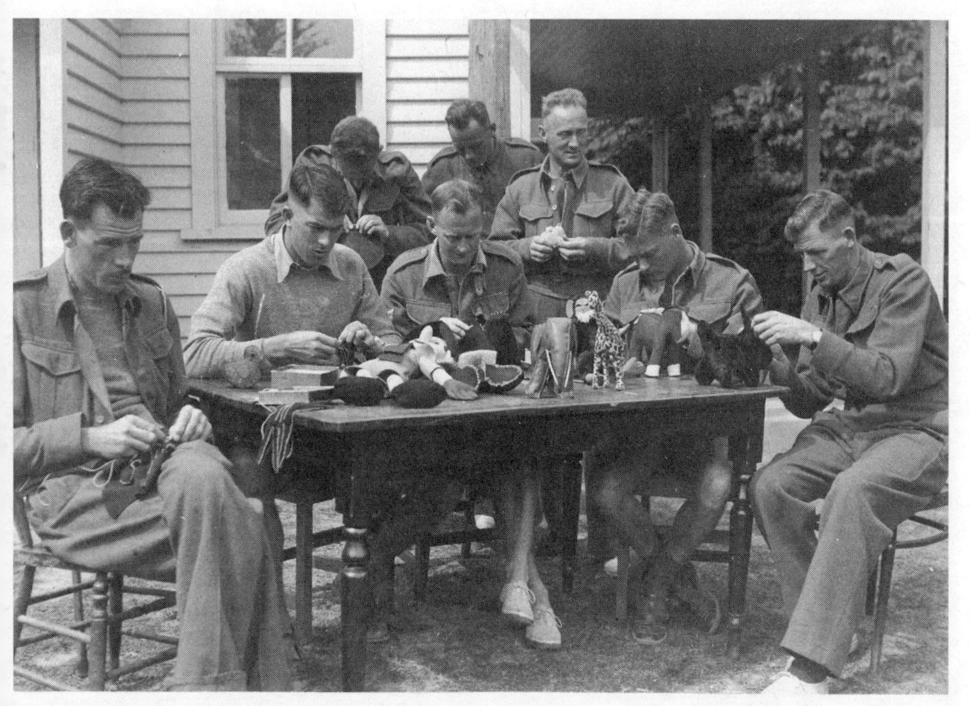

Figure 5.2
Queen Mary Hospital at Hanmer Springs returned to its role of a treatment centre for war-traumatized soldiers in World War II. Courtesy of the Hurunui District Libraries.

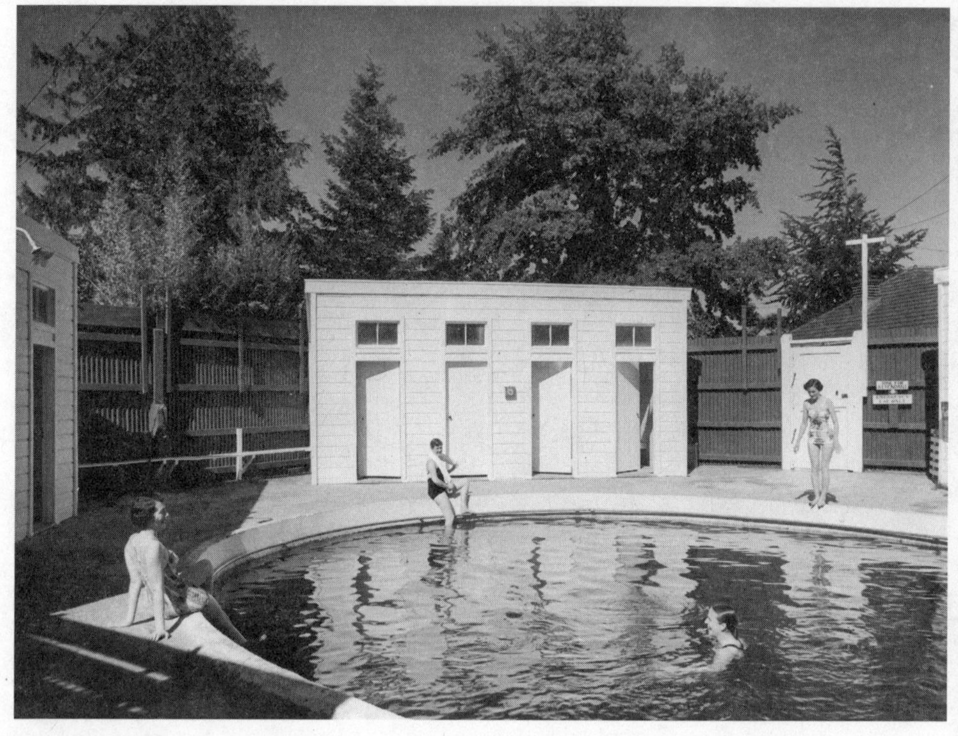

Figure 5.3
From the 1920s until it closed, Queen Mary Hospital at Hanmer Springs dealt with depression and alcoholism. As this picture of the Ladies Swimming Pool shows, there was an effort to reduce the stigma of hospital treatment. Courtesy of the Hurunui District Libraries.

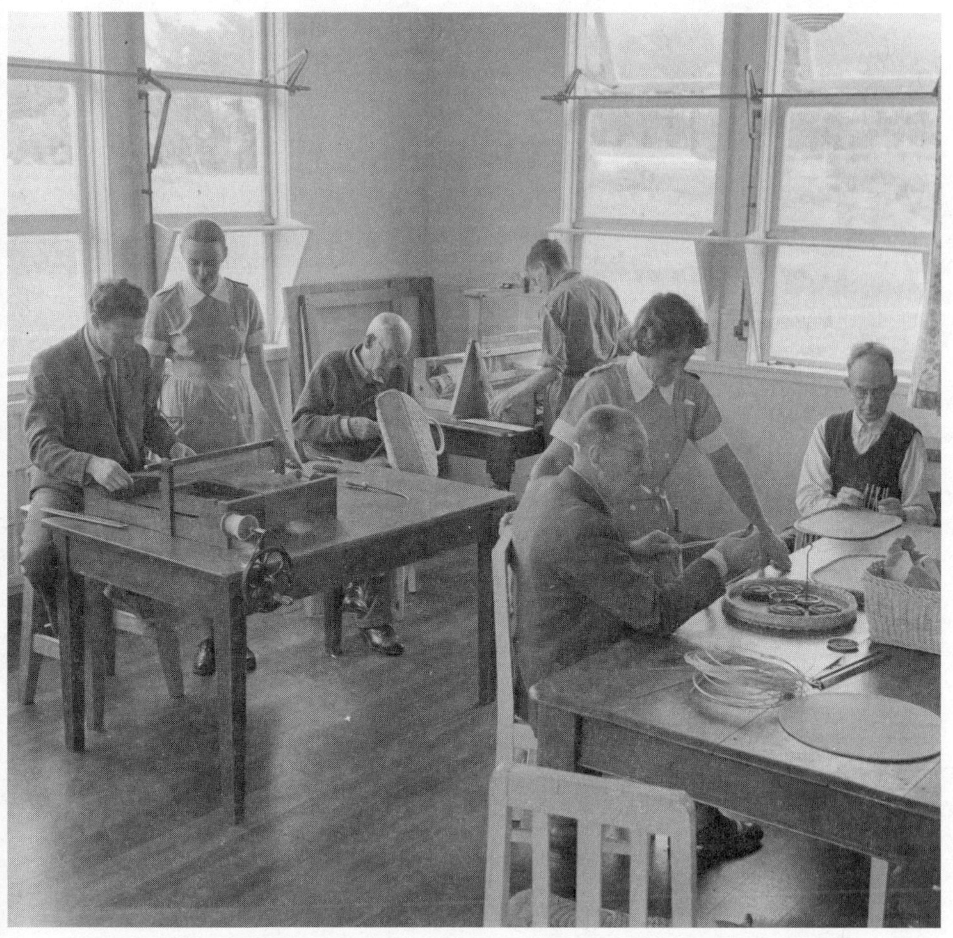

Figure 5.4
Occupational therapy had been a mainstay in the repertoire of psychiatric hospital treatments in New Zealand for most of the twentieth century. This picture was taken in 1956 at Porirua Hospital near Wellington, one of New Zealand's larger psychiatric facilities. Image courtesy of Alexander Turnbull Library, National Library of New Zealand, Te Puna Mātauranga o Aotearoa.

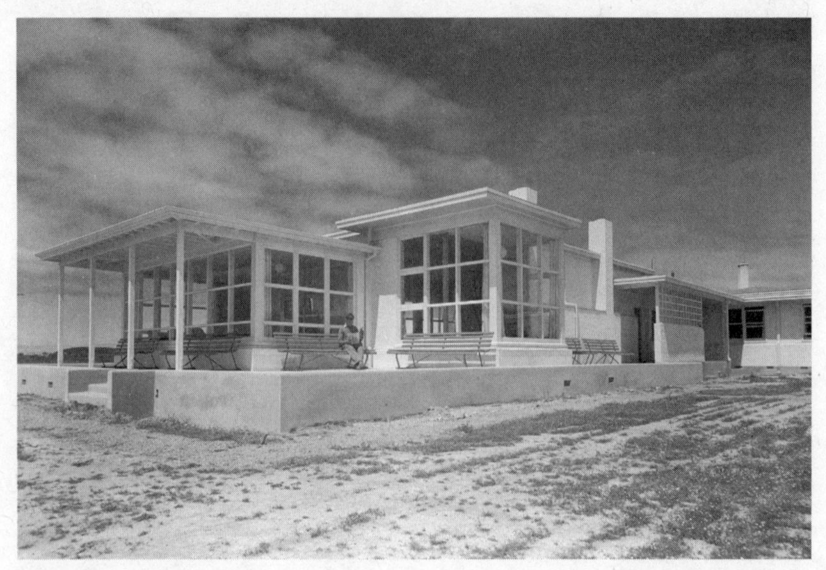

Figure 5.5
In the early 1900s, New Zealand's psychiatric hospitals began to establish villas or small hostels for patients with light symptoms or recovering patients about to leave on "parole." The use of villas increased as the mental health department attempted to create a more congenial atmosphere for treatment. This villa was built at Cherry Farm Hospital (Dunedin) around 1958, at the moment when Chlorpromazine was being introduced in the hope of reducing the numbers of patients in psychiatric hospitals. The photograph was taken by a New Zealand government publicity department. Reference AAQT 6539 A29, 455. Courtesy of Archives New Zealand, Te Rua Mahara o te Kāwanatanga.

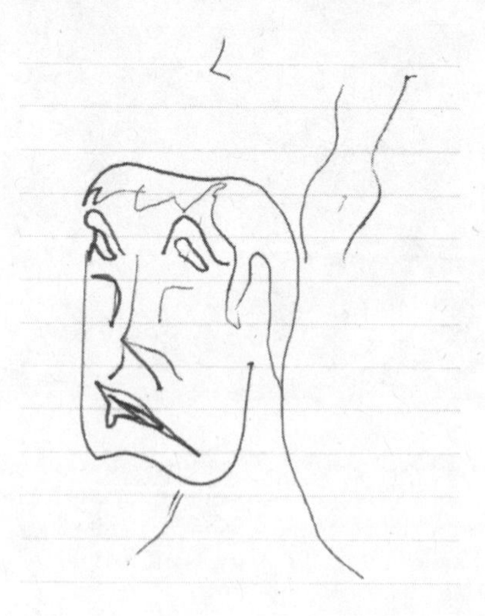

Figure 5.6
This self-portrait from the diary of a young man diagnosed with schizophrenia was intended to convey a feeling of detachment that he described in a diary entry. "Uncertainty coupled with lack of conviction about issues which should affect me dog me until I regard myself as a something akin to a blob of oil in a stream or water, tumbling along but completely separated bumping into people and things etc. but never totally integrated. What I would give not to be different." Courtesy of Archives New Zealand, Te Rua Mahara o te Kāwanatanga. Coroners' Inquest File, J46, 1976/389.

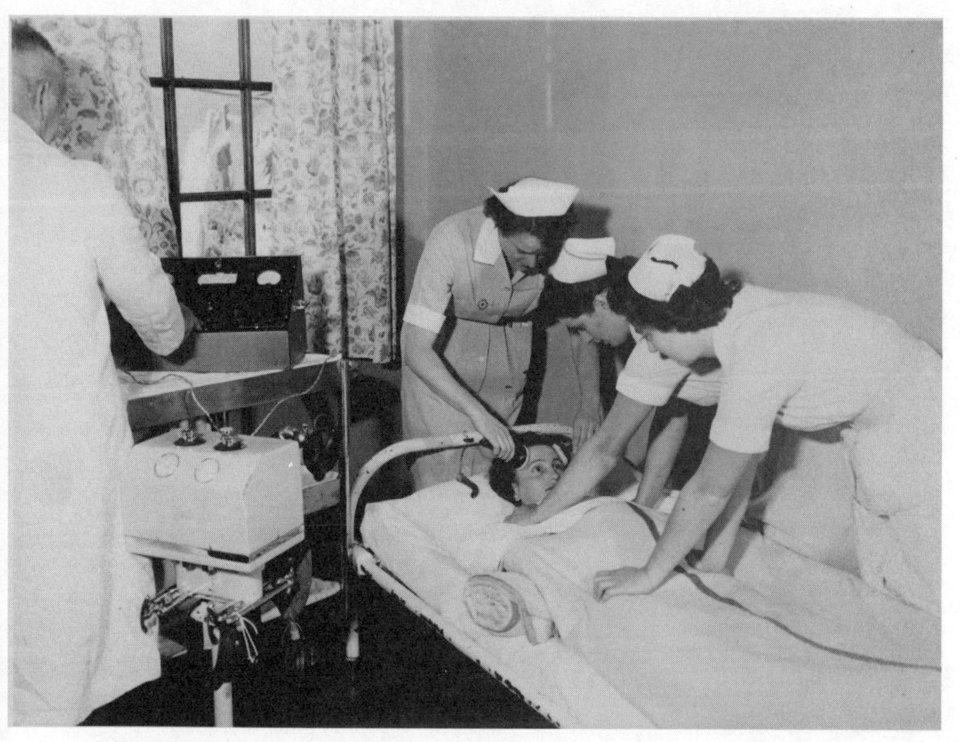

Figure 5.7
ECT Treatment at Porirua Hospital in 1956. A nurse plays the role of patient. In more recent years, a modified procedure uses an anesthetic and muscle relaxant. This picture illustrates the practice at an earlier time. Courtesy of the Porirua Hospital Museum.

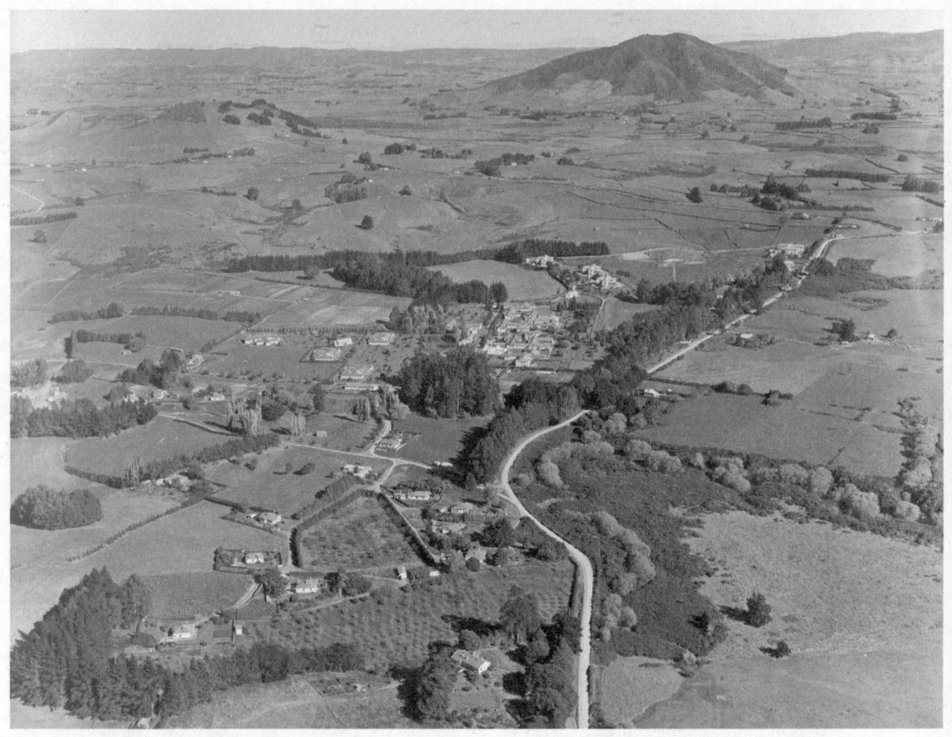

Figure 5.8
Tokanui Hospital, which opened near Hamilton in 1912, exemplified therapy through fresh air and outdoor work. Along with other psychiatric hospitals, it expanded in the 1950s. Its location meant that it treated and employed Māori. In the late 1950s, the Department of Māori Affairs promoted the recruitment of Māori nurses to serve in psychiatric hospitals; a number trained at Tokanui. On account of the distances families had to travel to see patients and due to the trend of de-institutionalization, the number of patients peaked in the 1970s. The hospital closed in 1998. Patient files (1912 to 1956) remain restricted but preserved; they form an immense potential source for a future social and medical history. Image courtesy of Alexander Turnbull Library, National Library of New Zealand, Te Puna Mātauranga o Aotearoa.

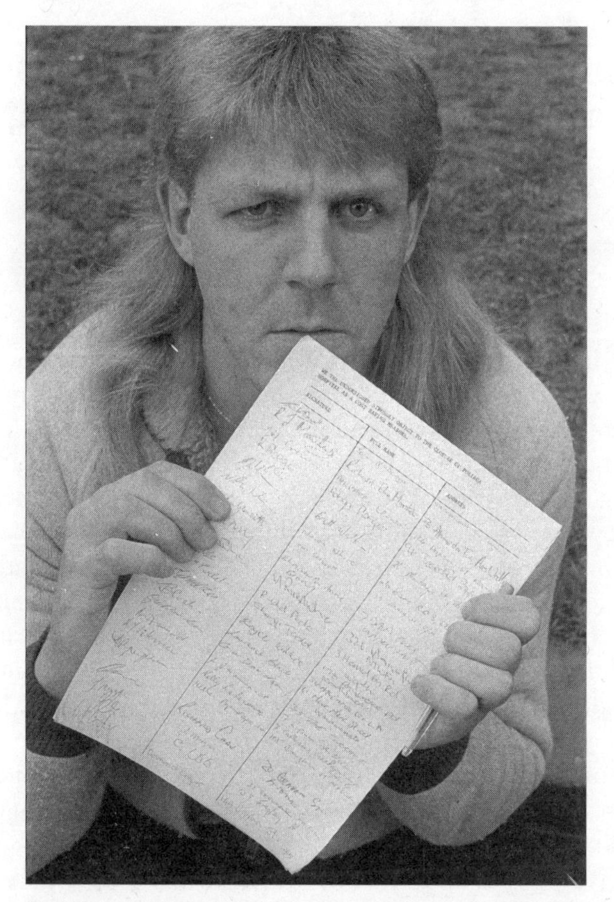

Figure 5.9
Despite criticism of conditions in the country's psychiatric hospitals and controversy over institutionalization, there was opposition to the closing of several of these hospitals. Within days of the announcement in 1989 that Porirua Hospital would be closed, a petition opposing the closing was signed by about 2,000 people, including members of a patients' support group. Courtesy of Alexander Turnbull Library, National Library of New Zealand, Te Puna Mātauranga o Aotearoa.

6

The Youth Suicide Panic: Framing a Mental Health Crisis, 1988–96

If youth includes anyone under twenty-five, then youth suicide rates in New Zealand began to rise in the early 1980s and by the end of the decade had overtaken rates for the elderly, who historically had always been at greater risk. Poorly explained statistics made a bad situation appear worse. The absence of forewarnings about alternate definitions of youth and about the untrustworthiness of suicide data from other countries permitted a panic about New Zealand leading the world in youth suicide. Academic and popular commentators alike described youth suicide rates as "shocking," "staggering," and "disturbing." A contagion, an epidemic, a plague, a psychological virus had descended on the country.[1] The panic eventually led to an ascendancy of mental health characterizations of suicide.

The youth suicide rate accompanied wrenching economic adjustments in the 1980s; thus political topicality spiced the controversy. Depending on the political case being made, the suicide scourge was either attributable or not attributable to New Zealand's sudden encounter with high unemployment. Psychiatric and psychological perspectives, particularly when influenced by American scholarship, dismissed economic explanations.[2] Psychiatrists around the world in this period were in a state of flux about the scope and treatment of mental illness, about the role of compulsion in treatment, and about drug therapy. They may not have known where they wanted to go, but along with psychologists they pursued mental health leadership in the suicide field. In general, psychiatry had been moving for years toward pharmaceutical therapies, which made the study of the roots of disorders less important. One consequence was that many psychiatrists paid less and less attention to stressors in people's lives and more to prescribing for syndromes. But as noted in chapter five, there were competing viewpoints.

The economic crises of the 1980s and 1990s were of immense significance for New Zealand youth entering their earning years, but by and large mental health interests diverted the youth suicide panic away from a critical probing of these hard times and shifted discourse into medical channels.

PANIC AS A NATIONAL MOOD

The panic came in three waves (Table 6.1). The annual release of suicide statistics piqued media interest, but personal angles that accompanied sets of suicides in the same community truly promoted the panic. The first wave came in September 1988 after the deaths of two Takapuna students who knew each other well. Media attention was drawn to the fact that both they and a suicidal girlfriend of one boy were reputed to be "followers of a youth-based music cult known as '[G]oths.'"[3] A second surge in May 1989 originated with news that two young men had committed suicide in the Central Canterbury community of Ashburton. Rumours of a larger group subscribing to a suicide pact widened into damning descriptions of town life. These assaults provoked defensive reactions from community leaders who framed youth suicide as a national problem. Thus, the Ashburton deaths catapulted youth suicide into national politics. A third surge of media attention followed the release of a Department of Health report on youth suicide in early 1993. Several years later, the department's senior officials adopted a policy of silence respecting suicide, but in 1992–93, they wanted publicity so long as they controlled the story line.

Scattered across these years and beyond, there were incidents in an associated suicide controversy about deaths in police or prison custody. Young men in custody were at great risk. For a long time preceding the panic, the Department of Justice had maintained that psychiatric hospitals should treat "the criminally insane." It insisted on this practice during the troubled shift from nationally to locally managed psychiatric hospitals or psychiatric wards in general hospitals.[4] Tension over who had a duty to treat criminals with a mental illness played out for years. The Medical Association of New Zealand resented the fact that hospital services had to assess suspects and prisoners with mental disorders and consequently had

Table 6.1
Press coverage of youth suicide in Auckland, Wellington, and Christchurch, 1987–95

Month and Year	N *of stories*	*Approx. n of column lines*	*Comments*
November 1987	1	385	
December 1987	1	230	
July 1988	1	50	
September 1988	12	960	Takapuna suicides; panic about Goth subculture.
November 1988	3	185	
February 1989	3	215	
March 1989	5	235	
May 1989	18	1,000	Ashburton youth suicides; panic about suicide pacts; politicization of youth suicide.
June 1989	2	120	
February 1990	1	60	
June 1990	1	60	
December 1991	2	95	
January 1992	2	155	
February 1992	5	415	Release of study on jail and prison suicides.
May 1992	5	245	Department of Health official advises Wellington *Evening Post* reporter on suicide data and who to interview. Two feature articles result and prompt the formation of task force and a report.
July 1992	1	25	
August 1992	3	190	
September 1992	2	35	
October 1992	1	75	
January 1993	1	40	
February 1993	21	1,150	Release of Health Department Report. In 1992–93, the Department of Health is the source of considerable publicity on suicide.
March 1993	3	75	
April 1993	5	250	
May 1993	2	100	
Gap in Clipping Service			
September 1995	1	40	
October 1995	1	35	
November 1995	1	60	
December 1995	4	225	Release of report on multiple failings of psychiatric health services in Canterbury.
July 1995	2	235	
August 1995	5	200	
September 1995	1	65	
October 1995	4	235	Cluster of suicides at Marton.
November 1995	1	15	

responsibility for security. Press criticism landed at the door of the hospital whenever there was a suicide or escape.[5] An initial step in downloading responsibility for psychiatric care from nationally administered hospitals to locally administered ones in 1972 intensified the problem. Oakley Psychiatric Hospital, under the Auckland board, took in patients from national prisons in the region; however, its doctors started to block committals in the early 1980s. Some felt that security was inconsistent with treatment, because, they claimed, patients needed to trust their therapists. A few staff members felt insecure with prisoners around. The costs of dealing with prisoners from outside Auckland were seen as an unfair burden on the local board.[6]

The hospital's management team and its supporters disapproved of treating patients in a secure facility, as locked doors allegedly corroded patient trust. Other psychiatrists dissented and felt that it was "ethically diabolical" to foster a particular climate for one set of patients by denying access to another.[7] Some nurses were at odds with doctors and wanted security. For years, prison and police officials clashed with psychiatrists over the best place to treat mentally ill detainees on remand and convicted prisoners. Prison and police officials felt that they did not have the facilities to diagnose or treat mental illnesses. Furthermore, alterations to psychiatric care put many at-risk individuals on the street where constables encountered them. Distrust and misunderstanding between doctors and criminal justice personnel played out in the press. Critics of the police denounced the appalling conditions into which "young offenders and disturbed young people" were placed. The police association responded that "if the police are going to be required to act as psychiatric guardians then police should be provided with psychiatric experts at police stations."[8] As a distinct yet related matter, the controversy went around and around during the youth suicide panic.

The prison suicides contributed to a general rise in the youth rate that led to alarmist reports. Commentators freely asserted that New Zealand led the developed world in the rate for young males. In 1988, a pivotal figure in the debates over the causes of youth suicide, Barry Taylor, justified school programs on coping skills and youth self-esteem, because "we have the second highest suicide rate in the world for young males (between 18 and 25)."[9] "Let's face it," said a school counsellor in 1996, "we're a world leader in youth suicide."[10] These remarks bracketed the period of the suicide panic. Based on the aggregate data reported by various countries, newspaper reporters claimed that New Zealand had the highest youth suicide rate in the world for males between 15 and 24. Grim pre-eminence was expressed in other ways. Dr Max Abbott, director of the Mental Health Foundation, claimed in 1988 that the suicide rate of young men in New Zealand was higher than that of Japan and triple that in England and Wales.[11] Rarely did anyone report sensibly that comparisons were foolhardy because "we keep better statistic than other countries."[12]

Assertions about pre-eminence became a mainstay in the panic about youth suicide. World leadership was "a cause of national shame."[13] Newspaper reporters covering youth suicide during the 1990s easily located authorities working with youth who were ready to proclaim that "our youth suicide rate is a national embarrassment."[14] The trouble with these claims – one of the few unchallenged assertions appearing in hundreds of speeches, memos, and newspaper articles from 1988 to 1995 – was that the country's suicide data was collected according to rules of evidence that did not accord with those of other countries, where public officials charged with investigating the causes of sudden death had political and religious reasons for rendering courtesy findings once foul play had been eliminated. International rates were not comparable; however, the rise in youth suicide in New Zealand was an embarrassment on its own. The claim to pre-eminence, not the rise in youth suicide per se, was what grabbed public attention and forced political action.[15] Since the panic started under a Labour government, National in opposition reacted first. Opposition leader Jim Bolger in late 1988 asserted that unemployment kills. He pointed to Mental Health Foundation figures which suggested that the country could expect a three to five percent rise in suicides and mental disorders for every one percent rise in unemployment.[16]

The bulk of the increase in New Zealand's youth rate came from people between the ages of twenty and twenty-four. For the most part, discussions about youth suicide in New Zealand during the 1990s combined ages fifteen to twenty-four. Youth had even been officially defined as reaching twenty-five and the Minister of Youth Affairs had a mandate to consider issues affecting people from twelve to twenty-five.[17] These aggregations were not standard practice among researchers throughout the economically developed world; rather, many restricted youth to people under twenty. More insight would have been gained if commentators had considered separately three age groups: pre-adolescents (up to fourteen), adolescents (fifteen to nineteen), and young adults (twenty to twenty-four). Richard Langford, a psychologist visiting from the United States in 1996, believed that New Zealand work on youth suicide had erred by not breaking down the age group fifteen to twenty-four. Studies needed to narrow their focus, he felt, because "the time between 18 years and 20 is a big transition in someone's life."[18] Apart from being good advice, Langford's warning reminds us that during the panic, domestic and foreign academics stepped into the limelight. Suicide researchers had serious public exposure for the first time.

A SCRUM OF EXPERTS

The three surges of press attention (Table 6.1) show media attention waxing and waning in harmony with unusual events (copy-cat suicides or suicide pacts), the release of alarming data, and eager prompting by interest groups and civil servants. The surges are noteworthy because they contained reports that captured conflicting theories among the academics who studied suicide and interest groups whose members dealt with suicidal individuals, as well as politicians, civil servants, police, coroners, and the parents of young people who had committed suicide. Suddenly, everyone in contact with self-destruction had an opinion that reporters could string together for a news item. On two big questions, experts stated conflicting outlooks. First, they disagreed about how much information in public debates was healthy. Second, they clashed about the degree of emphasis to be placed on sociological versus psychological factors in explaining the recent surge in youth suicides. They differed over whether youth suicide was best tackled as a mental-health or social-economic matter. Psychiatrists and psychologists tended to accent the former. However, some authorities remained idiosyncratic. Auckland University psychiatry professor John Werry shared his colleagues' attitude that public discussion of suicide might prompt copy-cat incidents, but was sceptical about the effectiveness of boosting national spending on adolescent mental-health services. "I am not saying it's totally useless, but the thing that's most likely to have an effect in the long run is social policies which aim to give children, adolescents, and their families a fair break in life." He went on to say that a first step would be to pay school teachers a decent wage, because "if you under-value education, you under-value children and adolescents."[19]

Academics had their spats, but surges in news coverage that kept the panic alive were reliant on more than quotes from PhD holders. They fed on human interest stories attending clusters of seemingly related deaths. Never far away were the country's suicide statistics. A two-year lag in official reports delayed awareness of the problem's dimensions. Coroners had a backlog of inquests, and thus some deaths were registered a year or more after they occurred. In 1988, the latest statistics covered 1986 when rates for age groups still showed the persistence of the long-established pattern of elderly men and women at great risk. Interviewed in June 1989, at the exact moment when youth suicide became a national concern, the co-ordinator of the Christchurch Hospital crisis team could comment accurately enough that "the highest proportion of suicides occurs among the elderly."[20] He wondered about a possible under-counting of the elderly and based his scepticism on field experience. Coroners, he believed, had trouble determining if older folk had deliberately or absent-mindedly overdosed on barbiturates.[21] If family members commented on forgetfulness, legal precedents recommended caution on the part of coroners when drafting their findings. Coal gas deaths among the elderly also presented a challenge for coroners determining intent. My aunt, a witness might say, was absent-minded and carelessly neglected to ignite the gas stove.[22]

Specialists who worked with the elderly might reasonably argue that 'the olds' remained at great risk, but employees at community agencies who worked with young people sensed that the data under-estimated the youth rate dramatically. Drug overdoses among the young, like barbiturate overdoses and coal gas deaths among the elderly, posed problems for coroners; for they left sufficient doubt for a ruling of accidental death or an open verdict. By 1989, official suicide data finally pointed to the replacement of the elderly by youth as the age group at greatest risk. In May 1992, the acting director of the New Zealand Mental Health Association, Barbara Disley, pressed the Minister of Health, Simon Upton, for action on youth suicide citing the 1989 data.[23] It was a fair demand. Yet, the comparatively good news about a drop in the suicide rate for the elderly was ignored.

Impressions increased that more young people than ever had serious emotional troubles. Youth counsellors noticed robust demand for a brochure that gave advice on coping with problems; university counsellors detected increases in feelings of low self-esteem and inability to cope.[24] Alarm about youth suicides erupted on the public scene in the late 1980s on account of a convergence of anecdotal reports, interviews with researchers, and pairs of suicides at Takapuna (September 1988) and Ashburton (May 1989). These two "outbreaks," accounting for merely four suicide deaths among hundreds, attracted excessive attention. Parents, teachers, and youth counsellors were in panic mode, partly on account of the morbid subcultures exposed by these deaths. 1989 was the turning point in the development of the panic, after which topics in youth suicide (including jail suicides, hospital suicides, and failings in psychiatric care) were seldom out of the news.

While a handful of suicides and their revelations of youth subcultures fed the panic, the annual release of data was getting wider attention. Lagged statistical reports had shown enough of an increase in youth suicide to alarm psychiatrists and psychologists. In early 1989 several pronouncements featured in newspapers. In February the Youth Mental Health Project published a report entitled *Swept under the Carpet*; it claimed that recently – a vague timeframe – there had been twenty outbreaks of "suicide virus," meaning a cluster of suicides in the same family, school, or social group.[25] Despite recourse to a medical metaphor, the report connected youth suicide to economic instability and unemployment, not to mental illness per se. In interviews about the report, project co-ordinator Barry Taylor mentioned the direct and indirect consequences of unemployment and economic pressures. Not only were young people pessimistic about their futures, but more of them encountered troubles at home where tight finances contributed to domestic upheavals. Taylor wanted the government to support public information. "Unemployment," he said on a prior occasion, "was the most dehumanizing problem facing young people and the southern South Island was a particularly bad area."[26] Over the next few years, Taylor publicized youth suicide at workshops and in study groups where he insisted that youth culture needed study and that young people needed to be consulted and empowered.[27]

In the same month that Taylor promoted his group's study, an American psychiatrist, David Schaffer of Columbia University, spoke to psychiatrists in Auckland and Christchurch. Consistent with his conviction that press reporting might encourage suicides, Schaffer met with colleagues behind closed doors.[28] Arrangements for his Auckland stay had been made by John Werry of the medical school, who was reported as claiming that "a large scale examination of suicide had much in common with pornography. It used young people for adult gratification."[29] He had an ally in Schaffer. Dismissive of press coverage, Schaffer claimed that most socio-cultural explanations beloved by the press were dangerously misguided. Paradoxically, there was nothing like a threatened veil of secrecy to stimulate attention.

In Schaffer's estimation, youth suicides, like all suicides, originated in mental illness. To deny this 'truth' was to advance the stigma of mental illness and deny its prevalence. In his opinion, it was "better to recognize a mental illness than to allow people to go around promoting the idea that suicide is a response to stress and its victims were weaker in coping with stress than others." In a deterministic fashion, he claimed "suicide victims are simply built differently."[30] Could that have meant they were built weaker in coping with stress? He appeared oblivious to the inconsistency in his claims. Shaffer's conception of suicide and psychiatric conditions exposed medical imperialism. Along with many psychiatrists and psychologists, he defined mental disorders broadly to include proneness to aggression, perfectionism, and depression. A survey of international literature in 1992 reported that, if mental illness included mood disorders, substance abuse, conduct disorders, personality disorders, adjustment disorders, depression, and schizophrenia, then possibly ninety to ninety-eight percent of suicides suffered from a psychological illness.[31]

The impression that mental illness explained youth suicide had been reinforced in New Zealand by Schaffer, who was unbending in his insistence that depression predated other factors. The aetiology of mental illnesses was not just invisible in his formulation, but any reference to a stressor was a retreat from confronting mental illness. Schaffer wanted the entire subject of suicide sequestered, claiming that prevention programs gave people dangerous ideas. It was best, he maintained, to let psychiatrists work with the mentally ill and for government to avoid addressing the problem through awareness and education.[32] In a matter of weeks, the broad outlines of an intellectual and policy debate on youth suicide had gelled. In opposition to those who sought to medicalize suicide and sequester discussion, there were social workers, youth counsellors, coroners, and educators; they accented socio-economic causes and advocated greater public information. Barry Taylor represented their outlook. Those who championed educational efforts included teachers and guidance counsellors, who found students fully aware of suicides. Realistically, how could talk be contained?

The emphasis placed on mental illness by psychiatrists and psychologists prompts questions about what constitutes or causes a mental illness. The medical experts on suicide cornered themselves. If youth suicides were largely committed by the mentally ill, as they alleged, and if youth suicide rates had suddenly escalated, were psychiatrists thus intimating that the frequency of mental illness among the young had recently soared? An affirmative answer was an inescapable corollary to their position. Could changing sociological factors explain an outbreak of youth mental illness? To concede that would be to downgrade the medical explanation.

At stake in these questions was a long-standing separation in suicide studies between sociologists and psychiatrists. The two approaches operated at different points on a time line: background causes and proximate expressions. Background causes favoured by sociologists were bound to be diffuse. Adherents to the view that life's troubles were important reproached the country's current economic and social performance as well as a few cultural attitudes. Meanwhile, the mental health approach held the promise of direct remediation through therapies. While we tend to link psychiatrists and clinical psychologists, it is important to note a distinction and professional strains. The former emphasized the disease aspect of some mental disorders while the latter tackled behaviour.[33] Both disciplines struggled for respect in the late twentieth century. Psychiatrists had to contend with the fact that fads in therapy had shifted often in the twentieth century. Meanwhile, as members of a newer field, clinical psychologists laboured to grab a seat at the medical table.[34] To maintain the public esteem for their respective members, advocates for these professions overstated the science in their day-to-day activities, and suicide was one field where exaggeration occurred.[35]

Psychiatrists and psychologists had to deal with cries for immediate help. In the late twentieth century, reflection on the roles of psychologists included the idea that in addition to modifying the behaviour of individuals, they might help make society more civil. This latter thought acknowledged the social and cultural bases of many personal troubles.[36] There was room in both psychiatry and psychology for recognizing the responsibility of material misery for many instances of mental illness, but attention to immediate needs and the disciplines' claims to science promoted a focus on suicide as mental illness. This inclination served politicians too.

By the late 1980s, youth activism (prominent from the late 1960s through to the early 1980s) was waning but not extinguished. Māori advocacy of Māori remedies and autonomy had acquired importance. It would surface now in government reviews of youth suicide. The youth suicide panic erupted in an age of consultation, but no longer an age of widespread optimism about solutions to difficult social questions. Newspaper stories and internal government memos reveal confusion, contradiction, and scepticism about intervention to reduce youth suicide. In reference to youth suicide, some of the complexity evaporated when officials in the Department of Health medicalized youth suicide. For the best of reasons – to secure resources to assist people – employees of the department and of medical interest groups that worked with them narrowed the official response to the panic. As a practical matter, it perhaps had to be this way. Yet, the full, complex, and unmanageable truth was sacrificed.

TAKAPUNA AND ASHBURTON RECONSIDERED: HOW THE LOCAL BECAME NATIONAL

In the mid-1980s, there had been a smattering of newspaper stories about the alarming number of youth suicides in New Zealand.[37] The topic lacked the human interest needed for press momentum until a pair of suicides by sixteen-year-old students from Takapuna Grammar in mid-1988. They were good friends and, what interested the public, they were in a group of about six who embraced the Goth subculture. The boys dressed in black stove-pipe pants and black jerseys; they wore Doc Marten boots. They displayed crucifixes and immersed themselves in morbid music. They withdrew from other social activities, retreated to their rooms, and fell behind in studies. Their assiduous separation from schoolmates fascinated the public; the Goth scene did contribute to the suicides in a way that will be explained later in this chapter. What the public did not glimpse in these cases were the aspects of the boys' lives that influenced their choice of a dark subculture. The loving mother of the first boy to take his own life, Jason Capner, described him as short, thin, artistic, sensitive, gentle, and affectionate. He wanted to be a hairdresser. "He wasn't your big Kiwi joker rugby player," she said. His parents accepted most of his choices, but wanted him to clean up his room and contribute to household chores. That led to tension.[38] The second boy, Marc Hitchcock, was deeply affected by Capner's death: "Don't blame what I'm doing on Jason. It is not totally a result of what he did. He was however the best friend I ever had and it hurt me a lot when he left." It is probable that the loneliness of this second youngster also owed something to his father's death; he wanted to have his funeral at a locale that was "a lot nicer than the place where dad had his."[39]

The boys were outsiders even before their Goth affiliation. They gravitated to the Goth identity because it gave them a place, although far outside predominant expressions of male culture. As well, they abandoned struggles for achievement at school. Marc Hitchcock wrote that "I haven't even done any school work for two months and I'm far too far behind to catch up."[40] Press coverage included a controversy about pressure to achieve at school. A new headmaster was moving the school away from its former emphasis on sports under the previous headmaster to a focus on academic achievement.[41] The idea that schools put inordinate pressures on students was countered by a community health specialist who argued that the crucial pressures came from parents who encouraged their children to accept the challenges laid down by the schools.[42] Marc Hitchcock did report stresses at school; however, they comprised just one of two sets of pressures on him. "Our school," he wrote, "puts too much emphasis on academic achievement and more work needs to go into teaching people how to get on in life and also teach people to do as they want to do and not be afraid of what others will say."[43] Additionally, he felt the pressure to conform. The world of work and the employment market had changed. Parents and schools reinforced what a few students feared. They would have to pull up their socks and conform to get on in a tougher world.

The Takapuna suicides fuelled the first surge of press attention, essentially by putting the Goths on display. It was partly to counter that coverage and a fear that Goths would be marginalized on account of bad publicity that David Schaffer had been invited to speak to New Zealand psychiatrists. Some psychologists insisted there was "no evidence linking [G]othic games and certain types of music to suicide."[44] Soon after the basic clashes of opinion represented by Barry Taylor and Schaffer had been aired in 1989, related teen suicides rocked Ashburton. If the two Takapuna deaths put youth suicide in the press as never before, the Ashburton ones thrust youth suicide into the national government arena, where it would stay.

The core facts were uncontroversial. After the death of a friend in a motorcycle accident in July 1988, six young men appear to have been parties to a suicide pact.[45] One killed himself in April. Six weeks later another died. Community reactions swung from immediate panic about youth subcultures to calmer but inconclusive discussions about nationwide troubles affecting young people. The immediate wave of reporting was sensational and reflected badly on Ashburton. Rumours flew about depraved small-town youth. The manager of the local youth centre circulated reports that the dead teens had participated in bizarre forms of substance abuse, devil worship, and sex for drugs.[46] He condemned parents for burying their heads in the sand. Adding to impressions that the town's young people were lurching out of control and parents were in denial, a senior constable who served as the town's youth aid officer disclosed that he had been alerted to a youth suicide pact. He contacted the parents of the alleged participants. On the strength of a rumour about a pact, the parents of two adolescents secured committal orders to send their sons to Sunnyside Hospital for mandatory assessment.[47] The boys reacted by describing Sunnyside as "a nuthouse" and claimed they were being punished, not helped.[48] Another rumour suggested that there had been a youth séance after one of the suicides, and that a message from the other side had called upon teens to join friends in the great beyond. Wild stories attracted unwelcome attention. Less sensational but also damaging to the community's pride, some commentators remarked on the high rate of youth unemployment in Central Canterbury. At a low point in community morale, a parent declared, "everyone is in a mess down here."[49]

Serious researchers at the time and subsequently sought a single tidy socio-cultural or mental-health factor that adversely affected youth.[50] Among those who favoured a mental health understanding of youth suicide, mental depression figured prominently. However, they could not agree on what touched off the presumed swell in depression-based suicides. Mental health professionals generally dismissed youth cults and suicide pacts, which had been blamed at Takapuna and initially at Ashburton.

To protect the community's reputation, the local Member of Parliament, Jenny Shipley, commanded the limelight and stressed that

Ashburton's troubles were not endemic but national, that the town was stable and caring, and that mental health studies had shown that smaller communities across New Zealand were at elevated risk because of a centralization of health services.[51] The trouble with her deflection of attention from Ashburton to the entire country via Labour's restructuring of medical services was that there were substantial regional disparities in youth unemployment, and if lack of work was a contributing factor to youth suicide then Ashburton was a high-risk locale. Its youth unemployment rate, at nearly seventeen percent for 1988, was the second highest in the country.[52] Shipley had thrown a life-line to Ashburton's self-esteem and concurrently transformed a pair of suicides, about a half of one percent that year, from a local to a national concern. In later years when other local clusters of suicides caught the attention of the press, politicians, school heads, and community leaders were quick to say they too were a national problem that needed to be dealt with by Parliament.[53]

Before Shipley's assertions, there had been sensible responses from several Ashburton citizens. After the first of the two suicides, citizens set the wheels in motion for a public information seminar that would include a psychologist and social worker from Christchurch. More than other locales, the garden city had the voluntary and professional personnel to deal with suicide bereavement. In June 1988, Women Supporting Women, a suicide survivors' support group, had been organized. Among its activities, it arranged for someone to attend coroners' courts to support survivors.[54] The second suicide at Ashburton assured that the local meeting to discuss suicide attracted considerable out-of-town attention.[55] Shipley shrewdly announced that she would open the seminar.[56] Far from being a sensational affair that advanced speculation about morbid youth subcultures, the public discussion at Ashburton quickly settled down and centred on intelligent representations of conflicting explanations. The press interviews and seminar indicated that while the town did not have mental health professionals on hand, it did have a youth aid officer attached to the police and it had school counsellors. Young people constituted a population for study and management in advanced welfare states, and New Zealand was no exception.

There was one development in youth culture that various observers agreed was disastrous. Alcohol, drug, and solvent abuse had become more pervasive among young people. Initial reports on the Ashburton teen suicides in 1989 cited the local police youth aid officer on his opinion that an upsurge of youth in crisis had to be seen against a backdrop of alcohol and solvent abuse.[57] Protecting his school, Ashburton College's senior guidance counsellor stated that solvent abuse was a problem among drop-outs; the school was not a centre of trouble but economic depression brought on by "dependence on the dole" was a serious problem.[58] There was a consensus about the pitfalls of substance abuse, but discord over the alleged hazards of youth subcultures and music.

The Goth subculture merits more serious consideration than it received after several medical experts dismissed its significance following the Takapuna suicides. During the late 1980s and into the 1990s, a few superficial critiques of contemporary youth culture accompanied press speculation about the reasons for youth suicides. Outbreaks of unconventional youth subcultures coincided with the rise in youth suicide. Parallel events became associated as cause and effect. The music of disenchantment plus the style statements of Goths attracted attention as potential 'causes' of a rise in suicides. David Shaffer's visit to New Zealand originated with the city's psychiatrists, who, among other objectives, sought to dispel the idea that three recent Auckland-area youth suicides, including the two at Takapuna, had been influenced by the lyrics from the bands that Goths followed.[59] At the same time that the mental health establishment waved aside suggestions that Goths and dark music played a part in some youth suicides, Goth values troubled the police constables who investigated suicides. They accepted the idea that morbid lyrics and corpse-like make-up indicated an unhealthy fascination with death. "What type of music did your daughter or son listen to?" officers asked at the scene.[60] In the case of one 1988 teen suicide, the police report stated: "the deceased was a follower of the GOTHIC cult, and one of their beliefs is that there is no life after twenty years of age."[61] If the police were excessively alarmed about Goths, academics were too blasé. Psychologists and psychiatrists dismissed the importance of a dark subculture, but they might have gained some insights by paying attention to the morbid content.

Another theme that surfaced from time to time pertained to copying. Some students of suicide proposed that a young person with low self-esteem might envy the outpouring of attention that a recent suicide had received at a school memorial service. In the estimation of some psychologists, publicity attending a suicide could promote its glamour, making it seem attractive. The rise in youth suicide prompted a running discussion about copy-cat suicides and press coverage of suicide. Those who felt that at least some young people could be impressed by the suicide death of a celebrity or a popular student wanted to ban reporting about how a teen idol or admired local youth died, although it is hard to imagine successful censorship among fans or in schools. Moreover, advocates of restraint in reporting never reconciled the alleged glamorization with the ghastly irrevocable character of the act. Many details, if released for publication, would have undercut the glamour or fantasy of escape. Escape to where? School-based grieving kept attention at an elevated level; students close to the deceased acted as pallbearers.[62] In one respect, newspaper reporting did fail. The Takapuna and Ashburton teen suicides were picked up because the youths involved seemed to have participated in prior bizarre activities. Other clusters went without notoriety, possibly because the young people involved were poor, lived in more remote areas, and had distinctly mundane motives such as romantic break-up. Their deaths were not deemed puzzling like the deaths of so-called talented youths or sensitive boys.[63]

Explanations that centred on youth culture or on adulation deflected attention from society and family. Potentially, details about a premature death could indict the community, schooling, peer pressure, family, and even the deceased. Such a stream of intimate explanations would not have been comforting news for grieving friends, relatives, and school authorities. Sensitivity may explain why information about circumstances, motives, and suicide notes were rarely mentioned in public. When broken down on a case-by-case basis, motives for suicide include some disturbing things about some families' conduct, the raw sensitivities of youth, and evidence of immature individuals catapulted by their own actions into situations demanding maturity.

Professional observers came to the topic with disciplinary biases. Psychologists who attempted to understand the rise in the suicide rates of young people wrote off the idea that a trend in popular culture could lead to self-destruction. On several counts, they were right to be critical. First, suicide could not generally be caused; it usually involved a decision based on a path of reasoning that led from problem to solution. Second, not many youth suicides involved clear evidence of a morbid turn of mind influenced by a subculture; but there were some. The disquieting fact is that in a few cases in the late 1980s and into the 1990s, there was an association between a dark subculture and a few youth suicides. Interestingly, if the case files are any measure, it had vanished by 2000. But for more than a decade, a subculture and its music were significant. As one fifteen-year-old expressed it in his suicide note, "they say that music doesn't have an influence. It does."[64] It did in his case. Morbid postures continued beyond death, because Goths left instructions for funeral music by their favourite bands.[65]

DARK MUSIC

Discerning the nature of the association between a youth subculture and suicide is challenging. Was the subculture for some young people a carapace to deflect pain, in which case the subculture masked real motives? Police officers conducting investigations were transfixed by the morbid darkness in and of itself. Even if the subculture was an expression of something else, it still may have played a critical role in a few youth suicides. It could have contributed to a relaxation on the hold of life by normalizing the idea of death at an early age. Suicide seems to involve two steps. First, there are the motives that make individuals miserable; second, there are the reasoning processes that raise death as a solution to the problems or make death less frightening. Consider four youth suicides from 1992. A fifteen-year-old student kept his clothes in a coffin and listened to music by Suicidal Tendencies.[66] A seventeen-year-old student with a record of irresponsible conduct had turned to cannabis, heavy metal music, and denunciations of authority and family."[67] A twenty-five-year-old who had been involved with heavy metal music was listening to it prior to killing himself. He had written the words of one of the songs, "Fade to Black," along with a suicide note that commented on a song written by Obituary called "Internal Bleeding." He had written "Satan" and put marks and crosses in what appears to have been his own blood on notes.[68] In these cases, evidence suggests that a Goth environment made death unusually pervasive in these boys' routines.

In the fourth case, there was evidence of treatment for mental illness. An eighteen-year-old who had been treated for two years for "a major depressive illness with psychotic features" had become "increasingly preoccupied with death and suicide, and with the Gothic music cult."[69] References to a Gothic or Goth subculture surfaced in at least ten inquests in 1988, 1990, 1992, and 1994. The subculture originated in the late 1970s in the United Kingdom as an offshoot of Punks, but with lots of black clothing, lace crucifixes, and white makeup. Lyrics about "meeting on the other side" were popular with a string of Goth-favoured bands, mostly from the United Kingdom. They included The Mission, Sisters of Mercy, Kingdom Come, The Cure, The Jesus and Mary Chain, The Smiths, and Bauhaus.[70]

The Goth outlook presumed an early death and an afterlife. Death notices placed in newspapers by friends said "catch you later" and "be with you soon."[71] This idea of life after death needs to be recognized and situated alongside mainstream belief systems. In the first half of the twentieth century, many mature men and women who took their own lives left messages that indicated how they reasoned their way toward death by making it a step toward a family reunion. In the late twentieth century, a few young people arrived at a comparable position through affiliation with a subculture. The earlier expressions of faith by suicidal men and women were accepted, for they matched the Christian belief in heaven and the deceased were seldom young. Goths were not only young but challenging conformity while accepting the existence of an altered state that did not mean an absolute end. At the conclusion of a long farewell letter, an adolescent who was immersed in dark music told his parents, "I won't say goodbye because I'm not really leaving, just going to sleep."[72]

Panic over music was not new. Billie Holliday's "Gloomy Sunday" – the so-called suicide song – had been blamed for a string of suicides in the United States during the 1950s. Self-styled Satanist Ozzy Osbourne was accused of contributing to suicides with his single "Suicide Solution." Anxiety about music extended to more than the Goth subculture. A study of suicide ideation among students in Adelaide, Australia, in the early 1990s found that nearly a third preferred heavy metal music, but many also came from broken families and experienced the associated sadness of loss.[73] A 1998 inquest noted that the sixteen-year-old was into "heavy metal music emphasising suicide."[74] By the end of the twentieth century, there were additional suspect influences. There were misgivings about gangster rap. It was more than a coincidence that an eighteen-year-old took his own life a year to the day after Tupac Shakur was shot. No claim is made here that strains of popular culture induced young people to commit suicide. There was no Pied Piper. Instead, violent lyrics and a commitment to a related subculture could have habituated a very few to death or a wobbly faith in a transition to another state of being. Death may have seemed less frightening, less premature, or less final on account of fatalistic messages. Critics of morbid popular music had a point when they said that "the lyrics send the wrong message."[75]

The vast majority of young music consumers were impervious to self-destructive or violent messages, but for a handful looking for a solution to their woes, the messages not only proffered a remedy but accustomed them to death. It is curious that a few psychologists would insist on press silence while a strand of popular culture, described by them as benign, projected fatalistic messages directly to young people. A seventeen-year-old Goth, interviewed by a newspaper reporter, described the communication power and message of music that went unappreciated by scholars who attempted to know young people and protect them from a glamorization of death. "Death is fascinating. We don't know anything about it so it can be romanticized ... Music let's [sic] you know your [sic] not the only one who felt like this [depressed]."[76] It was easier for psychologists to criticize mainstream media pitched at adults than to explore the counter-culture bands and life histories of ill-fated stars that in point of fact reached the vulnerable. Morbid young people could and did check out biographies of James Dean, Freddie Mercury, and Jimi Hendix from libraries.[77]

Some psychologists were aware of vague associations between subculture and morbid thinking and recognized too that "the general well-being" of young people was intrinsic to mental health.[78] Nevertheless, the profession increasingly accented mental illness *tout court* and shunned nebulous references to general well-being.

THE MENTAL HEALTH AGENDA, 1992–93

During the years of panic (1989–2000), socio-economic explanations were challenged by Department of Health officials and academics based in psychiatry and psychology. A deep split in explanations acquired a political dimension when the Department of Health established management over suicide prevention. Caught in budget retrenchments in the late 1980s and early 1990s, senior departmental officers and spokespersons from related non-governmental agencies believed that they could stem the rise in suicides; they could also see that by characterizing the youth suicide crisis as a mental health problem, they might restore funding. Public and private mental health analysts acted from a belief that practical intervention to stem suicides required placing mental health services at the core. In relation to the times, there was a case to be made, if we accept that a substantial amount of mental health effort was required to deal with the fallout from socio-economic stress. Soaring redundancy notices during the 1980s had strained mental health services and social counselling in resource communities and cities. In chapter seven, more information is given on the origin, nature, scope, and consequences of unemployment.

From the beginning of the panic, the Mental Health Foundation's staff members were vigilant and proficient when it came to securing press attention and slipping in a line about under-funding. During the turbulent 1980s, the organization produced admirable reports on mental health facilities, violence, Māori and Pacific Island issues in mental health, and women's mental health.[79] Commenting in July 1988 on the rise in youth suicide rates, the deputy director of the foundation, Hilary Haines, remarked to a *New Zealand Herald* reporter that "the mental health system does not have enough money to help adolescents in crisis."[80] As would be the case throughout the panic, the foundation's spokespersons asserted without hesitation that suicides were largely connected with mental illness and prevention required more funding for mental health. An initial budget submission by the department to fund a study on youth suicide failed to survive a trimming exercise for the 1991–92 budget. Shortly afterward, suicide prevention groups, politicians, and journalists picked up the pace of public commentary. Articles depicting New Zealand as leading the world in youth suicide rattled politicians, and so did contemporaneous reports on the suicides of young men in custody. In January and February 1992, prison-cell suicides became the focus of attention. During these months, the leader of the left-leaning Alliance (New Labour) Party, Jim Anderton, demanded a commission of inquiry into prison suicides.

Reports that the rate of prison cell suicides was among the highest in the world shocked Prime Minister Jim Bolger, who followed the suicide reports and soon acted to rein in bad publicity.[81] The Department of Justice released a thoroughgoing suicide prevention report in 1994. Recommendations included redesigning cells, providing special clothing and bedding, selecting sensitive prison personnel, arranging emergency response training, and developing better communications among staff handling prisoners.[82] Meanwhile, on the youth suicide front in 1992, spokespersons for the suicide prevention group the Samaritans as well as the Drug Foundation gave interviews that insisted there was a national crisis. They called for more funding.[83]

In May 1992, a reporter from the *Evening Post* was working on a feature story claiming that New Zealand's youth suicide problem was the worst in the developed world. The Department of Health assisted by supplying data and suggesting that she contact the New Zealand Mental Health Foundation. "If I were you," Velma McClellan of the department wrote to Lindsay Morgan, "I would look at the rates to do the comparisons." The advice went further. "I would suggest you contact Barbara Disley [of the Mental Health Foundation]." [84] The first instalment appeared on 15 May and the second on 18 May. The second mentioned the unfortunate prominence of New Zealand's youth suicide rate internationally. The claim upset Bolger, who wanted the Department of Health "to investigate the issues surrounding the high New Zealand youth suicide rate."[85] The possibility that the Reuters news service would pick up the story animated the prime minister's office. Meanwhile, four interest groups lobbied for action. The New Zealand Mental Health Foundation, the New Zealand Drug Foundation, the New Zealand Medical Association, and the Samaritans requested a meeting with the Associate Minister of Health to discuss mental health services for adolescents, the shortage of research on adolescent mental health issues, the lack of specialist training for dealing with disturbed adolescents, and the possibility of convening a ministerial committee on adolescent health. The youth suicide issue was being defined as a medical matter by a major department and the non-government parties with whom it had a working relationship.

The delegation was granted a meeting for 27 May 1992; in preparation Kaye Saville Smith, Manager Responsible for Women and Young People's Health Policy, briefed the associate minister, Katherine O'Regan. Saville Smith presented clear ideas about what the ministry could promise. The Minister of Youth Affairs, advised by Barry Taylor, put an oar in the water and suggested a national youth suicide strategy that consulted youth. Youth Affairs participated in the subsequent meetings, but the Department of Health ran the show. O'Regan met the delegation with a plan in hand. First, a budget item for youth suicide intervention would have to be restored. The wave of publicity and prime ministerial angst made that a good bet. Second, the delegation's idea of a ministerial committee was rejected. The department wanted a "scoping exercise" involving the country's experts. Third, the department replaced the committee idea with a four-phase scheme: collection of data and information on crisis services already in place; a two-day workshop attended by no more than twenty experts with a report to follow; the formulation of an intervention and prevention pilot study; and an evaluation of the intervention.[86]

By mid-June the government had approved funding for the first year, and soon afterward the department contacted twenty experts who would be brought together on the "neutral ground" of Burma Lodge in the Wellington suburb of Khandallah.[87] No government department claimed to be in charge, hence the neutral location; however, the Department of Health managed the lead-up to the meeting and supervised the report. The twenty experts consisted of six clinicians, five community or interest group representatives, five policy specialists, two psychology researchers, and one Māori representative. Medical personnel, widely defined to include psychologists, had a majority. Nevertheless, the group fragmented and no consensus emerged from the meeting held on 28–9 September 1992. However, since the Department of Health sought the medicalization of suicide, that is what it delivered.

A shrewd and forthright contract researcher, Helena Barwick, was secured to write the report, based on the workshop. In her "Youth Suicide Prevention Project Workshop Report," Barwick cautioned that suicide literature was substantially written by psychiatrists.[88] In a note to the project manager for the youth suicide prevention project, Velma McClellan, Barwick confided that "somewhere there needs to be a repeat of the caution that I have made in the introduction, that most of the literature in this review [of the literature] is written by psychiatrists, and the bias that that gives the report must be acknowledged."[89] Her forthrightness surfaced in the report's conclusions, which accented a lack of agreement at the workshop.

Few specifics were supported by the whole group. However, the majority placed youth suicide more firmly in the mental health area than was warranted by current international literature. The literature "tended to discuss suicide as a discrete event with its own unique causation." If mental health was the key, then logic dictated an improvement of mental health services to all youth as an intervention strategy. However, to accept the idea that each suicide had a unique causation would lead only to a policy nightmare and a government admission of impotence. Apart from mental health initiatives, the report mentioned other preventative measures. Access to means of self-destruction needed to be closed (surely a chimera, as we point out in the conclusion to this book); crisis call lines needed to be increased, and so too awareness of their existence. Schools needed to give attention to achievement levels and self-esteem, a healthy school environment, active parental involvement, a greater connection between schools and workplaces, teaching social and life skills, and more staff training.

The recommendations were diffuse. However, the mental health message, a deceptively simplified theme, was pursued by the Department of Health. In February 1993, the department released its report. The Associate Minister of Health admitted that each case was a tragedy that had many factors behind it. "It is clear, however, that the problem should be addressed with the broader context of youth mental health and that major psychiatric disorder, primarily depression, is one of the key risk factors in youth suicide."[90] This statement sounded reassuring and placed youth suicide in the hands of medicine by evading a pair of linked questions. What was depression? What was behind depression? Moreover, based on a review of the international literature, the report from the workshop noted that studies in Denmark and the United Kingdom in the 1960s concluded that "the introduction of psychiatric services had no impact on the suicide rate." These negative findings preceded the introduction of anti-depressants, so medical professionals dismissed them. New developments in psychiatry, they assumed, would work.[91]

At the Associate Minister's mention of "it is clear," alert readers might have wisely suspected that there was confusion in the ranks. If youth suicide was connected with depression, why had that illness afflicted young people so suddenly at this moment in history? Witnesses at suicide inquests had often linked depression to life circumstances, including but not limited to economic woes. Responding to the report, the opposition Labour spokesperson for employment proposed that the new government had to share the blame for the tragedies of youth suicides, "as it had done little to encourage employment opportunities among young people."[92] A debate was in play.

The 1993 report stirred up unprecedented reporting, an ironic outcome given that some participants in the workshop had wanted a lid put on reporting. In 1992, the government's newspaper clipping service assembled forty-one stories on suicide; in 1993 there were seventy-three plus thirteen letters to editors. Assessments of the prevention report included one from the Secondary Principals Association that wanted curriculum developments to contribute to happy, well-balanced teenagers.[93] The association's president, Brother Pat Lynch, further recommended that "the spiritual dimension of life needs examining and putting before young people." He added that Spain – presumed by him a country of superior spiritual sensitivities – had a higher youth unemployment rate but a lower youth suicide rate that New Zealand.[94] On countless occasions since the collection of the first national suicide statistics in Europe in the early nineteenth century, spirituality was proclaimed a remedy, and non-comparable data from several countries was adduced to sustain this preconceived argument.

The accent on mental health that accompanied the department's report did not pass without sharp partisan political criticism of the drift toward medicalizing the problem. Opposition leader Michael Moore articulated Labour's stance that suicide was connected to unemployment. In opposition, Bolger had done the same. "The issue is jobs," Moore declared; "people need a reason for getting up in the morning."[95] He had support from mental health expert Dr Max Abbott. Abbott, then dean of Health Studies at Auckland Institute of Technology and president of the World Federation for Mental Health, agreed with the report's statement that youth suicide had "multifactoral causes, but he was disappointed that it downplayed the effect of unemployment."[96] Abbott had a long-standing interest in how the end of New Zealand's years of full employment (roughly 1940 to 1975) affected mental health. In 1982, he edited a collection of academic papers on New Zealand's sudden encounter with unemployment. He mentioned that unemployment was a product not just of redundancies, but of the imposition of barriers to school leavers, tertiary students, and married women. They could not get into the workforce. In the 1960s, the parents of the young of the 1980s and 1990s had easily found employment and had faith in a future.[97] Their children were not all so lucky.

MORE OUTBREAKS, ARGUMENTS, AND ACTION, 1993–2000

Clusters of youth suicides continued to receive national attention. Over a twenty-month period in 1992–93, there were four teenage suicides in the Upper Hutt, and four in Bulls in 1996.[98] In late September of that year, six ministers conducted a "spiritual cleansing" of "the suicide bridge" in Bulls where the four suicides had taken place.[99] Coroners could not help but note clusters of suicides in their jurisdictions. At the same time, there was evidence of planning and action by local and national officials, action more substantial than the ceremony at the bridge. Preparation for helping "suicide survivors" represented a different, earnest stage in the panic. By the middle of the decade, when several suicides came from the same school, a team from Special Education Services moved in to deal with "the cluster suicide phenomenon."[100] Schools had emergency plans for informing and counselling students.

The Department of Corrections joined the list of institutions that studied suicide after the 1993 release of the Department of Health report. Corrections and its research partners – Te Puni Kokiri (the Ministry of Māori Development) and the prison parole board – identified young Māori as a group at elevated risk.[101] In the mid-1990s, nearly half of Māori remand detainees and four out of ten Māori sentenced inmates were under twenty-five years of age. Young Māori suicides in custody were now projected as part of a more general and gloomy turnaround for Māori. It was alleged that Māori used to have a much lower suicide rate than other ethnic groups.[102] That Māori prisoners were at high risk is not in question, but the claim that in prior decades Māori overall had a low suicide rate constitutes another misunderstanding founded on flawed data. No Māori rates before 1950 are reliable on account of under-reporting of Māori deaths generally; in later years and in urban areas, Māori identity was not always indicated on documents.[103] Only in the 1990s, when autopsies and witnesses more routinely identified ethnic background, are counts likely to have been more credible. The entire subject of race and identity when applied to counting people is strewn with pitfalls.

At the same time that schools adopted contingency plans and that young Māori and youth offenders surfaced in discourses about youth suicide, suppression of discussion in the press gained ground. There was a renewed denunciation of public discussion similar to that introduced by David Schaffer. In fact, since the Coroners Act of 1951, coverage on suicide could not mention the method; reports were confined to name, address, occupation, and the coroner's finding.[104] Nevertheless, objections to coverage continued, and they produced ironic consequences. A suicide researcher at Princess Margaret Hospital in Christchurch, Annette Beautrais, alleged that "shutting up" about suicide was a practical step to reduce it. She worried about lurid or dramatic accounts which, based on American research, she felt projected self-destruction as a solution to problems.[105] An episode of the New Zealand soap opera *Shortland Street* featuring a teen suicide was allegedly followed the next day in Christchurch by six suicides rather than the usual one. She took this as a demonstration of the harm of dramatization while remarking, opaquely, that the deleterious influence did not always happen immediately. Her remarks led to more publicity.[106]

Silence became official orthodoxy by the mid-1990s and was accompanied by pious pronouncements that showed how ludicrous it was to attempt to stifle discussion. The Associate Minister of Health with responsibility for the youth suicide portfolio, Katherine O'Regan, stonewalled the press in mid-1996 to deflect criticism that silence was akin to sticking one's head in the sand. She insisted she was exemplifying the idea of silence as prevention. Her press secretary, putting her foot in her mouth, responded to reporters that "Ms O'Regan feels it would be irresponsible to comment because 'the more you discuss it the more people throw themselves off bridges.'"[107] The New Zealand Press Council had itself opposed publishing statements such as "Boys Hang Themselves."[108] Initiatives to silence responsible media discussion were self-defeating and based on contested scholarship that had focused on celebrity suicides.

Annette Beautrais, who had attended the crucial youth suicide meeting in September 1992, had given an interview shortly after the release of the ministry's report in which she challenged the notion that unemployment was responsible for the rise in youth suicide. "If you are psychiatrically ill," she suggested, "you are more likely to be unemployed. It becomes a chicken-and-egg argument."[109] Would psychologists and psychiatrists accept the full dilemma implied in that "chicken-and-egg" puzzle? Would they also accept that "if you are unemployed, you are more likely to be psychiatrically ill?" That is the other half of the problem, as we have suggested in chapter four. In fairness, Beautrais spoke sensibly about the rising youth suicide rate. The reasons "are not clear," she said. Simplistic explanations could not be expected from serious research.[110] During the next fifteen years, her research publications, often based on structured interviews with individuals in Canterbury who had suicide ideation or had attempted suicide, exemplified psychology's best research methods.

In early 1996, following the suicides of two girls at Tuakau College, south of Auckland, television journalist Paul Holmes wanted to broadcast an investigative report. A motion from the school and the Commissioner for Children for a court injunction to bar such a show was upheld by a High Court judge. Opponents of coverage cited the risk of copy-cat suicides. A special education services official told the court that some friends of the deceased students "wanted to join their dead friends."[111] A lack of critical thinking made this position sound plausible; however, the background incidents, as witnesses' statements showed, were well-known to students without media exposure. By keeping details from public view, censorship did protect the families and the school; it also shielded from criticism the idea that more and better counselling could save lives. The facts in the two linked cases actually illustrate how difficult it was to discipline or counsel youngsters when drugs, rebellion, family tension, and juvenile violence were involved.

The first girl, thirteen, experimented with drugs. She told her cousin that "she was 'popping pills.'" The specific incident that most upset her, judging from a suicide note, was a teacher's discovery that she maintained "a friendship book" that "had really disgusting stuff in it about teachers." A teacher also caught her and friends reading "an explicit magazine." None of this was terrible conduct, but she was to be punished. "I HATE THE TEACHERS," she wrote. There was more. In her note, she expressed hatred for an auntie: "I hate her guts." She despised her sister; she wanted to finish with a boyfriend but was intimidated by his older brother. A picture emerges of a vicious environment without a shred of glamour but with every reason to fantasize about escape. A threat to come back and haunt her enemies discloses a casual attitude toward death and the element of vengeance.

Not mentioned at the time was a third related suicide. In the previous year, at the age of fourteen, the first girl's cousin had hanged himself; he had been sexually abused by an uncle, was called a "poof," fought with his parents, experienced "hidings" and verbal abuse, and thus was described as "a sad little boy."[112] At the time of his death he was receiving counselling by a therapist with the Children and Young Persons Service. Acquaintances engaged in so-called "bulk fights" that pitted the young men from Tuakau against others from Otara. The first girl had witnessed this fighting and considered getting a gun to help her brother.[113] Coverage of the second girl's suicide would have disclosed more unpalatable truths, primarily about how drugs had unglamorously possessed her, and how case workers could not get her to clean up. This girl had attempted suicide a year earlier when her father left the family for Australia. She took up petrol sniffing. Her mother had her see a psychologist; a family member wanted a Māori counsellor. The psychologist agreed and stressed the importance of acting promptly. At this point the girl, profoundly uncommunicative, refused to meet with anyone.[114] Censorship may have protected lives, although this is disputable, but it definitely kept from public scrutiny tales of dysfunctional families and the insuperable challenges that sometimes defeated therapists and counsellors. Knowledge of suicide within family and community circles, not public reporting, had promoted the idea of suicide as a solution.

The limitations of attempting the management of youth suicide by psychiatrists and psychologists were apparent to coroners. Several South Island coroners in 1996 felt that the youth suicides that they examined were not adequately explained by the mental health model and they distrusted the notion that suppression of public discussion could serve any good purpose.[115] Their concerns exposed again a clash between medical professionals and informed personnel in the judicial system. Each looked at suicides from a distinct position. Focused on immediate suffering, often mental anguish, medical clinicians and researchers stressed mental health. Listening to witnesses describe social and cultural background problems, and well aware of the shortcomings of medical services through the evidence they saw at inquests, coroners wanted to know more about the lives that the individuals had led, more about peer pressure at school, and more about home life. Ian Smith, coroner for Nelson, wondered if "New Zealand's macho male image" had contributed to some male suicides.[116] It was a bold conjecture, but on the basis of evidence from the files it was a defensible position only requiring refinement. Some self-destructive male conduct was macho, although this was not unique to New Zealand. It developed from a combination of basic biological drives and cultural factors.

Neither the mental-health nor the unemployment explanations satisfied the clergy, who saw suicide as a sign of spiritual emptiness. In mid-1996, the head of the Anglican Church in New Zealand,

Archbishop Brian Davis, indicted "economic wealth and technological progress" for their fundamental materialism. "Material wealth is not enough to nourish the deep needs of human beings." Churches needed to help re-establish community. Capitalism was here to stay; government could not do everything to soften its hard edges. As he saw it, young people were questioning authority, morality, meaning, and purpose. Without Christian values to guide them, some arrived at the wrong answers or simply did not care about any answers. "They get their kicks where they can."[117] In the next chapter we develop the last point about getting one's kicks, but the prelate underestimated the morale-sapping impact of unemployment. In the materialist culture, material rewards counted toward a satisfaction with life and their absence promoted dissatisfaction.

CONCLUDING OBSERVATIONS

New Zealand's youth suicide panic suggests trends in the country's social, medical, and political history. First, even before the panic, many careers were associated with addressing the troubles of young people: social workers, psychologists, psychiatrists, youth-aid police officers, church ministers, school counsellors, and youth advocates. Psychologists had been increasing their fields of activity since the 1960s; in succeeding decades their appeals that society take more notice of their behaviour modification skills increased.[118] When newspaper reporters looked for people to comment on an apparent rash of youth suicides, they had no trouble finding well-read and often experienced authorities. Second, many psychiatrists and psychologists simultaneously favoured containing public discussion, dismissing the impact of culture and economics on suicide, and elevating a mental-illness understanding of the act. The epistemic models of these disciplines advanced the idea of explanatory frameworks rather than sensitivity to the context of individual cases. As a result, suicide research became statistical and remote, and that was the way medical professionals wanted it. They may not have owned up to it, but secretiveness kept them safe from questions about therapies and their effectiveness.

Third, there was political capital to earn from getting out front on the topic; Jenny Shipley did that capably. Politicians afterwards were in the frame; some wanted to speak and were heard; others wanted to speak and were ignored; and some wanted to remain silent but then faced embarrassment.[119] In a significant political development, the Department of Health took over the subject. Fourth, there emerged a divide between those researchers who accented the effects of New Zealand's economic crisis and those who highlighted mental illness. The latter were ascendant. Fifth, people familiar with many cases of youth suicide asserted the individuality of motives and the distinctiveness of the individuals' reasoning processes. Despite such unpromising terrain for the medical and social sciences, there was an outpouring of sophisticated research on youth suicide and suicide in general, and the launching of a series of suicide prevention programs. Finally, the panic showed the country's incorporation into the geographically distant but culturally close "Western world." So-called developed countries provided the standard of comparison; experts from abroad offered opinions. New Zealand was among the affluent countries that provided counselling and therapy.

In an unpublicized step, the New Zealand police were advised in a 1985 study by a psychologist and a police chief superintendent that "it would be helpful if regular procedures for the documentation of personal and social factors in suicide were given the same structured attention as the legal and medical."[120] Some police officers working with coroners responded and inquest files ballooned. The next chapter uses the more extensive inquest evidence to explain the rise in youth suicides.

7

What Is Happening to Our Children? Youth Suicides 1980–2000

In this chapter we explain the upsurge in youth suicides by analyzing witness statements and suicide notes extracted from more than a thousand youth suicide cases (males = 924; females = 218). The explanatory argument is that rising rates of youth suicide are best studied in relation to deep changes to the culture and economy which coalesced in 'a perfect storm' bearing down directly and suddenly on young people. New Zealand, along with many "Western societies," had moved toward consumerism after World War II. Where materialism had strengthened but the economy was faltering, the moral disorientation and nihilism of some young people is understandable. The increase in youth suicide that alarmed so many people at the time, provoked public controversy, and advanced the medicalization of suicide was a particularly cheerless summary of epic cultural and economic changes.

Before going further, it is important to establish what is meant by youth, and to indicate how many cases were found in even-numbered years for each component age group. Youth comprises three phases on the life-course: pre-adolescents (up to and including the age of 14; 45 cases), adolescents (15 to 19; 415 cases), and young adults (20 to 24; 682 cases). Youth suicides are best understood by keeping these phases in mind. Unfortunately, New Zealand studies and statistical reports generally have not followed the practice of researchers in the United States, who concentrated on fifteen- to nineteen-year-olds when writing about youth suicide. New Zealand reports included twenty- to twenty-four-year-olds, the age group with the highest suicide rates in New Zealand during the 1980s and the 1990s (Graphs 7.1 and 7.2).[1] By defining youth to include what were really young adults, researchers introduced a bias that connected youth suicides to mental illness. Mental illness cases were over-represented in this mature youth group relative to the other two age groups. There is another age-related observation worth mentioning. Seldom were pre-adolescents discussed in the New Zealand literature. Academic studies and press reports truncated the concept of youth at one end of the life-course and stretched it at the other.

Our data disclose that mental illness was a prominent motive for young adults, but less so for adolescents (Table 7.1). Mental illness per se had been and remained disproportionately an older person's burden. A substantial portion of mental illness motives among youth suicides consisted of their suffering what appeared to be clinical depression; additionally, witnesses described a substantial number of young people as depressed. As we have seen in chapter six, depression covered symptoms that could originate from assorted stresses. For young people in the 1980s and 1990s, anxiety included failure at school, unemployment and under-employment, and the trauma of parents separating. Competition played out in school hallways and on playing fields, with physical appearance, unpopularity, and rejection humiliating a few students.

Studies by psychiatrists and psychologists packed substance abuse, delinquency, and disruptive behaviour into their big hamper of mental illnesses; however, we coded substance abuse as a separate matter, and placed outbursts of temper, impulsiveness, evidence of extreme jealousy, low self-esteem, youth rebellion, unhappiness at home or school, and social isolation into categories other than mental illness.[2] We branded some of these latter motives character and adjustment issues, and resisted the tendency of psychiatrists and psychologists to identify many kinds of conduct as mental disorders, including alcohol or substance dependence and anti-social behaviour. Labelling depends on perspective, not an exact science. Thus, in a report on a patient in 2000, a general practitioner wrote that the man "had no mental illness to my knowledge but was a heavy drinker."[3]

Advocates of the clinical approach inverted relationships between social stresses and disorders. "Life events in the year before death," asserted the authors of one study, "must be examined with caution: separation, change in habits, and moving can all be attributed to personality disorders, depression, or substance abuse. They may even be helpful at the clinical level, serving as possible suicide risk indicators."[4] If suicide stems from disorders of an autonomous or biochemical origin, why was there a sudden change in age rate late in the century? Moreover, most motives that we identified could not be deemed mental illnesses by any stretch of the Diagnostic and Statistical Manual. It is possible to argue that self-destruction is *ipso facto* a sign of mental illness, but such a simplification obscures the meditative processes undertaken by many suicidal people and removes from scrutiny the conduct of people around the deceased.

It is useful to break down the clusters of leading motives into constituent parts. For adolescents in the 1980s and 1990s, the leading alcohol and drug abuse problems were heavy drinking, heavy drinking with violence, drug abuse, and drug and alcohol abuse combined. The most important work and finance problems were unemployment and attendant worries, financial difficulties, and anxiety about job security. Additionally for this age group, there were school pressures. A fair number of males aged fifteen to twenty-four were reported as unemployed or as welfare recipients. The percentage described this way at inquests soared in the 1990s, but it has to be added that young adults were not alone in suffering during an economic crisis.

The end-of-century economic and cultural transformations affected mature men too, and they deserve attention before we turn to youth. To personify numbers captured in a summary table (Table 7.2), we can cite examples. To represent men in their prime experiencing the woes of economic adjustments, there was thirty-three-year-old Kevin Wilson, who lost his job on the docks in 1999. He went for months on unemployment benefits and "was finding this frustrating." But there was more. His alcoholism – "he could not get off the piss" – and a failed relationship are reminders that problems accumulated. He had been prescribed Prozac for depression; the diagnosis and medication call to mind the derivative nature of depression in an untold number of mental health cases.[5] His problems – no work, alcoholism, a failed relationship, and depression – were consistent with the leading troubles for men in his phase of life. We can mention too forty-seven-year-old alcoholic George Parsons. Driven home from a pub by his wife, he broke down and cried, because "he couldn't pay his bills anymore and was fed up with working."[6]

Economic distress was on the increase while romantic disappointment persisted as a leading motive for suicide among men in their prime. Looks depressed some young adult males. Geoffrey Howard

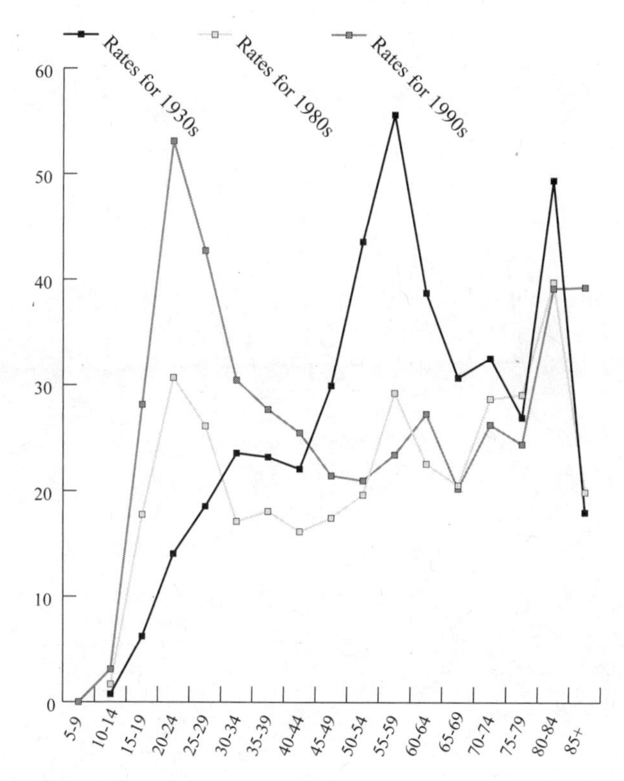

Graph 7.1
Rates of male suicides by age groups, 1930s, 1980s, 1990s

"would talk about his physical appearance like he was very unhappy about it." To compensate he drank and smoked to excess.[7] Living on his own, thirty-year-old Toby Agnew wrote to his cousin that "I don't know if you can imagine what its like to never to have anyone fall in love with you. I hate every night. I have to go to bed alone and every morning I wake up alone." "Severe cystic acne lesions" left him feeling "ugly and inadequate." He mentioned four women as "such good friends."[8] Once we pass beyond men in their prime with their array of troubles, the pattern of suicide motives shifts to difficulties that had bothered seniors throughout the century. Older men, such as seventy-year-old Brian Rivers, faced serious illnesses. Rivers was taking morphine on a daily basis for lung cancer and was understandably described as depressed.[9] Depression persisted as a troublesome term, an effect that could have diverse concrete origins.

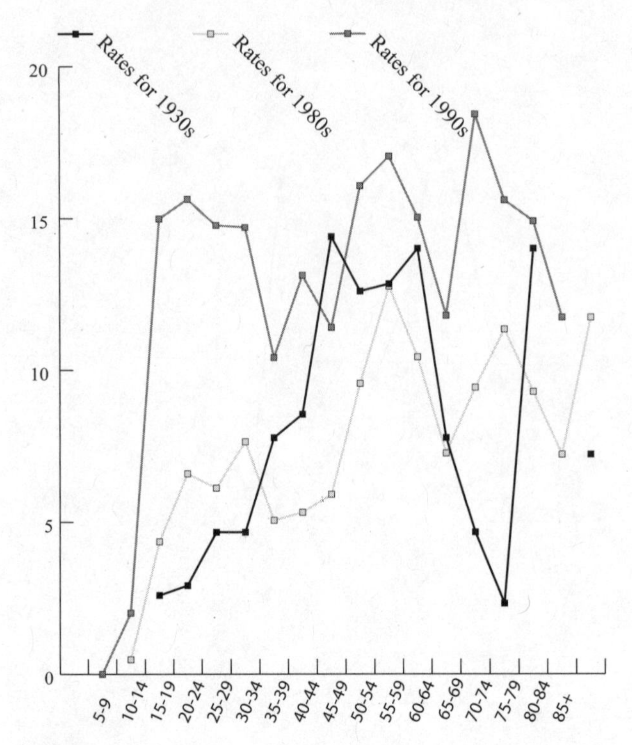

Graph 7.2
Rates of female suicides by age groups, 1930s, 1980s, 1990s

OUT THE DOOR IN A BURST OF PASSION: PRE-ADOLESCENT MALES

Suicides by pre-adolescent males were rare in the late twentieth century and always had been. As in past decades, their motives mainly pertained to arguments with parents or setbacks contributing to low self-worth.[10] Thomas Joiner in *Why People Die by Suicide* proposed that "the facile explanation that parents are responsible for their children's death by suicide because of high demands is hardly worth considering."[11] Yet, the enforcement of high expectations and poor parenting did appear in the case files. Joiner adds that the young people already perceived themselves as not measuring up. What is left out of this portrayal is the path to low self-esteem. Somehow these individuals acquired feelings of emptiness, perhaps from well-meaning volleys of prior criticism. The sudden rise in youth suicide

Table 7.1
Motives for male youth suicides, 1980s and 1990s (* = over-represented)

Motive cluster	*1980s* 9–14	*1990s* 9–14	*1980s* 15–19	*1990s* 15–19	*1980s* 20–24	*1990s* 20–24	*1980s all other ages*	*1990s all other ages*
Alcohol and drugs	2 (18.2%)	1 (4.8%)	17 (13.1%)*	7 (3.7%)	12 (5.6%)	15 (4.2%)	49 (4.6%)	85 (5.7%)
Work and finance	0	1 (4.8)	22 (16.9%)*	24 (12.8%)*	19 (8.8%)	38 (10.6%)	115 (10.7%)	169 (11.3%)
Marital and romantic problems	1 (9.1%)	0	21 (17.7%)*	39 (33.5%)	36 (25.0%)	111 (34.8%)*	178 (16.6%)	303 (20.2%)
Physical ailments	0	1 (4.8%)	5 (3.8%)	2 (1.1%)	12 (5.6%)	11 (3.1%)	188 (17.5%)	202 (13.5%)
Mental illness	0	0	16 (12.3%)	21 (11.2%)	54 (25.0%)	90 (25.1%)	343 (31.9%)*	412 (27.5%)*
Character and adjustment	4 (36.4%)	2 (9.5%)	23 (17.7%)*	28 (14.9%)*	14 (6.5%)	21 (5.9%)	36 (3.4%)	78 (5.2%)
Law and order	0	1 (4.8%)	7 (5.4%)	24 (12.8%)*	19 (8.8%)*	26 (7.3%)	52 (4.8%)	123 (8.2%)
Death of someone close	1 (9.1%)	1 (4.8%)	3 (2.3%)	6 (3.2%)	6 (2.8%)	7 (2.0%)	45 (4.2%)	40 (2.7%)
Family issues apart from marriage	0	9 (42.9%)*	5 (3.8%)	17 (9.0%)	6 (2.8%)	7 (2.0%)	9 (0.1%)	28 (1.9%)
Unknown	3 (27.3%)	3 (14.3%)	11 (8.5%)	20 (10.6%)	27 (12.5%)	30 (8.4%)	67 (6.2%)	59 (3.9%)
Total	11	21	130	188	216	358	1,074	1,499

Table 7.2
Motives for adult male suicides, 1980s and 1990s (* = over-represented)

Motive cluster	*25–54 (Prime of life)*	*55–64 (Transition years)*	*65 plus (Seniors)*
Alcohol and drugs	122 * (6.6%)	19 (4.7%)	9 (1.7%)
Work and finance	214 * (11.6%)	58 (14.4%)	19 (3.6%)
Marital relationships and romantic	456 * (24.8%)	40 (9.9%)	19 (3.6%)
Physical ailments	106 (5.8%)	67 (16.6%)	248 * (46.4%)
Mental illness	556 (30.3%)	132 (32.8%)	118 (22.1%)
Character and adjustment	74 (4.0%)	17 (4.2%)	18 (3.4%)
Law and order	139 (7.6%)	25 (6.2%)	17 (3.2%)
Death of someone close	134 (7.3%)	36 (8.9%)	65 * (12.2%)
Family issues apart from marriage	13 (0.7%)	3 (0.7%)	15 (2.2%)
War-related troubles	0	1 (0.2%)	1 (0.2%)
Unknown	24 (1.3%)	5 (1.2%)	5 (0.9%)
Total	1,838	403	534

rates at the end of the century puts the ball back in the court of material conditions and concrete situations. Case files show that anxiety about the future in a period of economic troubles could contribute to despair, while altercations within the family over work and parental expectations could be precipitating events in the suicides of pre-adolescent and adolescent males.[12] There was also a special circumstance operating in a few cases during the first half of the twentieth century. Some farmers adopted boys for their labour and worked them hard. Ted Driscoll adopted Brian Roland through a newspaper advertisement.[13] When an adopted son refused to clear scrub, his farmer father told him "to pack his swag and look for another job."[14] Biological sons were also told to get out. One Māori farmer "got into a temper" when his son neglected the cows. He told the boy to clear out.[15] Joiner's admonition to focus on the low self-esteem of victims and avoid bringing parents into the dynamics of situations has problems; from a professional standpoint it steers aspirations for prevention toward the clinical treatment of the individual.

By the end of the century, the altercations between farm lads and supervising adults had given way to volatile confrontations in urban homes. The late-twentieth-century case files showed instances when parents rebuked a son or daughter at mealtime in front of the family. Events then flowed in a continuous outburst without interludes for reflection. In the late twentieth century, the explosive sequence began with a parental condemnation of laziness, a theft, a lie, an unauthorized party, a sexual encounter, the harassment of a sibling, or a lapse in school studies.[16] Maurice Hill's father told the coroner that "I once suggested that he take a job." The tone of voice can be imagined. Maurice's report card noted that he could "try harder."[17] Impulsiveness frequently stands out; harsh words precipitated a sudden flight. Robbie McLay had ignored his mother's instructions and "became cheeky." She slapped his face. He dashed from the house. He may not have intended to kill himself, but conceived of an attempted hanging in hope of a timely intervention and an outpouring of a mother's remorse.[18] A family altercation precipitated Gregory Mahler's sudden act. His father had "chewed him out" for holding a party against family rules while his parents were away. He was given "a good telling off," grounded for two weeks, restricted in his use of the telephone, and sent to his room.[19] The mother of fourteen-year-old Shaun Grey argued with him about his friends: "he went to his room."[20] Nine-year-old Graham Goodwin hanged himself directly after an argument with his brother. He placed a suicide note next to his baby picture and wrote that his family would find his body but not his spirit.[21] He thus expressed a notion of a soul that was not unusual among suicides.

After a dressing-down by his father for snatching something from his sister's room, an action that greatly upset her, thirteen-year-old James McCullen shouted a reply, dashed into the garage, slammed the door shut, and hanged himself.[22] The father of another thirteen-year-old, a Polynesian, wanted his son to succeed at school and scolded him at dinner for missing classes due to sports. "Dad never hit him and we gave him the best any parent can give."[23] On account of his failure to complete farm chores, the father of fourteen-year-old Tim Muir reprimanded the boy for wasting time at his computer. As a disciplinary measure, the father removed the keyboard and mouse. Muir was younger and smaller than his classmates, who had mercilessly bullied him. Unbeknownst to his parents, the computer had been his solace.[24] A strict disciplinarian, the father of fourteen-year-old Alec Stokes could get "very angry" with his sons; he barred Alec from seeing his girlfriend. A social worker felt that the boy's "wish to see the girlfriend was the major issue for him." For the parents, alcohol, drugs, and burglary were issues.[25]

Fifteen-year-old Daryl Johansson took a stern lecture from his father about poor school results in mathematics and English; then an argument erupted over dereliction of domestic chores.[26] Daniel Campbell was sixteen when he shot himself. His rashness reminds us of the immaturity of some adolescents. He had argued with his parents over skipping school.[27] Precipitating events in the suicide of sixteen-year-old Jason Capner at Takapuna, a death mentioned in chapter six that touched off a youth suicide panic, conformed to a tragic pattern of over-reaction to a scolding. His parents accepted his Goth affectations as a stage he was going through, but his mother criticized him about his slovenliness and he ignored her. His father gave him a telling-off. If he wanted to go out with friends, he had to work around the house and get his hair cut.[28] When his close friend Marc Hitchcock committed suicide two months later, he gave directions that his dreadlocks remain for the funeral.[29] Assertions of independence clashed with parental ideas of responsible conduct. Suicide was the ultimate defiance.

The suicide of sixteen-year-old Greg Maclean in 1996 is notable. He was not a pre-adolescent; however, like many pre-adolescent cases, his act occurred in a successful, loving family. The boy's parents were teachers; another son had excelled at school, now he had to do so. They pressured him to break off his association with a girl to concentrate better on studies. Maclean told a friend that he really liked this girl, but he could not go out with her again. He added: "If I killed myself it wouldn't be because of her." He put the responsibility on his parents.[30] The preceding suicides were by immature boys whose parents acted like many others in common situations; they rebuked their sons for conduct that upset the household. Ill-calculated bids for sympathy or blows to parents were mixed into motivations for a fair portion of youthful rash acts. Similar motives were behind a handful of adolescent suicides as well.

In a few cases, boys came from dysfunctional families that had inflicted emotional damage. The life of Michael Mains introduces an array of delinquent events that hint at the harm meted out by his mother's abandonment and his father's violence. A child welfare case worker felt that Michael "has seen and been involved with violence all his life." At the age of eight he orchestrated a dog attack on a constable; at eleven he robbed a Melbourne bank with a sawed-off shotgun and was so small that he could barely haul away the loot. When he was thirteen Michael set fire to his school and was sentenced to Weymouth Boys Home. Teachers and youth counsellors described him as amoral, cold, vengeful, and ruthless. One of them "greatly feared for what he might become." Nevertheless, in keeping with the anti-authoritarian attitudes in psychology and counselling at the time, his case workers pleaded with him to stop putting them in a corner where they had to be "disciplinarians." Michael had few opportunities to develop goodness. According to one assessment, he had a "long-standing fantasy that his parents will get back together and he will live with them." To help achieve this flight of imagination he conspired to break up new relationships entered into by either parent. He craved an exclusive embrace that could never be proffered. Frustration and his father's example contributed to his sociopathology.

In late 1988, at the age of fourteen, Mains hanged himself at a residential home for socially and emotionally disturbed youths. Several witnesses wondered if he had been playing at hanging himself and had merely slipped. This perplexing case merits attention.[31] First, it is flush with evidence about a habituation to violence and pain. In this sense, Mains' suicide has more in common with some by older men. He had grown up fast and hard. Second, upheavals in Mains' family and his apparent longing for his parents to live together with him suggest nurturing denied. It surfaced often at youth inquests. Unable to access case-level information, some sociologists have employed aggregate data on church attendance as a surrogate variable for family dissolution and have conjectured that the latter is a determinant in youth suicide.[32] We have entered broken homes by the front door.

If suicide follows from combinations of social and psychological factors, then these crucial circumstances can frequently be located in the family. The economic crises of the late twentieth century are only part of any consideration of a loss of self-worth. On occasion, even prior to 1980, academic aspirations combined with an unexpected setback led a youth to feel worthless.[33] However, this phenomenon appeared relatively more often in the era of economic crises. Driven by parents to stand first, a brilliant student with an IQ of 149 wrote, "as for my being brainy, I've never heard anything so ironical. So far this year my work has been extremely shoddy."[34] Many of the rare pre-adolescent suicides disclose precipitating arguments that could erupt in any caring family. Radically different were the instances of exceedingly dysfunctional families such as that of Michael Mains. Less extreme cases of bad parenting and love denied were not common but did appear. The tragic case of twelve-year-old Kelly Morrison illustrates vividly emotional pain and its likely parental source. His Samoan father had died in a street fight ten years earlier. "I had a few rocky relationships," his mother admitted. She disciplined Kelly by yelling and smacking him; at school he drew a picture symbolizing his plight as he saw it (Figure 7.1).[35]

THE ECONOMIC HYPOTHESIS FOR YOUTH SUICIDE

Placing pre-adolescents in a separate category clears the way for an evaluation of adolescents and young adults, and a test of the proposition that there are social costs attending a sudden shift in government policy to address a sovereign debt crisis and to stimulate growth. Clearly, pre-adolescents were not entering the workforce. New Zealand provides an appropriate setting for a study of the consequences of retrenchment, because in the span of roughly two years it went from the most regulated and protected OECD economy to the least controlled.[36] The male suicide rate, which climbed during economic restructuring, rose most for young adults, suggesting but by no means proving a connection (Graph 7.3). We judge that bleak economic circumstances had a demoralizing effect on adolescents and young adults. A straightforward argument blaming economic restructuring for the rising suicide rate is unachievable, however, because retrenchment and restructuring coincided with a period when the sexual revolution and youth autonomy were working their way through the country's domestic culture, when hard drug and cannabis use were increasing, when young offenders were prominent in remand centres and prisons, and when mental health services were in upheaval.

To sort events and pose an argument, this chapter first reviews the highlights of restructuring and conventional evidence for retrenchment's adverse impact on the young. It then considers the impact of the following: the sexual revolution and youth autonomy;

encounters with the law; mental health factors; and hazardous living and the drug abuse scene. We then reintroduce the economic crises and conclude with several pessimistic observations about suicide prevention efforts.

From the late 1940s to the mid-1970s, New Zealand experienced an intermittent boom, writes Bronwyn Dalley, "and it lay behind much of the comfort of this period."[37] Farm exports were the key to this period of "the golden weather." New Zealand had little recent experience with unemployment until the late 1970s. The hiring practices of large state enterprises, including insurance, railways, and communications, helped mop up unemployment. An array of trade controls and industry subsidies, including price supports for agricultural commodities, had originated with the First Labour Government, elected in 1936 and especially active after re-election in 1938. The managed economy with its many state enterprises had worked well enough in periods of high farm prices and low production costs. Farmers received subsidies to offset tariff protection for manufacturers. A combination of external shocks hit the county hard; these jolts included the 1973 oil crisis and the end to the United Kingdom's preference for New Zealand produce, a change that started when the UK entered the Common Market.[38] Farm subsidies evolved into income support to an unsustainable extent.[39]

By the early 1980s, the number of jobs for unskilled and semiskilled workers on farms, at freezer [meat] works, in forestry, and coal mining declined (Graph 7.3). As for alternative work, a 1987 regional report described conditions that applied to several other areas: "employment developments have not developed."[40] Urban labour markets were awash with rural and city unemployed. Auckland was especially affected (Graph 7.4).[41] Social impact studies reported that health workers had increased stress-counselling case loads.[42]

The dollar came under pressure and inflation climbed in the early 1980s. An interlude of state-financed industrial diversification schemes, the "Think Big" projects (1981–84) of National Party Prime Minister Robert Muldoon, and assorted make-work projects postponed a severe employment crisis but increased foreign borrowing and expanded government departments unrealistically (Graph 7.5).[43] Pessimism and cynicism among the young erupted in the early 1980s.[44] In 1981, the government-financed National Youth Council published a booklet to inform young people about unemployment

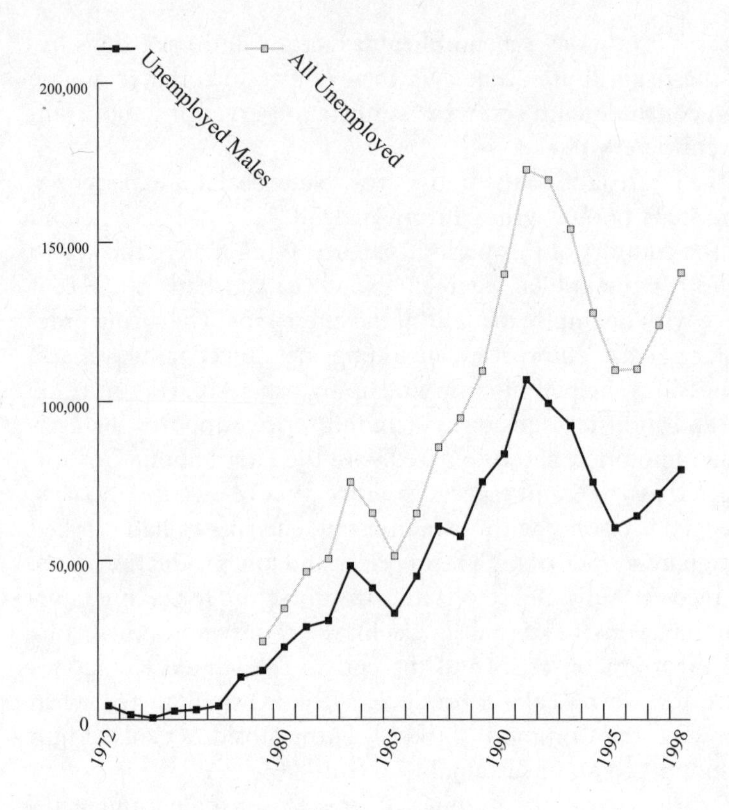

Graph 7.3
Unemployed males and all unemployed, 1972–98

benefits, but its covert goal was to blame the government for greater job losses than officially reported.[45] "Will you be staying on in school or going straight into redundancy?" asked a character in one of the publication's illustrations.[46] Grounds for sardonic remarks increased after the Labour Government came into office in mid-1984.

This new government confronted multiple economic crises by abruptly adopting neo-liberal economic policies. Retrenchment plus restructuring continued into the mid-1990s under a National Party government.[47] Criticized as a "blitzkrieg" of insensitive liberalization that brought no swift improvements, or defended as a revolution that established the basis for later prosperity, the new path remains controversial.[48] It was initially the handiwork of Finance Minister Roger Douglas, whose program became known as "Rogernomics."[49] Rogernomics affected young people materially and emotionally. The

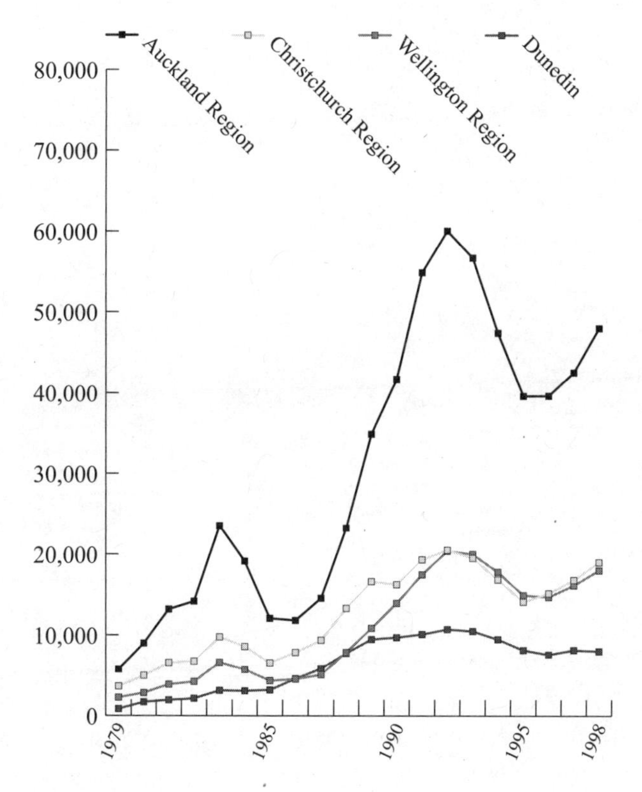

Graph 7.4
Unemployed in major urban areas, 1979–97

reorganization of state enterprises put these entities on corporate operating principles.

Alterations hurt youth employment, because school leavers previously could have expected a position with a state company or government department. New state-operated enterprises placed a premium on the balance sheet, not on national full employment, which had been part of the remit of the former government departments.[50] The closing of post offices and reduction in public works meant several years of job losses.[51] Coal mining and forestry included substantial government operations that soon shed jobs. Not surprisingly, resource-based communities reported that half their registered unemployed were under twenty-five.[52] In remote North Island regions, it was claimed that "the majority of Maori people, young and middle-aged, are in Labour Department

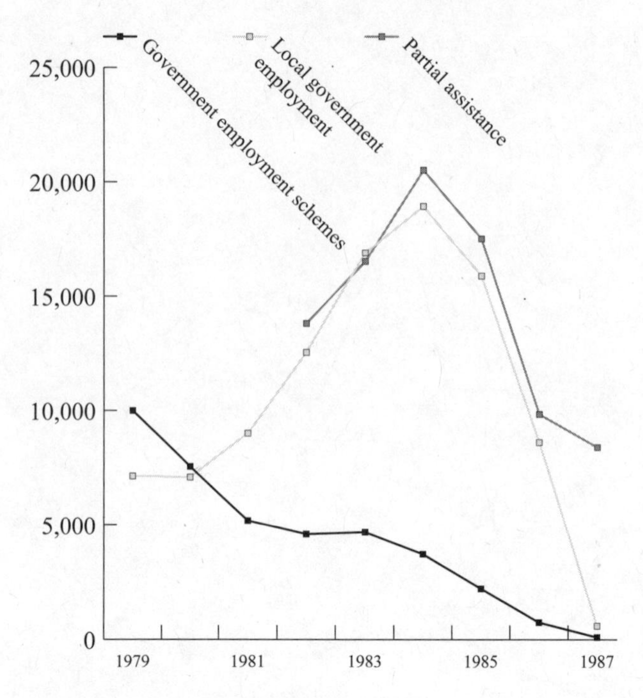

Graph 7.5
Numbers employed by government assistance programs, 1979–87

funded work schemes."[53] Labour curtailed these programs (Graph 7.5).[54] Private companies, meanwhile, worried about the future and deferred hiring. Retrenchment in government departments, corporatisation, the termination of make-work projects, and private sector caution worsened the circumstances of young people coming into the employment market.[55]

Before we go further, the long-running gender difference in suicide rates for New Zealand requires a warning. The gender gap in suicides does not measure relative gender suffering. Male suicides expose the alarming capacity of men to harm women psychologically and physically. On account of an entrenched attitude that men were breadwinners, the close association of completed male suicides to economic booms and recessions is noteworthy. There was public discussion about the origins of the rise in youth suicide. Government critics blamed the economy or restructuring (Figure 7.2); psychiatrists and psychologists alleged it was almost wholly a product of mental illness.[56]

The economic crisis in New Zealand at the end of the twentieth century was the worst since the Great Depression, but the traits of suicidal people and of their misfortunes differed. The age data for male suicides in the 1980s and 1990s (Graphs 7.1 and 7.2) accent the youth aspect. There was an occupational shift too. During the Great Depression, the population most at risk consisted of middle-aged rural males. Farmers and farm labourers then had a suicide rate double that for all other males. Rural men were less prominent among the suicides of the 1980s and 1990s. Social security beneficiaries, absent in the 1930s, appeared prominently, particularly in the early 1990s when the initial reforms were pushed further.[57] The impressions of distress from the 1930s are of older farmers anxious about their debts, and older farm labourers facing destitution and coping with work-curtailing ailments or injuries.[58] At the end of the century, the image is of young men and a few women dwelling in urban flats, surviving on social assistance, and losing hope about the future.

At century's end, inquests disclose the striking phenomenon of suicides among unemployed yet financially assisted youths. Older men facing redundancy notices had ways of coping with a downturn unavailable during the Great Depression. Some could retire with pensions and redundancy payouts; some hard-pressed farmers could sell assets. Unlike in the Great Depression, mature men affected by the late-twentieth-century crises had more opportunities for avoiding destitution or charity, but redundancy notices left bitterness. Forestry and coal mining communities were hit hard.[59] The government's policy was to assist with adjustment, not to compensate. As for young people, the economic crisis inflicted psychological setbacks that welfare could not cover, because young men and women could neither look back on the enjoyment of good times nor sense short-term improvement.

Work figured in self-esteem. As a psychologist working at a Child and Family Centre in 1988 expressed it, "most of the kids ... worry a lot. They fear not getting a job which they believe gives them an identity in society."[60] Work provided the money, beyond welfare, to attain goals, but there was more to work than that. In 1988, a feature newspaper article on youth unemployment mentioned "the need people have to work. It is how most of us define ourselves – and also how we achieve social status as well as a reasonable living standard."[61] Witnesses at inquests repeated analogous sentiments.

Getting a first job had become difficult, a fact that adds to the list of differences between this crisis and the Great Depression. Traditionally, career days at schools put employers in contact with young potential workers. School and university guidance counsellors in the late 1980s noted that more students than ever signed up for sessions with employers, but the number of employers arriving with jobs was falling. A school counsellor in 1988 expressed the consequences: "I get a lot of lost souls ... who don't know what they're going to do."[62] Without a job and a girl, claimed one desperate young man in 1996, "my life is fucked."[63] His sentiment and language were not unusual among youth suicide notes.

Secondary literature, conventional documentary sources, and qualitative evidence extracted from inquests support the idea that a serious crisis in morale was a social cost of retrenchment and restructuring. However, when we analyzed suicide motives based on our coding of the case files, a complicated picture emerged. To understand motives better, we considered that youth could comprise three groups: pre-adolescents (up to and including the age of 14), adolescents (15 to 19), and young adults (20 to 24). Pre-adolescents had distinct problems of identity, independence, and schooling. Their suicides were rare; work was not an issue. Adolescents, however, confronted broken relationships, work and finance difficulties, and trouble with authorities. Young adult males had the highest suicide rates in New Zealand during the 1980s and the 1990s.[64] The most startling increase in the proportion of suicide motives for this substantial group involved marital or romantic factors. Mental illnesses, always a prominent but problematic factor, remained important although essentially unchanging in their prominence (Table 7.1). Complications and nuances merit attention before we return to unemployment and propose that it often underlay or exacerbated other troubles. We quote from well-documented cases in order to project sounds and language. A mere "for-instance" method is avoided by citing the graphs and tables to address the bias of selection when choosing statements.

THE COMPLICATIONS OF THE SEXUAL REVOLUTION AND YOUTH AUTONOMY

The ongoing sexual revolution, a liberalized divorce law [1970], and newly created family courts [1982] touched the intimate lives of many.[65] It became easier in these decades to dissolve a marriage or acquire rights in a de facto relationship. By 1990, forty percent of the country's marriages ended in divorce or separation; the proportion was higher among Māori and lower among the conservative Christian Pacific Islanders.[66] Divorce upset young people's home environments. Concurrently, the sexual revolution altered youth relationships and extended young people's sense of autonomy. Some adults were freed from failed marriages, but men and women still suffered piercing emotional trauma from separations and, pertinent for this chapter, dissolutions added to adolescents' emotional burdens.

Marital separation left young people in the lurch or witnessing households of bitterness. This generation was the first to grow up amidst a substantial number of fractured families. With that came a weaker sense of security. David Prince, fifteen in 1990, told a school friend that "he got on really well with his father but thought that his stepmother was a bit of a bitch." "He wanted his real mother around. It was like he resented his stepmother taking his real mother's place."[67] "Dad this is not your fault," wrote Bill Weston. "I may not approve of your dizzy, bimbo, BONK, but that is obviously none of my business. I'm just sick of shit happening to me."[68] Derek Snell's drug and alcohol abuse with attendant mental illness began in 1992 "when his parents were separating and he began to present with unusual behaviour."[69] Outbursts of obscenity and contempt seem vastly more common in these decades. Ex-girlfriends were bitches; parents were arse holes; the world was shit; talk was shit; and the attitude was fuck you.[70] Coarse language accompanied rage. "Fuck my parents," wrote one youth who insisted that a Bleeding Hearts song entitled "Obituary" be played at his funeral, "cos' its Fuckin HEAVY."[71] Citing the lyrics from an unspecified song, biker gang member Lane Walters asked "Fuck, Fuck Fucken world, why do you treat me this way/What's in store for the next day/Is it glory or is it pain?"[72]

Low self-esteem began with under-achievement at school, a circumstance unmitigated when a household was in turmoil. A few parents were distracted with their own lives. When a loving parent was missing, the emotional battering from self-criticism over failure to clear hurdles at school or work penetrated deeply. Young males looked for maternal love, and wanted their fathers to be proud. Separation and divorce upset nurturing.[73] Brian Street's parents separated.

He definitely missed his mother, but she refused to see him "every second weekend because it was straining her [new] relationship."[74]

Many adolescent males in the 1980s and 1990s took on the challenge of locating a mate or sex partner. Some grossly mishandled these relationships, threatening, verbally abusing, or beating teen partners.[75] By the time he was thirty in 2000, Kevin King had "had several unsuccessful female relationships and fathered three children by different mothers."[76] At the end of the century, a coroner who had seen many youth suicides remarked that "it is sad to see such an intense relationship at such a young age. A break-up of such a relationship could have tragic circumstances as it has in this case."[77] A relationship's dissolution precipitated rage. Troubles had a straightforward makeup. Time after time, young men could not accept a break-up (Table 7.1; Figure 7.3).[78] Seeing his girlfriend with his best friend was more than Wayne Tuckett could stand.[79] Nineteen-year-old unemployed Māori factory labourer Graham Craig spent his days drinking, watching videos, and "continually talking about the break up with his girlfriend."[80]

A few young men threatened suicide to retain their girlfriends or de facto partners.[81] One young woman's testimony held a common refrain. "I told him that I would leave him if we couldn't get over our problems, and he told me he would kill himself if I left him."[82] When threats failed, young men acted rashly to impose a burden of pain and guilt on the other party. In another case, a young woman declined renewing a relationship. "He said, 'well I'm going to kill myself.'"[83] Men seemed prone to using suicidal gestures, then some followed them by action to show they meant it.[84] Break-ups and their fatal consequences were evident in prior decades, but the end-of-century increase in frequency is important.

The sexual revolution combined with the durability of traditional gender roles to establish a distinct pattern of crises for young women. Marital relations, romantic misadventures, character and adjustment issues, family disputes, and mental illness were the principal motives for their suicides. Troubles could often be assigned to a headlong pursuit of young men. During this quest, young women could be upset by a self-assessment of their looks, by the conduct of their boyfriends, and by parental discipline. Older values were maintained by some parents in the midst of the sexual revolution. For most of the century, virginity was a quality of importance to girls, and certainly to parents.[85] By the 1990s, a few girls were dating and having sex almost as soon as they reached double-digit years. The looser attitudes that gathered steam through the 1960s and 1970s left young women painfully aware of their appearance. They could fall for the message from commercials and films that a better body meant a better life.[86] A few felt that looks accounted for their rejection by cliques of girls and, as they grew older, by boys. Fifteen-year-old Susan Harper, who had changed schools, found it difficult to make friends, and rebelled by wearing "way out sort of clothes" and smoking cannabis. She hoped that when the dentist removed her braces she would look completely different and life would change. The results disappointed.[87]

Loneliness, self-criticism, and hope for a reshaped body were common, and there were additional romantic hazards. A number of girls and young women pursued boys and men with an ardour that placed them on noisy collision courses with parents. Where parents were missing, neglectful, or in conflict, young girls turned to intense relationships outside the home. Once these dissolved, they had little to fall back on. That was the case with fifteen-year-old Elizabeth Williams, who came from a broken home and clung onto her boyfriend. She told friends that "she hurt too much to go on without Ryan."[88] A friend of a recently jilted Polynesian girl told police that she "has tried to commit suicide before. It was about the same thing. It was involving another guy." She fell for them completely because "her mother didn't seem to care for her." Another witness said she "really needed her mum to show her some love."[89] In their haste for love, a few women accepted unworthy mates. With revealing insensitivity, Joyce Bailey's boyfriend described their tempestuous relationship as one in which she became upset, drank until she became "blotto," and then "you know going on about me not loving her and that sort of thing."[90] To improve his relationship with his twenty-one-year-old de facto, an argumentative and violent man alleged that "he had cleaned up his act." "I gave up sport, my job, and drugs to please her." He did not give up violence.[91]

Pre-adolescent and adolescent males had fiery encounters with their parents concerning their studies, violations of house rules, and relationships. Parents of young women living at home had different concerns. They worried primarily about the way their daughters pursued men. Sixteen-year-old Alice Fleming had a violent encounter with her mother over her boyfriend "Bubbles," whom she insisted she loved. Her mother slapped her and screamed "you slut."[92]

Seventeen-year-old Maria Upton's diary contained twenty entries on clashes with her mother.[93] Rebuked by her mother for spending time alone with two boys, Joanne Castle "sounded really upset and afraid of what her father would do."[94] Carla Norfolk's father condemned the way she dressed. "Some hurtful comments had been made." She dressed the way she did to retain her boyfriend.[95] Behaviour management for men in the late twentieth century involved anger control courses; for young women, the counterpart was counselling to stem rebellion or promiscuity.

Among the population of European origin, young women accounted for only about one in six female suicides (16.0 percent). The suicides of young Māori women were by comparison far more prominent relative to mature Māori women; astonishingly, young women accounted for nearly half of female Māori suicides (49.7 percent). Relationship problems, character and adjustment issues, and mental illness were the clusters of motives that had escalated for young Māori women. One conjecture that may explain the vulnerability of young Māori women was the disruption to the rural economy that affected young men and forced many men and women to leave for the cities and miss the support of extended families.[96]

TIME, TIME, TIME IS ON MY HANDS

Work was essential to the self-esteem of young males. Work also filled time that otherwise allowed space for self-criticism. The unemployed, prisoners, and jilted boyfriends or ex-spouses each had time to consider failures and their sinking trajectory.[97] The mother of an unemployed nineteen-year-old said that her son became depressed about once a week and complained "about being lonely and thinking that no one liked him, about being on the dole and not having a job, about not having any money to pay his bills; he complained about having too much time on his hands."[98] Nineteen-year-old apprentice mechanic Tony Alexander lost his girlfriend and without much money he stayed in at night. He told his employer "that he was very lonely at night with nothing to do."[99] After his live-in girlfriend left him, Ryan Henare Regan "just moped around the house and said very little."[100] Following a bust-up with his de facto, twenty-year-old Adrian Derby also "moped around." According to his sister-in-law, "he used to listen to a lot of music all the time, drink, and he didn't appear to be himself, really strange."[101] Twenty-four-year-old Dalton

Robertson, divorced for twelve months, lost his incentive to work, stayed with his sister, and spent most of his time "hanging around the house." He brooded but refused to talk about his problems or seek help.[102] Insomnia accompanied self-reflection, and vice versa.

Young men in prison carried a mix of problems that incarceration intensified: loss of income, gang pressure, substance addiction, mental illnesses, and shaky relationships on the outside.[103] Impulsiveness, a disinclination to think about consequences of actions, poor impulse control, and a low threshold for acting violently, the very personality traits that led some young men to wind up in prison, were attributes that raised the risk of suicide. In the 1990s, adolescents who had broken the law were unusually prominent among suicides. There had only been two adolescent suicides in jails or prisons during "the golden weather," but several dozen in the 1990s. Most of the increase came from young Māori. Younger prisoners, notably those heading to prison for the first time, entered the distressful unknown. Men in remand custody were at great risk because remand facilities were the dregs of the legal system and individuals placed there lacked the benefit of prisoner programs.[104]

First-time prisoners were observed for a while to assess their risk of suicide.[105] Assignment to prisons that were distant from family added stress. Robert Finchley was low-spirited because he could not understand why the classification board had declined his request for transfer to another prison to be close to his family "who had always been supportive."[106] All prisoners could see a prison psychiatrist, but access was no sure benefit. Prison psychiatrists in the late 1970s and early 1980s prescribed sedatives – mist-chloral – so generously in one instance that a prisoner managed to take a fatal overdose.[107] The prison subculture impeded the efforts of conscientious prison psychiatrists. An assessment unit set up to deal with prisoners with mental illnesses at the maximum security prison at Paremoremo was shunned by prisoners who ridiculed "the weaklings" at the "psycho unit."[108]

Younger prisoners had time on their hands to consider the shame they incurred, or more likely, to worry about the faithfulness of spouses or girlfriends. In retrospect, prison officers should have recognized a crisis for Māori prisoner James Eden when he made twenty-nine telephone calls to his partner "in a short space of time."[109] To facilitate the dropping of assault charges, twenty-four-year-old Grant Curtis had agreed to take an anger management course, but the girlfriend he had battered was not going to drop her complaint.[110] A series of petty crimes by nineteen-year-old Paul Fogerty helped to alienate him from his parents, who were separated. His father "had sort of disowned him and really didn't seem to care what Paul got up to." He was wholly reliant on his girlfriend and "desperately sought her assurances that she loved him," but her reactions to his pleas to arrange for their life together after his release did not ease his mind.[111] Twenty-year-old Shane Buck, a violent prisoner with heavy debts and a record of alcohol abuse, had a morbid attitude toward a girlfriend who had died in an auto accident; in prison, he learned that his current girlfriend would not wait for him.[112]

MENTAL ILLNESSES AMONG THE YOUNG

Case-file data disclose that mental illness was a leading motive for young adults, but not close to a majority of cases, let alone the ninety to ninety-eight percent claimed at the time by some empire-building psychiatrists (Table 7.1).[113] Moreover, as a motive for suicide it did not increase for adolescents and young adults during the period of economic restructuring. It is nevertheless worth mentioning how mental illness did contribute to suicides. The clear majority of mental illness motives among youth suicides consisted of depression, which could originate from concrete problems. When providing evidence for coroners, a few New Zealand psychiatrists referred to "reactive depression" and elaborated on sources of stress.[114] For pre-adolescents in the 1980s and 1990s, the sources of stress included failure at school and the trauma of parents separating; for adolescents and young adults, the sources could include these problems as well as unemployment, failed relationships, and substance abuse. The surge in youth suicides was unlikely to have been a product of endogenous mental illness, because the abrupt rise in adolescent and young adult male suicide rates rules out biochemical-neurological explanation based on genetics alone. Incidents of neurological harm due to anxiety about the future or due to drug abuse likely had increased, but these causes had associations with social and cultural factors.

The restructuring of health care points to another association between the economic crisis and mental illness. Here the illness deserving attention is schizophrenia. Young people with schizophrenia who committed suicide often did so in their twenties. During the

1980s and 1990s, one hundred and sixty men of all ages who took their own lives had either been treated for or presented as having schizophrenia; their average age was thirty-one and half were under twenty-five. At the age of twenty, Phillip Howe poisoned himself with psychotropic drugs. A manic-depressive with a schizophrenic undertone, he had been told that he would be on medication for life. This awareness and his ongoing unemployment upset him, but his condition imposed a further tragedy. His girlfriend, who had been supportive, "found that he was more than she could cope with and broke off their relationship." "He was very distressed by this," reported his mother. "He had been talking to me daily about how depressed he felt." Mental illness could disturb people's ability to live the life they expected; their relationships suffered and that wounded young men. Phillip Howe wanted a normal life of work and companionship.[115] Another young man, twenty-three, "desperately wanted treatment for his illness but felt local doctors did not give him assurances of any cures."[116]

There were a shocking number of instances where the hasty de-institutionalization of mental health care allowed young people with schizophrenia greater freedom but less protection. Internal hospital investigations and coroners' inquests exposed under-funding that contributed to releasing patients prematurely; an embrace of relatively new drug treatments permitted an increase of out-patient activities and consequently the disappearance of patients.[117] Until the late 1970s, few individuals who suffered from schizophrenia committed suicide. The number of suicides involving schizophrenia rose substantially beginning in the 1980s (Table 5.6). The timing coincided with de-institutionalization. During the youth suicide panic, schizophrenia suicides commonly took place in homes and public places. Previously, they had occurred in the rooms or on the grounds of psychiatric hospitals. The many failings of the mental health regime that replaced national psychiatric hospitals impacted the youth suicide rate, but so too did neurological damage due to excessive alcohol consumption, cannabis smoking, and substance abuse among teens.

Coroners required documentation if there had been a history of mental illness, because it was vital that they know the deceased's intentions in order to make a finding of suicide. Reports noted instances of "acute psychotic episodes which were drug induced."[118] Among young adults, less so adolescents, substance abuse in the

1980s and 1990s involved cannabis or alcohol and cannabis together. More young men were alleged to smoke cannabis than tobacco.[119] Remarks at suicide inquests about "bong and booze" plus medical reports referring to "major depressive illness with cannabis dependence" supply background for the government's refusal to legalize cannabis.[120] Use of pot and alcohol by adolescents affected cerebral development. As early as 1976, doctors suspected cannabis of contributing to mental change, although many New Zealanders seemed locked into the belief that it was harmless.[121] Cannabis use fused with youth socializing and rebellion. Family members detected changes in behaviour; doctors reported psychoses induced by alcohol and cannabis abuse.[122] A parliamentary committee inquiring into the mental health effects of cannabis use in 1998 concluded that it "may accelerate the onset of schizophrenia in predisposed persons, and cannabis use by people with schizophrenia may complicate the management of their symptoms."[123] Case files support this conclusion, and with it the idea that the ties between cannabis use and psychoses were more than a parallel association.[124] De-institutionalization, gaps in the new mental health system, and cannabis contributed to schizophrenia suicides.

THE HAZARDOUS LIFESTYLES OF MARGINALIZED YOUTH

A youth-centred culture appeared in the affluent "West" after World War II and was thriving by the mid-1960s. It was taken for granted by the 1980s, at which time very young people routinely embarked on moral decision-making. Males had hitherto unheard-of opportunities for unsupervised mixing with females. The change was well under way in the late 1970s. There was unprecedented liberty, but also performance measures that included formal education. Worth included economic prospects in a time of diminishing opportunities and evidence of promise in securing consumer goods. These were not new assets for the mating game, but had risen to prominence in a post-war consumer culture.

A tight labour market put more young men under greater pressure to finish schooling than in previous years. Those who struggled with learning were disadvantaged in the competitive job market. An eighteen-year-old lad, "a slow learner" according to witnesses, was "a lonely guy" who had "an extraordinary low opinion of himself and was very mixed up."[125] Low self-esteem afflicted early school-leavers.[126] One mother said that her son "wanted to do better but had not done well enough at school. We could not get him interested in anything and I felt he had lost his dynamo. He was slowly dying within himself." He left school at seventeen after failing English and that held him back for jobs.[127] Another mother remarked that her son "was a bit behind others his own age in reading and writing. He had trouble with his school work. He could not resolve his hurts." He turned to cannabis.[128] An investigating constable reporting on a nineteen-year-old male's background stated that

> the company was very impressed with Michael's performance over the first year of his apprenticeship. However, his work performance fell off both at the place of employment and with his studies. He fell behind with assignments and received a warning from the Technical Institute. This was nothing unusual but Michael did become visibly upset and did not want his father to be informed.[129]

Finding work shrinking in rural New Zealand, young men left family and girlfriends behind to come to a city where a number lacked intimate support. This wrench was sharp for young Māori, for whom the economic crisis was especially severe. For example, a young Māori man left his grandparents who had raised him and moved to Auckland, which he disliked. He asked his girlfriend to join him. She told him "I couldn't go up because I had an interview [for work]."[130] His loneliness was a new, unsettling experience. Witnesses in this case remarked on the further factor of his parents' separation. Years later, a young Māori woman would repeat over and over, "Auckland's too hard. I just need to be with my whanau [extended family]."[131] Strong cultural ties meant that many rural Māori faced entrapment in areas of declining employment, while flight to "refuge" towns and cities led to cultural dislocation and encounters with economic prospects as bleak as those back in their home regions.

A few young men were preconditioned to feel romantic let-downs acutely while the surrounding culture beckoned them to enter into relationships. The interconnected shocks of failure at school, social isolation, romantic rejection, meagre parenting, and disappointments in the quest for work contributed to status compensation through risky conduct. Some marginalized young men pursued dangerous pleasures that conferred reputation. Diversions such as binge drinking, drugs, wild driving, or reckless motorcycle riding could accelerate a decay of prospects.[132] According to a witness who knew a suicide victim well, "he became depressed from time to time due to his age [sixteen], the unavailability of a job, and his involvement in a couple of motor accidents."[133]

Youth autonomy permitted young males and females to flat together in the cities. Flatting was a strategy for hard times and relocation, but for some young adults it had the consequence of bringing together unhappy individuals with idle time. In an expression from the times, "they were all *doled* up with no place to go." Or "booze battles boredom." Flatting and youth parties disseminated knowledge about securing prescription drugs by purchase, guile, or theft.[134] Addiction clinics liberally distributed methadone starting in the early 1970s. Some of it entered illicit markets and turned up as the instrument of suicide.[135] Soft drugs, hard drugs, and prescription drugs assumed a casual prominence among young people who took their own lives. Binge drinking entered the mix. Abysmal living conditions, shattered health, and young people's "stoned" condition made it difficult to determine if they intended to commit suicide. Hazardous pleasures, miserable work, and rage combined in the case of a twenty-three-year-old man locked in a dead-end job. He drank heavily, smoked a lot of marijuana, and had a string of sex partners. "When he got pissed off he used to do stupid things like kick windows."[136]

Marginalized young men were attached to cars and motorcycles; wheels were flash property and fast driving demonstrated prowess. In her statement about the death of her jealous boyfriend, Brenda Black stated that "Robert sat in the car revving the motor and looked at me with a stupid expression."[137] According to his mother, Donald Halton "lived for his motorcycle."[138] Chris Wilson's Falcon was "his pride and joy" and "he desperately wanted a relationship with a girl." Cannabis use, debts, and auto accidents undermined his prospects.[139] Eighteen-year-old Justin Grant was despondent about demolishing his car when intoxicated, and facing the loss of his license. Alcohol abuse was not a leading direct factor as it had been in the past, but its impact could be indirect, affecting the right to drive and relationships. When his girlfriend Cheri rebuked him for drinking and demolishing a car, David Mitchell responded: "no one tells me what to do."[140] Disgusted by his alcohol-induced persona, Cheri left him.

Some young men could not abide condemnatory lectures that infringed on their already-limited autonomy in a flagging economy. After Colin Paterson's brother told him he was drinking too much, the younger man took his own life, partly to strike at his family. "FUCK YOU ALL. PS. May be this will stop me talking and drinking too much since I talk and drink too much."[141] Alcohol abuse had been prominent among the motives of male suicides for much of the twentieth century. Its debilitating impacts struck men in their forties. In the 1980s and 1990s, drug and alcohol abuse affected males and females in their twenties and thirties; the young binge drinkers rarely displayed delirium tremens or brain damage, but had a reduced threshold for rage and irrational acts.

ECONOMIC FACTORS REPRISED

The occupations of young male suicides were diverse, but most fell into groups with cause for pessimism in hard times. Many came from an underclass of the unskilled or semi-skilled; they included welfare and medical beneficiaries, students, and prisoners (Tables 7.3 and 7.4). Many resided in inner-city neighbourhoods or low-rent suburbs.[142] Their work status and residential locations suggest a connection between youth suicides and the economy. True, the array of motives that surfaced from our data set diverged from a pure work-related-troubles category, but unemployment had compound consequences. When a government working group in early 1991 studied the impact of reducing social benefits, it discovered that recipients of sickness benefits had risen by fifty percent "and this increase seems to be linked to rising unemployment."[143] Insecurity contributed to mental depression. A concurrent break-up of relationships added stress.[144] "Jobs are hard to get," wrote one young Māori male, and "my father does not like me and my girlfriend don't love me."[145] By 1990 roughly a quarter of Māori aged fifteen to nineteen received an unemployment benefit.[146]

Beneficiaries tended to associate with other beneficiaries and drifted deeper into a rut. Reductions in unemployment and sickness benefits in 1991 led to a migration to invalids' benefits and may have increased flatting.[147] For a number of young men, even the reduced benefits helped in material ways, but assistance signified stagnation in the paramount culture of consumption where welfare recipients could see others enjoying life. Failure at school, poor employment

Table 7.3
Ten leading occupations of male youth suicides

Occupation	*1980s*	*1990s*	*Total*
Welfare beneficiary	8	165	173
School or college student	48	89	137
Labourer, unskilled	42	29	71
Unemployed (no prior occupation cited)	37	7	44
Tertiary student	5	27	32
Sickness beneficiary	16	23	39
Inmate of prison or jail	9	18	27
Farm labourer	13	13	26
Patient (out-patient or in hospital)	9	7	16
Total (all young males in data set = 924)	198	398	586

prospects, hazardous conduct including cannabis and hard drugs, distraught partners, exasperated girlfriends, and encounters with the police were associated in various combinations. They undercut expectations for a good life.

For adolescents, work-related problems and unemployment were rarely associated with maintaining a family as had been the case in the Great Depression, but rather employment was now tied into consumption, and struggles for independence and respect. In 1990, at the age of nineteen, Martin Klein was dismissed by his employer for a work-related infraction. He had told his father that he never wanted to be without work again; he hated feeling worthless, useless, and powerless. He experienced these empty feelings on the dole. "His job was intimately related to his feelings of self-worth, financial independence, and control over his life."[148] Nineteen-year-old Jim Duffy had a different combination of work and character issues. His position as a low-level sales clerk left him humiliated. He thought he was being used as a "general dog's body." At a shop party, he erupted in anger when teased about his failings. Upset and drinking to excess, he drove his car through the shop window. The following day, he telephoned the shop in an emotional state and spoke to a constable.[149] Shame and fear contributed to his suicide. Education, work, and relationships were knotted together in the emotions of adolescent and young adult males.

A lack of self-esteem could originate out of parental criticism over a failure to find work or live up to parental expectations. "Just think of the things you wanted me to be," wrote John Riddell to

Table 7.4
Mean ages of men by selected class and types of years, 1900–2000

	Lower white-collar mean age (n)	*Skilled-labour mean age (n)*	*Semi- and unskilled labour mean age (n)*	*Students mean age (n)*	*Inmates mean age (n)*	*Unemployed and no occupation mentioned mean age (n)*
Early rural prosperity	43.4 (50)	44.4 (117)	43.0 (236)	14.5 (6)	49.7 (3)	45.0 (7)
War and recovery	41.9 (20)	47.0 (102)	43.5 (197)	14.0 (3)	44.5 (10)	42.2 (5)
Great Depression	37.8 (38)	44.4 (103)	47.2 (160)	18.3 (7)	50.4 (9)	48.3 (22)
Long Prosperity	43.7 (58)	47.0 (143)	44.2 (246)	16.0 (27)	47.8 (23)	35.1 (19)
Economic crises	39.6 (103)	38.0 (492)	33.5 (711)	18.0 (196)	29.8 (106)	29.2 (131)
Recovery begins (2000)	42.1 (20)	37.9 (33)	33.3 (47)	22.8 (26)	31.2 (5)	34.2 (51)

his parents, "now think how I turned out. Lazy." His thirteen-page note indicated that school assignments were "the bane of [his] life" and that he would rather get out of life now "than have to worry about jobs."[150] Some parental lectures about work were hard-edged. One twenty-one-year-old unemployed male who, in the words of his father, "was getting into a lot of trouble" was rebuked by his mother. "She told him he was a disgrace."[151] Fifteen-year-old student James Leslie "had a big blow up with his dad about September last year. He doesn't get on with his dad at all." Cannabis smoking, violent temper, and defiance of the law meant that Leslie fought with his father "almost every day."[152] The half-dozen letters of denunciation that William Gill's mother sent devastated him.[153] One father told his son that "you will become a blob. You know what happens to blobs."[154] The generation that raised the young people of the 1980s and 1990s had little experience with unemployment, thus some parents could not relate to their children's troubles.

Low self-worth due to an absence of work, learning disabilities, and caustic parental remarks could feed damning self-assessments. Even if guidance counsellors, psychologists, and psychiatrists penetrated surface observations, they could not address fundamental needs, because what some young men wanted was not the ability to cope but another life. One fifteen-year-old wished his body could be frozen for forty years and some money invested in gold so he could awaken to a carefree life.[155] Like many mothers, Ronald Saylor's thought that her son's problems arose from "his difficulties in learning at school. He fell behind at school and believed he was different from others."[156] It was not just failure at school that affected young men, since it is unlikely that a greater proportion of students were failing. The worsening job market also dashed plans for the future.

For young men who did not complete schooling, good employment prospects were very limited. The mother of an eighteen-year-old farm labourer said that she knew he was "not happy about his employment." The money was poor and payment irregular.[157] Dyslexia held back Thomas Dawson's progress at school and work. His frustration erupted in rage that led to criminal charges and that cost him a girlfriend. When he took his life at age twenty-two, he left a note that simultaneously displayed his learning disability and unhappiness. "I love all the ones how haev [sic] helped me but I allways [sic] shit on them."[158] Dyslexia contributed to Ian Garnett's truancy and the chip on his shoulder.[159] Roger Wesley's girlfriend commented that he left a suicide tape "because he was not very good at writing things down." He spoke about his inability to progress. "I wish life was not so hard living. Bloody trouble to get anywhere in life isn't it? Has to struggle."[160]

The concern about learning was mostly, but not exclusively, apparent in the suicides of males.[161] At the age of thirteen, James Markham's parents broke up; he took it hard and left school at age fifteen. At sixteen, he wanted to enlist in the Navy but needed an elusive school certificate.[162] "Slow learner" Peter Brown had been bumped from boarding school to boarding school by parents who took little interest in him. In the estimation of his head of school, "he had an extraordinarily low opinion of himself." Following his death, "the school could not immediately contact his next of kin."[163] According to Blain Houston's father, Blain "had left school and had no luck seeking employment."[164] Pursuit of employment in a low-skill sector took young men out of familiar rural surroundings where jobs were fast disappearing and into expensive cities where they lived by credit, skimping, and flatting. Ryan Sydney dropped out of school in the fifth form. To find work he had to move to the city. His girlfriend reported that in addition to loneliness brought on by the move "he didn't like getting treated as a boy at work."[165]

After failing to secure a school certificate, Ralph Preston held assorted unskilled jobs; he had been sacked from one job and made redundant in another. His parents had separated and his girlfriend reported that "he would get depressed about how he looked and that he didn't have a father."[166] Due to a learning disability, Douglas Roberts "had problems with written English and Mathematics" and consequently had trouble finishing his carpentry apprenticeship. It did not help that his father was a violent alcoholic.[167] At sixteen, Scott Bernard decided that he could never achieve his school certification. A friend noticed his sagging confidence on the two fronts that mattered: school and sports. "His older brother achieved really well in marks plus sport at school. Scott was sensitive to this and also felt pressured to perform in Rugby which he eventually gave away this year." Scott had voiced his low self-esteem to his mother: "my life sucks."[168]

Sixteen-year-old Morris Eastman felt overwhelmed by his studies and lacked support from his parents, because they had just separated and his father was on medication for depression and anxiety.[169] An early school-leaver gave up when he felt that he was not academic enough. To his psychiatrist he admitted that he had "on-going thoughts about finding out about life after death so that he could have a second chance."[170] Seventeen-year-old David Wolf succumbed to exam pressure.[171] University exams put a strain on students who were also on edge about employment.[172] Seventeen-year-old Brian Stockton "had not been coping well with his school exams." Whether seeking school certification in order to attempt to get a decent job or to go to university, a stumble at the starting blocks could lead to despair expressed in petty violence, recklessness, rebellion, avoidance of people, and frank statements of misery. Sequences of troubles with authorities that had begun with school failure could undercut parental support where it had existed, although some young men had not the slightest prospect of loving support, because their parents were distracted by the trauma of separation or self-absorbed in new relationships, behaved abusively, or had died and left children in the hands of disinterested relatives.

Thoughtful testimony on schooling, employment, and the vulnerability of young men came from Shirley Noble, a guidance counsellor at a large urban girls' school and the mother of a young man who took his own life. Her son had had a number of setbacks during his secondary education. After leaving school, he drifted; he found casual jobs and experienced periods of unemployment. He was turned down for a professional course. A six-year relationship with a girlfriend ended.

> He didn't know where to turn career wise. He had a series of unsatisfactory job experiences. During February 1996 a short intense relationship broke up. Steve was deeply hurt. He was losing his way. He had two more relationships and the third was destructive. It shook him. He began to talk about being empty inside and stopped communicating with others. He was sleeping all day and up all night. He became immobilized by depression. He couldn't make a decision about the course (hotel management). I cancelled the course. He'd lost his chance at the job.

His mother made a number of wide-ranging observations based on knowledge of her son's difficulties and her experience as a counsellor:

> I think young men must be encouraged to talk. I think that the government needs to take some form of action, that the

> employment contracts act has damaged the job scene, that the government shows a callous attitude to the young and unemployed. Steve had a series of jobs. Driving jobs and kitchen jobs, and a number of places on courses. There's been a shift in attitude. I think young men are unable to compete with young women on the job scene. Girls do better than boys, both at school and university. Girls are moving into traditionally male jobs, where they do extremely well. I would like to see something done to help young men. I have two friends who lost their sons in similar circumstances to mine over a 10 week period. We are all counsels and have similar training. Something must be done.

Asked in court if she felt that unemployment was a factor in mental depression, she believed that it had affected her son and his friends. "Some have gone through university, but that hasn't prevented bouts of depression. I don't think they have as clear [a] view of their future as we did at their age."[173] The pursuit of credentials, unemployment, and failed relationships fused. Steve was depressed, but behind that end-state were years of setbacks. Shirley Noble was correct in detecting a generational shift. Males born in the 1960s and 1970s came of age in the era of downward adjustments in employment prospects and upward expectations for credentials. But when the economy picked up at the end of the century, youth's cultural drift persisted.

Youth suicide rates eased at the start of the new millennium, but only slightly.[174] In case after case in 1998 and 2000, alcohol and cannabis still figured in unwelcome behaviour and a loss of prospects. Seventeen-year-old Lloyd Blundell found a job in 1999, and then "moved into a flat with some friends. This flat led to a lifestyle of drinking, cannabis use, and the use of drugs." He was known to the police for theft and disorder; he lost his job; he alienated friends by "being a dick and saying rude stuff."[175] In the same year, a twenty-six-year-old who inherited a substantial sum squandered it all on drugs and alcohol.[176] Economic conditions proved hard to change, but cultural attitudes and conduct more difficult still. The effects of substance abuse echoed for years. It was in 1981 that John Carroll "got into drugs" and "he just seemed to spiral down into alcohol and drugs from then on." His mother believed "he may have had schizophrenia. When we approached various Health Agencies we were told 'Sorry, we can't say' and they'd quote the Privacy of Information Act."[177]

CONCLUDING OBSERVATIONS

Consumerism and the sexual revolution held out enticing prospects for young men as employment prospects faded. It was apparent from the early 1980s to the mid-1990s that in contrast to "the golden weather," not everyone could partake of good times. In the midst of setbacks, when some young people could have used an embrace, there were family break-ups, a derivative of the sexual revolution and faltering economy. Family dysfunction was important. A few young people found short-term compensatory satisfaction in premature relationships which presented some with painful rejection or unexpected burdens. Meanwhile, shifts in mental health practices left more patients than ever on their own. A reduction in formal committals, the encouragement of voluntary patients to leave hospitals, the privileging of freedom, and retrenchments put young schizophrenia patients at elevated risk.

Historians acknowledge the complexity of causal sequences; they accept the restricted understanding that comes from living within the values of their own times. By seeking general truths, psychiatrists and psychologists evade such thoughts. Inconclusive research in medicine rarely becomes a source of grave doubt, but rather works as an opening for forecasts that more funds, more projects, more training, and more medication will achieve progress. It would be a loss for wisdom if these voices were accepted without rigorous questioning, particularly now when more jurisdictions are engaging in fierce retrenchment and restructuring. Events in private lives during New Zealand's ten years of austerity suggest the morale-lifting importance of work and the quality of parenting. To regard suicide as a mental health issue is to focus on how people presented themselves at particular moments and to discount their life experiences in changing times. Where do these observations lead? Can they inform prevention strategies? These are the questions that we turn to now.

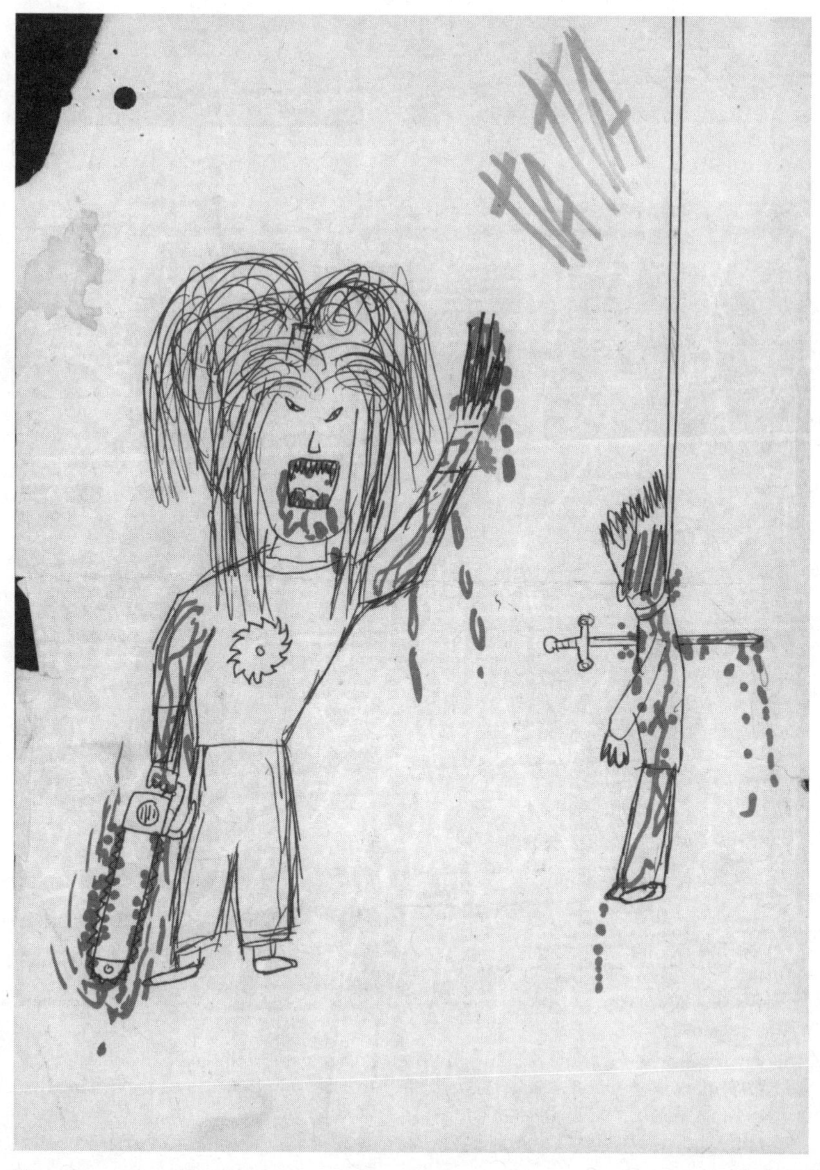

Figure 7.1
This drawing was found by a boy's teacher after he had taken his life. He had attended a summer camp for disadvantaged children and was reluctant to leave after being disciplined. Investigation into his death pointed to a dysfunctional family. Courtesy of Archives New Zealand, Te Rua Mahara o te Kāwanatanga. Coroners' Inquest File, ABVP [Number omitted for anonymity].

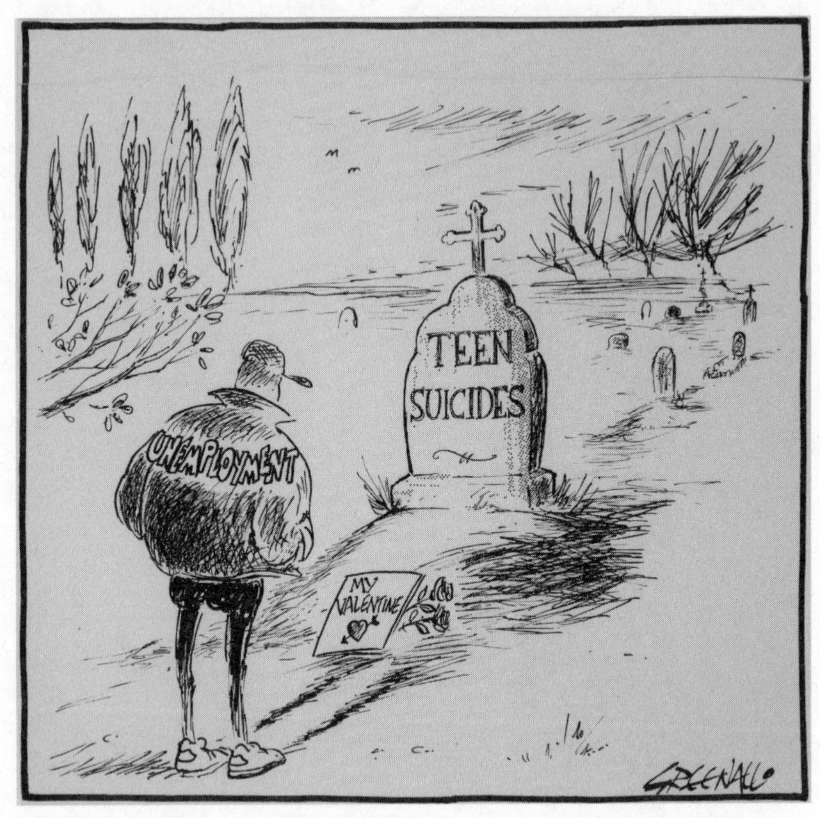

Figure 7.2
This cartoon appeared at the peak of the youth suicide panic and linked the crisis to unemployment. *Dominion Sunday Times*, 14 February 1993 [Valentine's Day]. The cartoon appears with permission of the artist, Frank Greenall. Courtesy of Alexander Turnbull Library, National Library of New Zealand, Te Puna Mātauranga o Aotearoa.

38

Ex3

These roses to you I do send
Such little time we did spend
my feeling's for you are so unreal
If only you understood how I feel
more than word's I needed from you
but sadly this you could not do
I needed your care and effection
but instead I only felt your rejection
Just like my love for you, this rose can not die
And now as my heart bleed's I say my final goodbye.
I will alway's love you

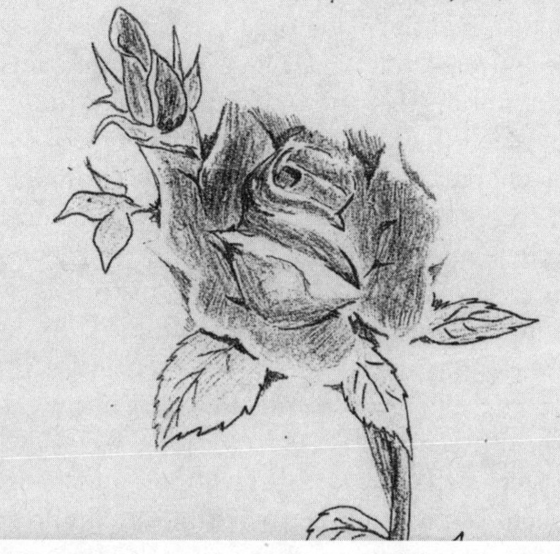

Figure 7.3
Poems and drawings occasionally accompanied youth suicide notes. This one was more sentimental and accomplished than most. Archives New Zealand, Te Rua Mahara o te Kāwanatanga. Coroners' Inquest File, ABVP [Number omitted for anonymity].

8

Decisions: Impulse and Reason in Historical Time, 1900–2000

How can it be that multitudes burdened with bad health, miserable work, and failed relationships have carried on, while others with no greater troubles ended their lives? In this chapter, our attempts to answer to this question follow the words of the exceptional few. The question just posed is the pre-eminent one in suicide studies. Our search for answers should take into account ideas from specialists who have dedicated their careers to understanding the suicide decision. They can assist with how we organize the case-based revelations about people's reasoning. Prior studies contain leads, but we challenge any assumption that the fundamental question of suicide can be studied by scientific methods to produce a theory worthy of that term. In this chapter, we caution against accepting claims that science can lead to a credible theory of suicide. Warnings are due because many individuals' reasoning for their actions had elements of popular culture that flourished in specific historical periods. A history of reasoning attached to popular culture is on display. To understand this reasoning and its variability over time is to go some distance toward comprehending suicide decisions, but without being able to explain them precisely.

At best, theorizers offer astute observations and insights. Not satisfied with such respectable contributions, ambitious writers in every generation have declared that their thoughts constitute a breakthrough or theoretical understanding so robust that it could lead to a reduction in suicides. They beckon, "follow my rainbow to enlightenment."

However, the resounding lesson from the inquests is that people are exquisitely complex with minds of their own. Therefore, epistemological difficulties intrude on all research that culminates in supposed theories. In 1967, iconoclastic sociologist Jack D. Douglas challenged his discipline and suicide studies. He wrote in *The Social Meanings of Suicide* that suicide originates in situations and that "*situated meanings* are significantly different from the *abstract meanings*."[1] His advocacy of research based on careful accounts of real-world events failed to catch fire, largely because the necessary case histories were elusive. Douglas hoped that an accumulation of evidence would ultimately assist with "the task of constructing more abstract theories."[2] He wanted suicide studies to proceed to theory by means of induction. While his accent on what people thought about when contemplating suicide inspires this chapter, his dedication to theory seems a recurring error in sociology and psychology. Reasons for this barbed judgement are presented later in this chapter.

While the individuality of the decision to end one's life is stressed throughout this book and while we take exception to the idea of suicide theory, we admit to shortcomings with our own material. Inquests were undertaken for a legal purpose, not for rigorous psychological or sociological examination. Inquests do not delve routinely and systematically into all important dimensions of personal temperament or social surroundings. Then again, neither can research based in psychology or sociology, for the dead make poor informants. That being said, prior chapters have demonstrated that inquests divulge a great deal about the crises in people's lives and about how distinct types of troubles appeared among different age and occupational groups in a succession of historical periods. Case files also give glimpses into inner lives.

A combination of insights from prior studies and statements from the case files will not produce sharply focused timeless answers to the essential question of suicide studies. Evidence gleaned from the cases nevertheless shows that the suicide decision cannot be narrowly described. At one extreme, a few individuals reached fatal decisions as an impulse during a flash of rage, in a state of inebriation, in the fatigue of illness, or through the haze of medication. Their reason was impaired.[3] Other individuals concluded after a long period of deliberation, including a reading of euthanasia literature, that on balance their suffering was too great to endure. Their reason was most decidedly not impaired. For some, a reasoning process included conjecture or conviction about a life hereafter. There were also men and women who shuddered at the thought of self-destruction but who acquired props to help them defeat their fear of pain during an act of self-harm or to purge thoughts of what, if anything, lay beyond. Others consoled themselves with a notion that their death would amount to a noble deed. They would endure, they reasoned, through survivors' remembrances. We should not underestimate the subjectivity of experiences, nor should we apply a label of mental illness when what has been uncovered (though it may strike us as odd) is in fact an intensely held popular belief.

The experience of suffering physical or emotional pain is subjective. Two suicide notes from three months apart in 1922 illustrate this point. They could have been written in any year. "No one knows but myself what pain I suffered," wrote ailing farmer Edward O'Brien.[4] Unemployed clerk Harry Thornton was separated from his wife when he wrote, "I am so extremely sad and unhappy."[5] It is their pain. A refined "experimental" search for the makeup and sources of subjective feelings that undercut the will to live would require a long-term and intrusive study that could survey multitudes of men and women as they confronted common problems. It is precisely the absence of any such studies about facing up to troubles that drew us to inquests in the first place, for they alone provide historians, psychologists, and sociologists with thousands of accounts of private lives. The historian's assumption is that inquests capture people's problems; these problems are not exceptional. Thus the pattern of troubles described by witnesses in different time periods fleshes out social history. Why individuals arrived at self-destruction as a solution remains a problem, but one beyond the reach of theory because of the scattered patterns of reasoning, patterns whose essential traits and frequency vary with people's ages and the crises of distinct eras.

The assumption that the visible burdens of suicidal people seem unremarkable has animated a few psychologists to search for deep character differences between survivors and the few who end their lives. In this pursuit, they opt for explanations that accent disorders. Thomas Joiner asserts that mental disorders, perceptions, and feelings are primary motives for suicide.[6] Concrete troubles and mean-spirited intentions are presumed secondary. Joiner's ranking of factors parallels an observation made in chapter five, namely that an inversion of causality crept into psychiatry and psychology when clinicians and researchers mentioned material difficulties like unemployment as products rather than causes of mental illness. An urge to rank factors with psychological ones on top imposes a discipline-specific idea of life. The fluctuation of the male rate of suicide in concert with broad economic trends is a firm fact that ought to give pause to enthusiasts for a mental-disorder and biochemical understanding of suicide. There is more going on.

The two-step approach mooted here – concrete problems and how they are evaluated by those who confront them – may be crude. It leads toward no theory and yields no findings about the consistent presence of disorders, but rather it stresses interactions between troubles and thought processes at an individual level where there are intimate perceptions, and sometimes evidence of mental disorders, although less commonly than has been claimed.

Returning to the question, if people's problems alone cannot explain suicide because others endure them, then what psychological traits might surface with further digging? How can these traits be discovered? For at least two centuries, suicide scholars have considered these questions and, although their answers are less precise and revelatory than they purport, their observations help us to sort evidence scattered throughout the inquest files. People's personal logic will be disclosed as far as possible in their words, but a description of this logic warns suicide scholars that a cultural conditioning of pain, suffering, and reasoning changes over time. Culture also provides materiel for people's thoughts about their immediate circumstances, their future prospects, and their bodies. Ideas about masculinity, self-image, relationships, injustices, vengeance, and a populated afterlife or a blank unknown are some of the culturally conditioned elements found in people's suicide decisions. They vary in importance and formulation across the hundred years.

Culture can change. Consequently, some matters that enter the minds of distressed people also change. Suicide must be considered historically. Additionally, the seemingly peculiar reasoning of some individuals should alert suicide scholars to the humbling fact that, because they stand outside someone else's skin, they will always have an imperfect appreciation of others' reasoning processes. We are obliged to think about culturally influenced judgements taking shape in active interior lives that can be remote from ours but that do not thus amount to a syndrome or a disorder. Theories fail because they conceal the intensity, imagination, and diversity of interior lives. The attendant loss of knowledge due to the strictures of theorizing is disadvantageous. By attempting to understand impulse and reason from the words of the people involved, this chapter shows how much has been lost when writers about suicide conceptualize to frame a theory. Douglas was right to highlight the real world; he was wrong about the feasibility of theory. This chapter shows how much can be recovered by a respect for narratives. The latter are sorted into rough categories. Before moving into the narratives, we need to examine theories and determine what can be salvaged.

AN ASPIRING PSEUDO-SCIENCE

We reject claims that suicide can be explained by theory. At their best, writers claiming to have developed a theory have assembled noteworthy observations, but despite their claims they have not advanced a theory as that word is properly understood. This section begins with a hard-edged critique of suicide studies; it then shifts to a consideration of recent survey accounts whose authors believed they were working with theory, but whose contributions are best considered as collections of loosely framed insights, some suggestive and illuminating. In particular we lean on a survey account of adolescent suicide sponsored by the American Psychological Association (2006) and then on two accounts of suicide by Thomas Joiner (2005 and 2010). By discounting their attachments to the notion that social sciences or psychological sciences can be exact sciences and by challenging characterizations of their work as theory, it is possible to retrieve ideas, not fog-clearing revelations but constructive contributions. This backhanded tribute means that reading suicide studies can strike a spark of recognition and help draw out more meaning from firsthand words. Presumptive theorists are in for a bumpy ride, although they are of greater value to us than as targets.[7]

Circumstances and latent motives have inspired theories of suicide. Primary among the circumstances is the general absence of numerous case files. This difficulty drove research onto particular paths of generalization because of the tempting availability of aggregated data collected and published by governments. Researchers followed Durkheim's use of data, just as he had followed a handful of late-nineteenth-century continental scholars who pioneered exploration of suicide by displaying aggregate data sent to them by clerks in nascent state bureaucracies.[8] The case files of inquests or the death certificates that government clerks counted to arrive at the annual figures that found their way into early studies were either destroyed or, in recent times, closed on account of confidentiality.

With little choice but to work with the data supplied in government publications, researchers turned uncritically, decade after decade, to these routinely published tables. Sometimes the suicide data was cross-tabulated with specific locales; sometimes demographic details were tabulated for the same locales, and that allowed crude linkages leading into explorations of suicide by age, gender, and marital status. Often the data was reported awkwardly using incompatible or changing jurisdictional boundaries or shifting definitions of attributes for vital information such as occupation. Published data in the past (and even now) has the allure of wide coverage, often at the level of the nation-state. The suicide rates of many countries are still contrasted as if the variations were real and expressed underlying cultural distinctions. Specialists seem loath to abandon aggregate data and superficial generalizations about national cultures and suicide, fearing perhaps that they could erode a discipline's foundations or downgrade its founders.

Published tables have tempted generations of writers into working with given categories, selecting those that appear worthy of exploration. The usual variables have included marital status, literacy, religion, occupational group, alcohol consumption, and employment status. Attempts to link published data on these variables to fluctuations in the numbers of reported suicides can be impugned on account of the ecological fallacy. The tables that report suicides and the separate tables that classify the population are not connected through the individual case but merely by the territorial unit in which the data was collected. Criticism does not end here. Suicide must be the dependent variable which is examined in conjunction with given independent variables, but the government-selected categories that supply the pre-sorted and compressed data for the independent variables are devoid of personal and situational complexity – devoid, that is, of the actual information most useful for studying the problem at hand.

The questions researchers have asked of such data have a deceptive veneer of profundity. Are the unemployed or divorced more likely than the employed and married to have taken their own lives?[9] As we have seen in several chapters, these questions are not insignificant, but affirmative answers do not take us far in understanding what it is about specific situations of unemployment or domestic separation that blights lives. Reasonable social scientists who have struggled to fill in these blanks admit in their conclusions that "some caution should be exercised." Inquests take us directly into the crises. They show that separation and divorce can be accompanied by acrimony and impulsiveness; that has pertinence not only for people in those states but for individuals whose marriages or relationships are in trouble.[10] It is situations in their fullness that deserve attention.

The unreliability of suicide statistics should cause concern. Curiously, even after listing the flaws, writers still have reported national differences. In a long goodbye to the Cold War, American texts mention the high rates in the former USSR.[11] Defenders of the value of published suicide data for national states could claim that even if there are distinct reporting practices in each country, aggregate data still has value because the data for a single jurisdiction will be consistent over time. However, the New Zealand inquest files show that rising standards of professional conduct by coroners in the late twentieth century led to increases in the numbers of violent deaths reported as suicides. When compared with reports from the early twentieth century, the reports from the end of the century are more reliable. The lessons are clear. National data is not consistent over time. Only a careful reading of case files can bring a measure of consistency to the data from even a single jurisdiction over a long period.

From its roots in the late nineteenth century, sociology has been the discipline most connected with and compromised by the use of aggregate data. Durkheim's *La Suicide* was filled with unreliable data and examples of the ecological fallacy. Yet Durkheim's generalizations have never vanished from the scene; a few sociologists continue the struggle to illustrate their utility. Durkheim's core observation about the risks of social isolation seem plausible, and its resonance with common sense helps sustain his enduring presence. Durkheim's so-called theory hypothesized an ideal state of society where people were integrated to the ideal degree; suicide rates went up when societies deviated from the right mix of integration and individuality. We can think here of the Goldilocks mean: not too hot, not too cold, just right.

Writers who followed Durkheim and generalized at a national or regional level attempted to confirm his insight by showing that suicide rates fluctuated in a correlation with some proxy for the ideal state of integration. An insuperable problem with his theory as well as the variations that followed is that key words such as integration or individuality can mean many things. Many conditions can be tucked into summary explanations. As well, such a pseudo-theory cannot provide guidelines as to when there is a real risk to a specific individual. Suicide, which is an individual and not a social act, is not really explained by social theory because non-suicidal individuals are also exposed to the social shortcomings in question. Non-suicidal individuals may feel alienated in a Durkheimian sense or, to take another of Durkheim's concepts, they may have an attitude of self-sacrifice derived from living in an altruistic society. It is possible to live an isolated life or to work in a self-sacrificing way and to die of old age by natural causes. On the one hand, individuals may work in a socially isolating industrial society but have social connections invisible to the census taker or researcher; on the other hand, they may carry hidden burdens that could be decisive. It is unhelpful to pretend that suicide is not the act of an individual. "Luck," as the iconoclastic psychologist Paul Meehl once argued in support of qualitative inquiry, "is one of the more important contributors to individual differences in human suffering, satisfaction, illness, achievement, and so forth, an embarrassingly 'obvious' point that social scientists readily forget."[12]

Troubles with aggregate data are not confined to the unreliability of published numbers, the ecological fallacy, vague capacious terms, a limited array of variables, avoidance of the individual, and failure to consider luck. Another barrier to understanding comes from the fact that the independent social variables taken from a census and employed 'to explain' suicide are far from revelatory.[13] The representations of the population supplied by census categories can never enable social science to advance past the construction of wooden caricatures. Real people engage with more experiences across more moments than can be captured in the bureaucratic snapshots that recent researchers call macro variables.[14] These austere variables supplied by censuses or found in other routinely generated government reports on a population do not expose desire, perception, satisfaction or dissatisfaction, judgement, or belief.

Psychologists have recognized this limitation, and thus some have endeavoured to establish research techniques that bypass aggregate data and overcome the scarcity of case files. In other words, historically they have appreciated individual mental states and laboured to explore them. Suicide specialists from this discipline with this point of view have contributed insights, but have overstepped the bounds of credibility by claiming to have produced theories and by associating their so-called theories with science, that powerful touchstone of modernity and government longing. They insist their work is a science or, better for media and funding attention, a medical science.

The two disciplines with the largest stake in claiming success in establishing a suicide theory, namely sociology and psychology, were founded more than a century ago by brilliant advocates who aspired to raise their work to the status of a science. Despite the production of dissenting internal branches, sociology and especially psychology maintain lines of training that presume an affinity with science even though experiments to test hypotheses are impossible when it comes to the phenomenon or action in question. For example, the so-called theories of suicide lack firm testable propositions about suicide. Claims to theoretical profundity are so vague and open-ended as to be impossible to test rigorously in accord with a well-understood conception of science, namely the expression of a theory in terms that would expose it to something directly testable. The circumstances of psychiatrists and psychologists have differed fundamentally from those of sociologists. The former have long focused on a very few instances arising from clinical work or admirably rigorous investigative research, but then they have a difficult time affirming that their limited observations are valid for a population. Meanwhile, in a discipline-wide trend to emphasize methodology and statistics, psychologists who assert that they are studying suicide have distracted attention from the fact that they are not studying suicide but rather phenomena that can be seen in currently living subjects. These probes, questionable even as a means to the end, become the end.

Pioneering sociologists and psychologists set out to privilege their fields as sciences. But what is a science and what is a scientific method? During the last four hundred years in the West, there have been and continue to be debates about the scientific method. The conception of science that we adopt is a powerful one pioneered in the 1930s by Karl Popper; it accents the obstacles to representing suicide studies as scientific. Consider first the deductive method, which involves the preparation of an elegantly compact theory, sometimes summarized in symbolic notation, and conveying predicative implications. Predictions can be tested and until they are falsified, the theory stands. Albert Einstein's theories led to testable predictions. No so-called theory of suicide has the notational precision or predictive capacity that can provide a testable question for the falsification standard. Thus, rather than attempt an imprudent and ultimately discipline-destroying prediction of who will commit suicide, psychological "theories" consider who might be at risk of suicide. A hypothesis might suggest that a certain type of person is at risk. In effect, the concept (risk) that might be subjected to a falsification test is not the actual phenomenon (suicide) that is the putative topic of investigation.

Time and again, psychologists looking to express succinct and profound conclusions about suicide have developed projects where a hypothesis may be rigorously tested but where the experiment operates at a remove from the prime subject of suicide itself. They have difficulty connecting the restricted operational conjectures of their research projects with a substantive theory about suicide itself. Studies of suicide ideation and attempted suicides employ statistical rigour to probe these proxy concepts. Suicide ideation index scores could be correlated with an index of social withdrawal, and then social withdrawal in turn could be associated with powerful events in a life history. Thus, a history of maltreatment in youth could be a source of isolation and, to use a common verbal escape expression, "the suicidal person" is seen as an abused individual. An unsuspecting reader could be forgiven for thinking that "the suicidal person" is truly headed for suicide or had in fact committed suicide. No such thing. In circular fashion, evidence for a cause becomes evidence for the phenomenon.

There should be loud disclaimers that an essential research step has been avoided. There is an absence of effort to confirm the inferred relationship between the proxies for suicide and suicides themselves. Parasuicide and suicide ideation are not the same as suicide, but by employing the term "suicidal person," this difficulty has been obscured. Distracting irrelevancies can be produced with the aid of sophisticated statistics, but in the end the onus falls on the researchers who subscribe to these techniques to show the relevance of their investigations to the fundamental subject. Authors should be forthright and admit that empirical literature linking assorted risk factors and completed suicides is limited.[15] They are bound by honesty to report, as some have, that "there is no agreed upon scale for establishing the severity of suicide risk, but clinicians tend to conceptualize risk on an ordinal continuum ranging from *no risk* to something akin to *high and imminent risk*."[16] In other words, clinicians are making rough but sensible decisions. That is distant from science and theory, but honest.

On rare occasions it has been possible to conduct interviews with suicide survivors who may have had serious intent. The numbers are small and restricted in time period to recent decades. Interviews with family and friends of individuals who have taken their own lives have been conducted by researchers but require consent. The motives of some parties volunteering statements may be suspect as they are offered in hindsight. Refusals to co-operate place in doubt the 'scientific' standing of those cases where consent has been forthcoming. What is representative about a self-selecting group? The authors of a major study of adolescent suicide published by the American Psychological Association admitted that they experienced "both limited observation of suicidal adolescents and significant methodological difficulties in adequately studying these youth." Nevertheless, they claimed remarkable results "in identifying empirically based risk factors." Moreover, they felt that "practical applications" were within their grasp.

What would validate achieving a grasp on the situation? It could not be merely accepting their list of risk factors, which consists of sensible but imprecise terms: a negative personal history, negative personality attributes, stresses, a host of asocial behaviour factors, isolation, self-deprecation, and availability of method.[17] Now then, was anything left out? How would these roomy circumstances guide intervention and avoid false positives? Theories of suicide seem pulled apart by two opposing flaws: the lack of breadth and the absence of specificity. Theories cannot encapsulate the complexity of individuals in the context of cultural and economic change. That is an immense flaw with theories. When writers try to describe risk factors as part of a theory, they employ terms too open to interpretation.

The legal requirement of an inquest ensures completeness of incidents, and evidence presented in open court under oath may make inquests a more reliable source. But they too contain statements made in hindsight. In the long run, psychologists may be able to follow the lives of a large cohort of individuals across their life-course, and that could yield worthwhile details about differences between the vast proportion of people who endure their troubles and the small number who do not. However, the effort will be prohibitively expensive, require patience, and demand the establishment of some constraints on how much information can be collected. At the conclusion of such a hypothetical study, it is probable that astute critics will point out aspects that had been ignored and that may have been important. There is no escape from presupposing the guiding ideas which will in turn influence findings.

There are many serious quibbles with assorted research strategies, but the towering obstacle to claiming affinity with deductive science is even greater than all that has been mentioned so far. A precisely expressed prediction of the phenomenon in question – actual suicide – will fail when anyone violates expectations and lives a long natural life. Vague terms cannot really be predictive, but clearer talk and firmer predictions would be catastrophic for a theory of suicide.

The inductive model of science is not one that suicide studies can attach themselves to for the purposes of claiming their affinity with science. Induction allows researchers to collect observations until the findings seem so overwhelming in number and clarity that generalizations with connecting arguments can be ventured. Naïve "inductivism" holds that enough facts may enable the spontaneous emergence of a theory with predictive power. The framing of experiments, however, sets the path to the theory. Besides, a theory from induction still has to pass the falsification test. Deduction presents the possibility of a prediction that can fail; induction presents the possibility of encountering abundant non-conforming cases that block summary or that force a cautious summary wrapped in loose language that anticipates and absorbs exceptions. In this latter relaxed form, so-called theories cannot truly be tested, because essential words bend to take on countless situations. A precautionary imprecision puts theories based on an accumulation of findings outside science. Verbal vagueness, as we have noted in reference to a publication of the American Psychological Association, allows suicide 'theorists' to evade the pressures of deductive and inductive science, but qualifies their work as pseudo-science.

When adopting the inductive technique, proponents of a science of suicide studies appropriate the paraphernalia of inductive science: they describe sampling procedures; they establish control groups; they apply confirmatory statistics; they measure responses to questionnaires; they speak of experiments. There is a good latent reason why some suicide writers present their work as scientific. Politicians in modern states harbour the idea that problems are capable of solution. What is politics without promises? Quality of life and life expectancy are important to citizens in affluent societies, therefore politicians understandably invest in medical research. Powering this political reality are tales of medical triumphs. The discoveries of insulin and penicillin feature prominently; the wild enthusiasm for chlorpromazine, mentioned in chapter five, is less familiar today due to its ambiguous ending. Proponents of chlorpromazine referenced insulin and penicillin as models, but their miracle drug ultimately did not join the others. Understandably, narratives with ambiguity are shunned by fundraisers and politicians. It is psychically satisfying and professionally rewarding to align suicide studies with science, or better yet, medical science, where progress has been presumed and universally desired. Unfulfilled miracles are washed from the media consciousness by a tide of fresh press releases about the latest promising marvel.

Studies of suicide would be more credible and valuable if authors in future backed away from claims to theory and science, and of course renounced aggregate data altogether. An insistence by scholars that original investigation files (not mere death certificates) be retained and made accessible, if successful, could do more to advance an understanding of suicide than all the analyses of published data from 1850 to the present. It can be countered that we would take a critical position such as this one in order to highlight our unusual information. This is true. We declare again our biases. The riches of case files have led us away from theory, models, and claims to science. Moreover, as historians we recoil from positivist projects for a variety of reasons. We are conscious of the values and prejudices of our own times, and thus inherently suspicious of claims to truth. As well, we look to the specific contexts of time and place to gain some purchase on human thoughts and actions.

In this closing chapter, we must investigate the big topic that enticed sociologists and psychologists to propose so-called theories. They investigated why some people with problems took their lives and others with comparable problems did not. For sociologists, either some social pressures or social omissions made the difference; for psychologists, character traits contributed to a fatal course. Sociologists and psychologists have avoided judging individuals. The long intellectual history on writings about suicide has many pre-1900 chapters on religious moral condemnation. Pretensions to science have secularized suicide. Additionally, if the qualifications for a scientific theory have not been met, there have been useable observations. Among them, we number the following: the idea of a lifelong pathway of risky conduct and troubles, deep emotional pain, feelings of guilt or being a burden, and a habituation to pain or death. Before we go further and show the validity but also the cultural complexity of these matters, it is necessary to question the psychiatrists' and psychologists' preference for branding most suicides as indications of mental illness. Clouded judgement is not necessarily indicative of mental illness, and there were other states including rational deliberation.

RATIONALITY, IRRATIONALITY, AND IMPULSE

In many cases, people's words plus physical evidence indicated preparatory thoughtfulness toward others. The act was deliberate and well-planned. These traits appear to have been commonest among mature and better-educated men and women, but that is purely an impression. Individuals acted out of a personal logic that testifies to their humanity, the culture of the times, and their urge to accent reason and not be considered mad. A young female clerk employed by the telegraph office in Auckland in 1922 had just been jilted – "it has broken my heart." She wanted it known that unhappiness made it impossible for her to go on: "I am not 'of a temporarily unsound mind' as the papers always insist on saying."[18] As she pointed out, rationality and reason were not favoured renderings of a suicide decision, and for good reasons. First, it would not do to have a society's failings or people's cruelty on display. Second, senility, alcoholism, mental incapacity, and some mental illnesses truly did result in poorly reasoned actions. But not all acts qualified. Turning back to rationality for a moment, it is important to consider suicide in conjunction with an appreciation for the shifting value sets that guided people. Thus to cite one major theme in the book, young people tended toward impulsiveness at all times, but in the late twentieth century many also evinced a tragic logic based on a youth culture and a pessimism attending the economic crisis. Times change; the patterns of suicide do too.

Coroners required information on the mental state of individuals to decide whether or not self-harm resulted from a deliberate act and thus conformed to definitions of suicide. Constables working under the coroners' directions gathered information about emotional states, degrees of sobriety, and mental illnesses. Beyond the major cities, coroners did not always have the resources or professional zeal to insist on the collection of evidence on mental states. However, plenty of files held pertinent information due to the professionalism and energy of city-based coroners. For the first half of the century, information on mental state was usually confined to a sentence or two in a witness' deposition. There were some exceptional extended medical reports in the first half of the century. Reports on mental health in the late twentieth century filled several pages and were the norm. In all periods, medical reports typically pointed toward irrationality in the suicide decision; however, mental illness did not always mean mental incompetence. Doctors were occasionally impressed by the considerable insight that patients with a mental illness had into their conditions.[19]

Furthermore, some individuals with a mental illness did not commit suicide during an acute episode of a mental illness when reason might have been impaired, but did so during an interlude when reflecting on what they considered a terribly diminished quality of life attending their illness and prospects for "a normal life." The police reported on physical evidence that could also apply to an assessment of the mental state; such evidence included descriptions of liquor bottles and drug paraphernalia. A few men and women contemplating suicide wrote about the rationality of what they were about to do. Evidence on the mental state is imperfect, diverse, yet more extensive than what might be imagined.

In chapter four we noted the exaggerated fear of cancer and suggested that from today's perspective a few pre-emptive deaths to escape pain seemed foolishly irrational, but less so when family histories and the then-current state of medical treatment were known. On account of this complication and the incompleteness of information in a number of cases, statistical breakdowns that identify rational and irrational states would be flawed. We have opted to reconstruct sets of mental states and reasoning processes without attempting to count the cases in each set. Intimate descriptions complied from the more revealing cases may have diagnostic and educational value, and for that reason revelatory phrases and sentences have been quoted. In sorting these remarks into arrays of reasoning, we followed the evidence presented in the files and acknowledge that prior studies suggested several categories.

Clusters of descriptions of rationality and irrationality amount to patterns, but patterns that necessarily convey imprecision marked by words such as "some" and "sometimes." Some individuals were not in a rational state, but some were. Sometimes the irrational state of insobriety resulted from a person's choice of an aid to assist with getting over the reflex to preserve life. Sometimes, courage flowed from bottles. An irrational state could have been a prior rational choice. For coroners, the amount of alcohol consumed could be taken into account to help determine if inebriation had deprived the individual of the intent to commit suicide.[20] As pointed out in chapter one, strict legal definitions of an act of suicide can differ from assessments by a reasonable observer. Alcohol clouded immediate judgement, but inebriation was often a planned preparatory step; its consumption was rational.

In studies of suicide where there is no attempt to explain the representative nature of instances cited as examples, the suspicion must be that the author has chosen items to argue a preconceived case. Thousands of cases have been read for this study and the data partly inform the selection of cases; however, we too have to go out on a limb – especially in this chapter. Additionally, we readily admit that we are unable to gain entry to the mind of the deceased. We can only suggest possible explanations and describe circumstances without making a claim to have found a neat answer to the question. This section of the chapter first considers the tragic instances of irrationality associated with mental illness and flashes of rage; it then looks at clouded reason due to alcohol or drug abuse. From reflections on fatal lapses of reason, analysis shifts to an array of reasoned events. These include instances of deliberate efforts to impair reason, reason emerging from values and beliefs, reason within a context of familiarity with death, and finally reason behind the timing.

Among seniors who committed suicide, dementia was reasonably common. Witnesses mention feeble-mindedness, senile decay, and acting foolish. The vague designation "old and unwell" occasionally represented this condition (Table 4.3). At the age of seventy-eight in 1910, farmer Frank Bolton was routinely "muddled" due to senility.[21] In the same year, "old man" Kelly was described by a family member as "somewhat childish of late."[22] Such characterizations of older men and women surfaced throughout the century. Chapter five, which reviewed mental illnesses, included examples of individuals who may have taken their lives in delusional states. As reminders, several additional cases can be mentioned. Betty Patterson was "troubled with delusions and a buzzing in her head."[23] Widower Lawrence Ball was being treated for paranoia. He had delusions of persecution from a religious sect.[24] The son-in-law of Emma Schmidt testified that "she has occasionally inquired as to the voices she heard when as a fact none had been heard."[25] When out for a drive with her brother, widow Ida Bothwell said that she enjoyed the outing but that "the devils were going to get her that day."[26] "Some great force is driving me," wrote Ilene Waugh; she had been immersed in reading the Bible.[27] The prominence of religious faith in the first half of the century receives explicit attention later in this chapter. There is no denying that senility and mental illnesses are evident in a substantial number of suicides. But clouded judgement could originate in other situations.

The influenza epidemics early in the century left people weak and despondent, particularly the 1918–19 epidemic. Witnesses and doctors alike wondered if influenza precipitated insanity.[28] At the very least, it left many people mentally delicate. The curious association of influenza and suicide has been explored in chapter four, and historically positioned waves of influenza should not be discounted. More commonly, it was alcohol that undermined judgement. Until World War I, drunkenness and drunken sprees abounded. The consequences of alcohol abuse showed up in myriad ways at inquests. Most directly, it appeared in the words of men and a few women who had wanted to shake the addiction and had failed. There were indirect effects. Destitution, family discord, probable brain damage, and premature physical decay were all motives for suicide that developed from alcoholism. Reading inquest files for the period before and into World War I, one is overwhelmed by the prevalence of hard liquor in the destruction of the lives of suicidal men, and of women as well. Alcoholism was more than a motive. It was also a factor in people's capacity for irrational judgement at important moments. By way of illustration, a doctor did not think that hotel operator Patrick Feeney was insane, just "enfeebled mentally" by heavy drinking during the heyday of booze.[29] Intoxication affected reason.

The most shocking instances involved investigations into deaths of people, mostly men, who had delirium tremens, also known as "the DTs," and literally fled their horrors by suicide. Numerous cases were summarized in chapter two; several additional instances will remind us of the damage of drinking sprees. Friends described individuals with delirium tremens as "out of their mind."[30] Whenever one man took liquor, stated a doctor, "he became an absolute lunatic."[31] Individuals with DTs believed they were being chased by enemies, the police, insects, or snakes.[32] To a layman, the symptoms of madness and "suffering a recovery" were easily confused, as Constable John Murphy discovered. Called in to testify at the inquest into the death of Neil Williams in 1902, Murphy mentioned that "when I arrested him two years ago I charged him with being a lunatic at large, but the medical evidence went to show he suffered from drink."[33]

Inebriation did not vanish from the hotels, houses, and streets of New Zealand, but it diminished during World War I and thenceforth remained less frequent and less memorable. Alcoholism accompanied by the horrors afflicted woman in the pre-war years, and that raises currently unanswerable questions about the types of alcoholic beverages consumed.[34] Women and men, not just men, suffered brain damage from years of drinking great quantities of distilled spirits. Mary Jane Cuthbert's husband knew she was an alcoholic "since the night of our wedding." She suffered the horrors and in a recent attack shouted "take that black bastard off."[35] Addicted to drink, fifty-year-old Catherine Freeman had a recurrent delusion of "someone coming to murder her."[36] John Kenny reported that his wife "had kept sober for some time until the last time she came out of gaol."[37] The waning of alcohol abuse as a motive for suicide appears to have been stunning after 1920 (Table 2.1). The destructive effects of excessive drinking still came to light. Although less common, instances now received more clinical portrayals. It was assumed that "brain damage through alcoholism" undermined Henry Shaver's reasoning ability in the 1960s, and in that same decade there were additional instances of "acute brain syndrome associated with alcohol."[38]

There were additional sources of irrational behaviour. War trauma erupted on the scene during and after World War I and less so during and after World War II; late in the century schizophrenia appeared as a diagnostic category associated with suicide. Hallucinations reported across the century may have originated in assorted insults to predisposed brains; therefore, the seemingly distinct sets of origins for hallucinations – alcohol or drug abuse, war trauma, and mental illness – may have been connected. Possible linkages were considered in chapter five.

Alcohol and drugs could certainly impair reason. Testimony in alcohol-related suicides often included remarks on an individual's weakened physical state and incoherence. Across the century, the striking feature of weakened reason in drug-related suicides was the downward shift in ages and the expansion in drug choices. Early in the century, drug addiction afflicted men and women in their prime, and the drugs were opiates.[39] A friend of Edwin Carroll asked why he was so shaky. He said it was his old craving, "morphia."[40] The physical degeneration of a divorced veterinarian, who had access to drugs, led the post-mortem doctor to conclude that "he must have been addicted to the morphia habit."[41] From time to time in the early decades, an alcoholic would take a nip of chlorodyne or methylated spirits. These were desperate supplements to chronic alcohol consumption, not elements in a new trend.[42] In the last quarter of the century, however, there were fresh developments. The pharmacological revolution expanded the means for getting high. Meanwhile, cannabis rivalled alcohol as a popular accessible intoxicant.

The states of irrationality that alcohol induced included blind anger, which featured in several fairly common circumstances, including domestic arguments that escalated into violence and extreme posturing by threats of self-harm. Heavy alcohol consumption could make individuals, mostly men, edgy and sensitive to criticism about – what else – their drinking. After consuming "a quantity of beer," Charles Baker argued with his wife and struck her. "You and I are finished," he shouted. "I'll show you what I can do. I'll cut my bloody throat."[43] In the last two or three decades of the century, incidents like this one included a growing number of younger men who intended to inflict emotional harm on girlfriends, spouses, or parents.

In addition to impaired reason, there were the associated mental states of acting on impulse or in a rage.[44] On a few occasions witnesses cryptically remarked that the deceased "was an impulsive man."[45] "My husband," stated one wife, "was impulsive by nature." He had warned her that "this will be the last time for these little arguments."[46] Harold Richards beat and threatened his wife, who said at the inquest that "I would not say he was mad, but when he was in a temper I often thought he was."[47] When wives testified to a husband's impulsiveness, they meant he was violent and blind to reason when angry. "My husband had a very bad temper and he often gave me a hiding," said the wife of a farmer who had threatened to use a shotgun on the family and himself.[48] Women too acted on impulse in the heat of an argument. During a domestic dispute in 2000, Theresa Dupuis suddenly walked away from her husband, secured a shotgun, and shot herself.[49]

There may have been more than meets the eye to impulsive acts, but plenty of suicidal acts do seem to have been suddenly determined. After drinking poison, George Flaherty stated, "God forgive me I did it on the spur of the moment." He had been a heavy drinker, ill, and out of work.[50] Suffering from influenza and facing a failed business partnership, a young carpenter drank acid alone in a hotel room. He survived in hospital for fifteen days, long enough to tell his former business partner that "he did not know why he did it, as he wanted to live."[51] Bankrupt accountant Fred McFarlane lived long enough to give a statement to the police in which he claimed that "I suddenly conceived of the idea of committing suicide under the influence of alcohol."[52] Unable to get his wife to agree to a divorce, Gareth Jones and his girlfriend jumped into Auckland harbour. His note claimed that "this deed has not been contemplated beforehand."[53] There were concrete troubles in the background.

Most cases of impulse fused with anger pertained to men, but there were some jealous and rash women. A couple who lived together "Māori fashion" clashed over his alleged infidelities. Witnesses concurred that "she was prone to violent fits of temper."[54] Decades later, a young woman argued with her husband about his speeding and threatened to jump from the car if he did not slow down. He paid no heed and on an impulse she executed her threat. It was men who usually threatened self-destruction if they did not get their way.[55] Some evidence indicating a sudden decision to act was physical. Immediately before taking a fatal step, a few individuals grabbed whatever was at hand to write a hasty note. The fact that they wrote on laundry bills, tobacco pouches, blank cheques, notebooks, sheets of cardboard, a piece of board, and so forth suggests a lack of planning.[56] A few witnesses' statements and fragments of physical evidence, such as long well-composed letters, indicate a hesitation and deliberation that are the opposite of impulsiveness.

HESITATION AND CHEMICAL COURAGE

Uncertainty showed up in an indeterminable number of instances of 'failed' attempts. The frequency of prior attempts cannot be estimated from the case files because the police did not ask a standard set of questions during their investigations and neither did coroners at inquests. Unsuccessful attempts, hesitation, and deferral surfaced in statements from time to time. The mother of a thirty-seven-year-old man reported that he had made eleven previous attempts; that was the most that we had seen mentioned by a witness.[57] Some rational men and women who reflected on the finality of death acted after days of deliberation. A Māori labourer wrote that he had planned his death for three weeks.[58] There were physical indications of hesitation. Faith healer James Leach, who lived in Auckland in 1906 and who was possibly gay, had numerous self-inflicted cuts indicative of prior attempts.[59] A few years later, injured farm labourer Patrick O'Malley was found with his throat cut. An autopsy showed "three little cuts near the commencement of the wound such as might have been made by a shaking or hesitating hand."[60] Mary Bristol made hesitant cuts on her arms and legs, then ran into a river.[61] A bystander saw a young man walking "to and fro" before he blew himself up with gelignite.[62] In the midst of writing a note in ink about not feeling well, George Williams stopped, possibly deliberated, and then completed the note as a suicide confession in pencil.[63]

Throughout the century, alcohol gave courage, or more correctly, it put people in a voluntary state of impaired reason. Some individuals explicitly mentioned that they considered themselves cowards and drink gave them courage. In a letter running to five pages, George Bowers warned his son, "don't hit the grog." Drink had ruined his life and, as he admitted, it now assisted him as he ended it. "Even to the last I was not man enough to do it sober I had to get Drunk."[64] Men who worried about "having guts" could access distilled courage. Bottles of gin and brandy assured that Emil Lasker "was in an advanced state of alcoholic inebriation at the time of his death."[65] Before an era of widespread car ownership and before the arrival of barbiturates, the use of alcohol to boost courage mainly occurred in conjunction with coal gas deaths in the home. Later, alcohol and drugs assisted with carbon monoxide deaths in vehicles. Describing himself to his wife as a coward to the end, Albert Dumfries turned on his gas stove and consumed a flask of brandy and several bottles of beer. These, he wrote, "have given me the courage to take the step I have taken."[66] In a long note to his parents, Henry O'Driscoll confessed that "if I get three parts Drunk I can do it right."[67] Alcoholic Willie Saunders was found "holding a bottle of gin."[68] By no means was the presence of alcohol a definite indication of a rash act taken in a moment of inebriation. The mix of alcohol and the arrangement of equipment to achieve a successful carbon monoxide poisoning showed considerable poise and deliberation. A rejected lover placed his golf trophies on his car's central console.[69] A couple found "holding hands" had planned their double suicide for some time. Their car contained bundles of letters written to friends and family. Their exact motive was obscure, but they had agreed that "there appeared to be no future for them."[70]

During the barbiturates decades, final cocktails were loaded for quick somnolence. James Calder drank a bottle of gin with Valium.[71] Psychiatric patient Margaret Taylor washed down Doloxene pills with sherry.[72] Recreational drugs appeared late in the century. Police found "a bag of marijuana and a number of beer bottles" in Peter O'Neil's vehicle.[73] The combination of carbon monoxide and intoxicants became commonplace in suicides during the years when carbon monoxide was an accessible means of suicide. Men and women eased their way toward death with alcohol. Chronic pain without the prospect of improvement depressed Tomas Vilniac. Described as "a solitary soul," he drank two-thirds of a bottle of vodka when ending his life by carbon monoxide.[74] Many factors made Alexander Malovich's life miserable, including psoriasis, business troubles, and domestic discord. He chose carbon monoxide assisted by alcohol. The police found a partly consumed bottle of whisky in his car.[75] The police report for the death of Allan Stanley noted a bottle of brandy one-third consumed on the front seat.[76] The report on George Pearson's death mentioned the empty bottle of rum in his auto.[77] Alleged sex offender John O'Shaughnessy was found holding a can of beer and there was a half-empty bottle of vodka on the seat.[78] Nigel Whitelaw apparently drank several glasses of port outside his car.[79] The prominence of alcohol in conjunction with drug overdoses or carbon monoxide deaths derived from the fact that other prominent methods of suicide required coordination that alcohol inhibited.

IMAGINING THE GREAT MYSTERY

True believers were convinced that their earthly demise would initiate a fresh beginning in a better place. In the 1950s and 1960s, American suicide scholars noted "that in suicide notes one frequently finds a reference to the self as being able to experience things after death."[80] New Zealand notes suggest how life as something nonessential to the real person was conceptualized. Obstructing ideas were dismissed. Thus, if suicide was deemed a sin by an individual's church, an all-knowing merciful God would forgive. "Lord Jesus rest my soul in heaven," wrote Robert Logan in 1900.[81] "Don't worry about me for God will forgive me," wrote Minnie James. She believed that life had been cruel to her and God would know this.[82] In a 1926 letter to the Catholic bishop of Auckland in which he described his suicide as an act of atonement, Thomas Dwyer concluded, "I believe in the resurrection of the body and life everlasting. Amen."[83] Ill health and financial worries at the outset of the Great Depression made farmer Albert Milligan despondent. His note captured a sincere religious belief: "Almighty and merciful God have mercy on my soul. I cannot live on earth any longer."[84] Another man in the same crisis year "talked about eternity."[85] "God alone knows the trial and tribulations I have been through," wrote another.[86] At mid-century, Harold Adams asked the Lord to bless his family; at the end of his farewell note he wrote, "so long folks, see you in Heaven."[87] Ruth Byrne declared around the same time that "I am not afraid to meet God."[88] "I am going to heaven," wrote another woman that same year. "I have been praying and I know God will take me."[89]

Rarely did anyone in the first half of the century express doubts about a happy family reunion in heaven. Church doctrine that established suicide as a sin was largely ignored. Poor alcoholic labourer Joseph Kelly was one of the few who took it seriously. He wrote in 1906 that "the World is hard and I am sick of it." At sixty-seven, he could not get work and his wife had died. To his son he mentioned, "I suppose that suicides don't go to heaven so I may not see your mother."[90] Faith unshaken, he questioned only his suitability for heaven. As late as 1964, a woman left a note asking "please God forgive me." She wanted to get to her loved ones.[91] The era in which the individual had been raised was important in terms of the intersection of faith and suicide. The youth suicides of the late twentieth century presented no evidence of 'old-time religion.' But there was a sense of entitlement. In his suicide note a violent abusive man who shot his former de facto signed with "see you's in the next life."[92]

As a presence in easing suicide decisions, Judeo-Christian ideas about God, angels, and heaven declined after 1950. The atrocities of Nazi Germany had earlier shattered the faith of a few individuals. A Jewish émigré who expressed his love for New Zealand as a "good and free country" nevertheless felt miserable and alone. He had had to leave his loved ones behind. To an acquaintance he wrote, "I am not able to share your lucky point of view of religious faith."[93] Yet concepts of an afterlife generally persisted, although as the century entered its last decades they expressed secular worldly attributes or betrayed cracks of doubt. A few people alluded to a non–Judeo-Christian faith. In a note for a war buddy who had bailed him out of jail, Talcott McClary said he would never forget such kindness "even in death if that is possible."[94] Here was a shadow of doubt.

A romantically smitten young man wrote at mid-century that "if you really love me we will find each other again somewhere."[95] No confident mention of a heavenly tryst! More than before, notes written at or after mid-century betrayed doubts or uncertainty about the soul's destination. A farmer with a lung tumour regretted leaving his large family, but the pain was too great to endure. A keen punter on horse races, he wrote with laudable wit that "my only wish is that they have a TAB [off-track betting shop] where I am going."[96] There was no mention of God, prayer, or heaven. Perhaps in this case there was no belief in immortality but rather sheer panache. Atheists and agnostics had to summon up extra courage. Conceivably, their growing numbers contributed to the fall in the suicide rate during the long prosperity. Not only was life relatively good then, but death was a decidedly unattractive proposition without a belief in heaven.

In the closing decades, non-specific or heterodox spiritual notions turned up. It was not unusual to see a simple final line "see you in the next life."[97] One individual gave the variation "see you in the new system."[98] Another wrote doubtfully, "wherever I end up I hope I have a friend as special as you."[99] Some people had written letters and diary entries addressed to a deceased relative.[100] A young man with an undiagnosed mental illness claimed to be conversing with his grandmother. On the morning of his death, he had been reading the chapter on "Experiences" in a book on Extra-Sensory Perception.[101] Underlying these remarks and practices was a vitalism that assumed the existence of an eternal life separate from the body.

Some of the increasing number of younger people who committed suicide in the 1980s and 1990s retained the idea of vitalism but were insensible to Judeo-Christian doctrines. A fifteen-year-old girl who had used cannabis in the past wrote that "this will be my last goodbye before I become an angel looking over you."[102] Unemployed labourer Hendrik Bilsma left this message: "See you in the next world. Keep hammering. I shall visit you one night."[103] The fusion of sacred and profane is arresting. The youth-specific Goth subculture, discussed in chapters six and seven, evinced a form of spiritual longing that assumed an afterlife. New characterizations of an afterlife were not all connected with youth. A victim of severe atherosclerotic disease longed for a better life and found solace in the idea of reincarnation. Her suicide note projected optimism: "I am now ready for my next Incarnation." Her hands were clasped peacefully, and nearby there was a 1987 magazine with a cover story on "Reincarnation: Fact and Fiction?"[104] At one level, it is hardly surprising that suicide and a belief in immortality were connected. The contemplation of death as a solution provoked thoughts about what might follow, and these reflections drew on consolations from folkways.

The desire for a reunion with people important to the deceased was a sentiment that persisted throughout the century. At times, it was mentioned casually in conversation. According to his daughter, Ronald Richardson had said not long before his death that "my mother was better off and it would be lovely to be with her." Mrs. Richardson had died three months earlier.[105] Comparable remarks appeared in numerous suicide notes. "Dear Mum, Dad, and Bill," wrote Arthur O'Toole in 1946, "I am writing you this note to say that when you get it I shall have gone to join my Sister Mary."[106] In her note fifty years later, Delores Shields indicated that she missed her father and several friends. "She wanted to be with them."[107] From time to time there was a tragic variation on the theme of a family reunion in heaven. Fearing that she would have to go to a mental hospital on account of psychosomatic symptoms, Katrina Black worried about her children. "Oh my poor little kids," she wrote, "I worry about them." In the end, she left two behind, but decided, "I am taking the baby."[108]

In the secular space expanding after mid-century, more individuals contemplating suicide had doubts about heaven, as they had about life's purpose. A few coupled doubts about life and immortality. "I can see no point in living," wrote Tony Sorger. "As I am not a religious man, I have no fear of death. I expect simply to go into oblivion."[109] Atheists were at least relieved of worry about Judgement Day. They could reason that a suicide was free from that risk. Agnostics could hold onto a thin hope that there might be something better. Convinced that he would "never make anything of my life," Wesley Bidwell told his parents in 1976 that "I will see you in heaven I hope."[110] In earlier times, individuals who mentioned heaven betrayed no such dithering, nor did they doubt their suitability for entry when God realized their full sad story. However, in the 1960s and 1970s, certainties were under siege and it showed. "I believed in God and Jesus Christ all my life," wrote one depressed woman in 1968, but she concluded, "I have been let down."[111]

Years later, a young woman with low self-esteem concluded her last letter with a mix of yearning and uncertainty. "They say it's a great life in heaven if you don't go to hell."[112] Made redundant by his employers and arrested for making violent threats, Jeff Upton wrote in 1994 to apologize to friends and relatives. He then went further and bared his feelings: "I am not afraid of death. It is fear of life which I find terrifying. Who knows maybe we'll meet again some day."[113] Drug addict Bill Mitchell, "Mr.Loser," admitted that he "had stuffed it [life] ... Hopefully, god can do something with me."[114] He was unsure about himself and immortality; God was now just a god. Through the words of final conversations and suicide notes during the last three decades of the century, we see and hear an age of imperfect doubt and imperfect belief.

If references to an afterlife provide a means by which mature men and women secured consolation, then notes from this age signalled not just doubt but a despairing shrug from young people.

Faith remained strong in some communities and with some individuals; with less frequency, faith continued to affect thoughts about suicide and beyond. Among the shrinking numbers of church-goers, heaven retained meaning. In a few notes written by the committed Christians from the Pacific Islands in the 1990s, belief endured. In one Islander home, alcoholism and domestic violence led to a police intervention. The man responsible wrote, "tell mum and your sister I will see them in heaven."[115] Religious faith soaring into mania infused the logic of a rare few. Matt Laidlaw thanked his parents for "giving me such a beautiful simple faith as a child" and then proceeded to explain that what he was about to do was not an act of suicide "but an act of surrender. The prize is great – wow, eternal life."[116]

There is no doubting Matt Laidlaw's sincerity. He worked as a volunteer for a Christian Life Centre. However, it is probably that some individuals drafted allusions to a life beyond as acts of kindness to friends and family. That consideration was occasionally explicit. In a long letter to family and friends, a man asked that everyone should "try to put it behind ... Think of me moved on to a place of peace, where there is no pain, no guilt, and no tears."[117] Kindness to others as well as faith could have inspired letters that ended with a reference to eternal life. Both possibilities – that is, thoughtfulness and faith – indicate that individuals had deliberated about their pending action. Through reflection, they built up resolve and displaced their anxiety by drafting statements to console others. By mentioning others, a prevalent feature of suicide notes, writers took their mind off the deficiencies of suicide as a solution. Mental exercises that envisioned a time after death put a portion of the act's reality behind them, while mentioning friends and family members helped detach the writer from the hand that held the pen.

Quite a few references to the possibility of an afterlife surfaced indirectly; the phrasing of sentences implied that existence continued beyond the act. Thomas Joiner usefully suggests that "imminently suicidal people fuse death and life."[118] The difficulty with such astute observations is the inconsistency of the appearance of the identified phenomenon, plus the great possibility that non-suicidal people share this idea of an immortal spark. Originating in hindsight, the concept has no predictive authority. Some suicidal people, often women, romantically elided life and death. In her letter to her daughter, Doreen Robins said she would "never cease to pray for you and Paul and the children." It was her wish that "may we all be re-united in a happier existence."[119] Valerie Porter told a friend that she wanted to be with Mark, "the person with whom she used to live. He was killed on 4 February 1974."[120] In a brief suicide note, a young woman mentioned her deceased boyfriend. "Where Paul McNeil is, is where I want to be."[121] The longing to be reunited could disclose objects of deep affection, but occasionally sources of pain. A sexually abused young woman despised her parents and hoped they would "rot in hell." She wanted to go back and "be with my Nanny who I know loved me." This young woman made a final request: "I want my white teddy to go with me."[122] "See you there," wrote one romantically disappointed individual.[123]

In the late twentieth century, "there" was not always heaven. A few letters conveyed hazy traces of belief in a future after death. One man wrote "good-bye for a little while."[124] In a note to a friend, a young woman declared, "I love you, have always loved you, and will always love you."[125] If time continued, so must she. A young man in 1986 addressed his relatives: "I will always cherish you in my heart."[126] A few years later, a young man assured family members that he loved them, "always have and always will."[127] It is impossible to know if these similar phrases of continuance expressed a wished-for persistence away from troubles or whether they showed once more that some individuals contemplating suicide were aware of the consequences of their pending action. Their rationality may have included a regard – admittedly imperfect – for survivors.

Apart from the belief that death transported one to a nicer place populated by all the right people, individuals with worries found additional ways to minimize a fatal act. Burdened by business troubles and suffering chest pains, travelling showman William Stewart considered a happy metaphor of winning derived from cribbage. "I think I am going to peg out," he told a friend.[128] People wrote about "crossing the border."[129] That phrase could have had an understated religious connotation similar to expressions such as "see you on the other side."[130] Death for some was the beginning of "a long journey,"[131] a trouble-free rest,[132] or a much-desired peaceful sleep.[133] A doctor who heard the last words of a war-injured veteran testified that he said that "he wanted to go off to sleep and seemed perfectly rational in his statements."[134] "Life," concluded a young man in 1994, "is no place for me so I am going to go from it."[135] These men and women had contemplated their troubles and the suicide solution; they blurred distinctions between life and death by trivializing the prospect that death meant irreversible oblivion.

The concept of an afterlife had an obvious attraction. It promised existence. There was more. It also meant escape from this fallen world. A few statements in every period included a critique of current world conditions or life in general. Old and out of work in 1902, Neil Horne told a friend, "It would be as well for a man to be out of the world."[136] Years later, an old age pensioner in bad health wrote, "may we all meet in a better world."[137] A poor widower in 1928 wanted his reason and reasons accepted. To the local coroner he wrote, "Sir, I am perfectly sane just fed up with poverty and ill-health, and am taking the short-cut out of it."[138] These sentiments had peak currency among older men before the establishment of the welfare state.

Late in the century, angry young people snarled comparable but less respectful remarks. Rather than a matter-of-fact disappointment with the world and its bountiful suffering, young men ranted about being hassled or applied harsh self-criticisms centred on their supposed unsuitability for the world as they found it. In addition to quoting lyrics from David Bowie's "Cat People," Martin Green wrote in 1984 that "the world is so false you only have to look at a place like America to see this."[139] For the first half of the century and more, the cultural representations of manliness had accented physical endurance, and with the body's failure, it was time for a real man to go. In the late twentieth century, the measures of success had become more complicated and included education and training. Young men who could not vault over the credentials barrier, for whatever reasons, were left to thunder against a hard world, to blame themselves, or to condemn both the world and themselves. One mode of expressing rage, tattoos, also habituated the body to pain and made a violent act against oneself commonplace.

HABITUATION AND THE SELF-ACCLAIMED SACRIFICE

Thomas Joiner suggested the importance of a habituation to pain in his efforts to theorize about suicide. Evidence from depositions and suicide notes suggest that there is value in this concept, although its borderless character makes it too vague to be of much use as a diagnostic tool or an ingredient in a true theory. There can be false positives, because plenty of people experience pain from a prior attempt or an injury, and do not then complete a suicide. Another problem with seeing a prior attempt as a habituation to pain and a near-death experience is that the sequence of suicide attempts had to begin somewhere; there is the possibility of regression back to an initial habituation-free attempt.

We recorded cases where witnesses reported that there had been a prior attempt, a clear threat, or a vague threat. These warnings were under-reported, because some witnesses felt that a failure to take notice of a history of attempts or threats might reflect badly on them. Thus, it was best to register surprise. In two-thirds of all suicide inquests (66.3 percent) there was no mention of anything that could be taken as a warning. The remaining third was composed of reports of prior attempts (10.1 percent), clear threats (18.9 percent), and vague threats or odd conduct (4.7 percent). We did not maintain a count of young men injured in automotive accidents who later committed suicide because evidence of an accident was not collected routinely, but likely the young men who committed suicide had had more accidents per capita than other young men. The difficulty with seeing them as habituated to pain or a death-like experience is that many were also disabled and contemplated how complete they had been before the crash. It is possible that war veterans who had known combat and who committed suicide had been habituated to violence and death, but it is also the case that many were disabled. Habituation is a possibility in some instances. Witnesses at an inquest into a 1950 suicide believed that returned soldier Joe Powers was "fearless and had a disregard for things dangerous." He shot himself with a rifle.[140] The impossible challenge for suicide studies is to discern when signs of habituation – combat experience and fearlessness – point toward great risk in specific instances. There will always be a call for more information and no chance of prediction without immense numbers of errors.

There were instances of a deliberate infliction of pain. The most extreme involved chewing glass. An alcoholic labourer with depression used to eat glass "by chewing off pieces of beer glasses and swallowing it."[141] A prisoner so violent that he frightened Mongrel Mob gang members chewed razor blades and light bulbs, swallowed the wire bits, and banged his head against the wall, gradually knocking all his teeth out.[142] More common were tattoos whose inscription by needle inflicted discomfort, particularly when crude tools were used in prison where tattoos figured in the subculture of defiance.

A few tattoos were reported at inquests in earlier decades of the century, but we can only be sure of thorough reporting on their presence at the end of the century, when an inquest document guided pathologists through their description of the body. Across earlier decades there are only sporadic references to tattoos, but they sustain the idea of a habituation to death. A sailor who jumped ship in Auckland in mid-1914 had a tattoo with a tombstone and the words "In Memory of My Dear Sister." Notwithstanding the incompleteness of earlier reporting on the appearance of bodies, it seems that tattoos became prominent in the 1970s.[143] They exploded into prominence during the 1990s.[144]

The proliferation of tattoos on the bodies of suicides in the late twentieth century may denote deliberate exposure to pain, a sign of resurgent Māori pride, or both and more. Māori brought some tattoo designs into fashion. Tattoos were extensive among gang members and prisoners, who covered their bodies. During the 1980s and 1990s, individuals were described as having multiple tattoos, being "extensively tattooed," "heavily tattooed," tattooed with numerous old healed scars, and "extensively tattooed over almost all skin surfaces." [145] An autopsy report near the end of the century indicated that "there were extensive tattoos covering the whole of the body other than the soles of the feet, the hands, head and neck, penis and scrotum."[146] The ability to withstand pain had limits.

The messages of many tattoos captured the nihilism seen in the actions and words of some young people during the century's final decades. Brain-damaged from an auto accident, John Cuthbert was angry; his knuckles displayed HATE.[147] The right forearm of another young accident victim carried the word MOB.[148] HATE along the knuckles was popular, and so too symbols of mob identity.[149] A nineteen-year-old prison inmate who sported the hate message also had tattoos of DIE and a sword. His brother had committed suicide.[150] In another case, the pathologist reported that the body had "multiple tattoos over the shoulders, collar, chest, abdomen, left forearm, left ankle, and a number of scars from incompletely removed tattoos and presumably from areas where there had been previous tattoos."[151] The manly occupant of a skin canvas was not to flinch but to endure pain as part of an identity-making experience.

Case files for the last decade of the century included autopsy reports with the following descriptions. A violent young man who threatened to shoot a neighbour's dog was covered with scars and tattoos on his arms and legs.[152] A Māori man whose drinking upset his wife and daughter had a dagger tattoo.[153] Another male sported a Chinese dragon and warrior over his shoulder blades.[154] Marijuana leaves festooned bodies.[155] These latter tattoos may have been painfully acquired, but were not indicative of anger. Others certainly were. An eighteen-year-old solvent abuser had swastikas below his eyes.[156] Prisoner Jeff Green had a gun, a snake, a dragon, a battlefield, and a panther skull with the statement "Kill 'em all, let God sort 'em out."[157] "Justice stinks," stated a message inked on another.[158] Satan made appearances.[159] So did the Grim Reaper.[160] The tattoos that covered the right arm of a long-time drug addict "mainly depicted skulls."[161]

The unemployed coward who beat his de facto carried "a snake, skulls, dagger, Viking helmet, and gargoyle."[162] Expression of anger and violence could be found elsewhere, for example among the sparse belongings of young men and women. A morbidly obsessed young man decorated his flat with the picture of a hangman's noose, a skeleton riding a motorcycle with the caption "Death Rider," and a photo of a Special Forces beret with the motto "Mess with the Best – Die Like the Rest."[163] The lyrics of songs favoured by Goths may have contributed to habituation, a point mentioned in chapter eight. Occasionally body art and music merged.

The body of an unemployed twenty-four-year-old man was covered with numerous tattoos. "Most were professional tattoos of symbolic medieval nature, flames and reference to a current heavy metal rock group, the Iron Maidens [sic]."[164] By imposing pain and representing violence and death, tattoos could habituate. Like other stimulating ideas in the field of suicide conjectures, habituation is a retrospective rather than a predictive notion. Very few people with an anti-social tattoo message are bound for self-destruction. But the pain and the message are a part of the psychic biography of those who did end their lives. Furthermore, along the same lines, there were rare instances of morbid themes in artwork. A sad and inspired student photographer who "felt very alone in the world" repeatedly photographed himself lying across a railway line. There he eventually died.[165]

It is difficult to pigeonhole every background event even when these events are reported. Uniqueness undermines theory; even the arrangement of cases in this chapter is too neat. One set of circumstances that has not been explored so far and that may connect with habituation is the certainty that some people grew up with knowledge of suicide. Since no standard question was asked on this subject at inquests, the voluntary statements are surely fewer than the unknown number of instances. The following revelations give a sense of the diverse means by which morbid knowledge was acquired outside media reporting. Two of Bessie Cooper's aunts drowned themselves, and she knew of this.[166] Schoolboy Billy Milton was raised by his aunt, who had reprimanded him about his bad conduct and warned him that, if it continued, she would have "to take him to Constable Wootton." Disciplinary action has already been discussed as a factor in some rare pre-adolescent and adolescent suicides; however, in this instance there was more. The boy had been abandoned by his mother, and his father and uncle had hanged themselves.[167] Unemployed teamster Graham McEwen had a friend who committed suicide, and he wrote, "I am going to meet Jim Thomas."[168] In her testimony on her husband's death, Emma Tomlinson mentioned that "some of his family have committed suicide."[169] Charlotte Kirk's "father committed suicide and one of her sisters is presumed to have done so."[170] Edmund Hayes told his foster parents that his father killed himself.[171] A former employer testified that Elizabeth Galtons' "mother's brother had committed suicide."[172] Before Gladys Albert hanged herself, "she repeatedly said her brother had hung [sic] himself and she felt as if she were becoming like him."[173]

Awareness of suicide could come through other channels. An elderly man with diabetes had recently received a letter from the wife of his greatest friend "stating that her husband had poisoned himself with prussic-acid."[174] In the late twentieth century, reports of suicide spread through public housing flats where the unemployed and medical beneficiaries lived in disproportionate numbers.[175] Throughout the century there were scattered instances of close friends or de facto partners unable to cope with the suicide of the other party.[176] It was folly to think that a suppression of formal news reporting could contain talk about suicide and methods.

Injury and illness caused men and women to think of themselves as a millstone.[177] They exemplified what Thomas Joiner called burdensomeness, or the perception of being a burden.[178] That perception of being a burden was repeatedly associated with a serious illness, and the need for nursing care. Perception had concrete foundations. Old pensioner Michael O'Connell told a friend, "I am buggered up and I don't want to go to the hospital. I don't want to be a burden on anybody."[179] John Carson had a lame leg from a World War I wound; he left a note explaining that if he continued as an invalid "I would drag on till I had to give up and that would mean you slaving your soul out to keep me and that would kill me."[180] Ian Alexander's wife said that her husband's lung cancer left him with no more than a year to live and she had no doubt that his death was a suicide, because "he would have taken his own life so he would not have been a burden to anyone during his illness."[181] Charles Buckley wrote that he had given his action "a lot of thought," because he "had a fear of getting old and a real burden."[182] Goitre treatment left Carlene Sharpe depressed and believing she harmed the family: "I want you all to be free of me."[183] With only slight changes, the phrases just quoted appeared time after time when there was a serious ailment or disability. 'Old Bert' Wilson did not want to be a burden and "he just chose to have his own quiet control over the situation." His arrangement of private papers and bills denoted a calm that contrasted with suicides of rage.[184] The insurance suicide to assist the family was a rare sacrifice event. A businessman wrote, "my dearest family, my insurance is not cancelled by suicide and it is better for me to do this than to reach that stage where I become a labourer unable to keep you in the position that I alone have accustomed you to." Then again, this declaration may have been fashioned to establish a favourable memory, for he did not want to be thought cowardly.[185]

The habituation to pain and death seen in tattoos emanated from self-centred outlooks; however, there were 'sacrifice suicides' far removed from the world of tattooed young people. Such acts were intended to help others. A few men and women who suffered from mental illness assumed that they imposed an awful burden of care on their families. Their thoughts repeatedly turned over a sentiment of unworthiness and the attached possibility of redemption. Writing to her husband, depressed alcoholic Iris Davis declared that she did not think it fair to live. "I can't bring you anything but worry."[186] Sentences like these, almost always addressed to a spouse, were a feature in scattered notes.[187] Notes included the words "cope" and "burden." The deceased said the family would cope better; the deceased did not want to be a burden.[188] Some messages reveal altruism and a remarkable look at life. Cancer was destroying Arthur Johnson's left lung. He wrote to his "dear ones": "My condition has forced me to contemplate bringing my life to an end. I see no good lingering on, in my own way and hindering others who can do much for others. An old man steps off this earth to help make room for a dear wee newcomer – and so I say farewell to you all. Poppa."[189]

Occasionally, one suspects that family members fostered or intensified low self-esteem, or at least did little to dispel the idea that the elderly were a burden free from which the family could better cope. These instances confirm the need for safeguards in laws that would permit medically assisted suicides. Aged sixty in 1972, widow Olive Charters was one of many older women who had become dependent upon barbiturates. Her note likely meant the opposite of what it started to say, namely, "don't blame yourselves children." She shifted direction by remarking that "life is so selfish and the old are a nuisance unless they are rolling in money."[190] Thus, not all declarations of sacrifice were what they seemed. When a spouse said 'I am leaving this world to free you,' as some did, the intent could have been to inflict guilt. "Goodbye Eva," wrote Donald Dodds, "I hope you find a bit better life without me since I make things so bad for you."[191] "I will not burden you again. You will be free of me," wrote Ann Olds shortly after her husband left her.[192] Depending on the all-important context, a self-acclaimed sacrifice could be quite the opposite.

Statements of sacrifice seldom, if ever, were found among the oddly loquacious notes of young people at century's end. For many of them, there was no one whom they wanted to assist, but some whom they intended to wound. The old culture of sacrifice had withered. In earlier times when knowledge of the fundamentals of Christianity had been stronger, the sacrifice of Christ would have contributed a model of behaviour. "He died for us." The two wars reinforced the idea of noble sacrifice. Heroes had sacrificed; families had sacrificed; the nation had sacrificed. If individuals could write themselves into uplifting narratives of sacrifice, they could more easily get over the will to live. On this matter of burdens and sacrifices, Joiner's observations have merit.

GOING NOW

In chapter two, we described suicides when the timing was related to a court summons or the appearance of a constable at the door. A few people were thrown into emotional turmoil by a powerful event that challenged their self-perception or expectations as to how life should have unfolded for them. The end of a marriage, the end of a relationship, and the end of a life's work were all occasions for self-assessment tinged with sorrow and regret. During the years of heavy alcohol consumption, a handful of men ended their lives when given the news that a spouse had contacted the clerk of the court for the papers required to initiate a prohibition order banning the sale of alcohol to the husband.[193] For a few women, the death of a baby was a final blow.[194] Two days after her three-week-old baby died, Alma Murdoch took her own life. In the estimation of witnesses, her death resulted from a combination of post-partum depression and grief. The latter was the precipitating factor.[195] The death of a beloved spouse could precipitate a suicide. Reginald Long had stayed by his wife's hospital bed until she died at four in the morning. He took his own life that day. "I promised mummy to stay with her and that is above all promises. We loved each other over ups and downs for 57 years. Don't let the coroner muck about with it. I want to be thrown to the wind with her ashes."[196] The approaching moment of exposure of a crime or debt also affected timing.[197] A dismissed schoolteacher who had falsified attendance records on which funding depended approached the local Member of Parliament to intercede, and when he declined she cut her throat. Her sister testified that she said that "she would commit suicide if she were disgraced."[198] A few individuals in every year feared the shame of exposure more than death.

Men and women occasionally wrote about their calculation of what constituted a reasonable lifespan. A fatalistic labourer with a probable case of syphilis asked, "what is a few years anyway it is only a matter of time and we all will be dead and gone?"[199] At mid-century one woman put it this way: "we all have to go sometimes, dear, and I would rather go now."[200] At century's end, an avid reader expressed the same idea, noting that "we've had some good times but they don't last forever." She expressed her thankfulness for the life she had had until her eyesight suddenly failed. "I'm thankful for reaching 80 with the good health I've been blessed with." Her letter went on to reflect on the frailties of age more generally and how those had affected her decision. She claimed to have seen many of her friends "pass on and find it a happy release from their sufferings." Her poignant enviable final sentence declared, "I have enjoyed life."[201] Similarly, Hal Clifford wrote that he had had "some good innings, three score and ten of good health and been there and done that."[202] Not nearly so fortunate were desperate single labourers in the years before the welfare state. In periods of economic depression, they did not select a moment but, to a degree, had it imposed. Alcoholic Ernest Otto's "means had come to an end."[203] "The deceased," stated a constable at a 1930 inquest, "was out of work and had reached the end of his resources."[204]

By the very selection of a time to die, there was an indication of planning. Christmas figured in timing, because people wondered whether to go before or after the holidays. Mary Murray remarked "that as it was nearing Christmas she seemed to think that no body wanted her."[205] An invalid widow during World War II explained to her family that she would go now, two weeks before Christmas, so that it would all be over and they could begin to forget her.[206] Or did she really intend to be the centre of their holiday thoughts? At her last consultation with her doctor about a nervous breakdown, Christina Miller mentioned that "she did not think she would be alive by Christmas."[207] Confined to bed, Alice Smith concluded that operations and medicine could not cure her "internal trouble." She planned to take her life but would wait until after Christmas.[208]

A date of significance to the deceased could trigger self-assessment by men and women with severe illnesses or lives that had not gone well. Birthdays are an obvious time for a review, and witnesses tended to remark on them if the suicide occurred around the same time. Cancer victim Lillian Horne killed herself on her sixty-third birthday.[209] When police found Winston Phillips' body, it lay near recent birthday cards and a package of cigarettes. His house reeked of tobacco smoke; he had long turned to cigarettes to deal with depression.[210] A widow with severe heart disease took a massive overdose of a painkiller several days before her seventy-fifth birthday.[211] The approach of two dates started Curtis Bruce reviewing his failed marriage. In a long recriminatory note directed at his ex-wife and children, he stated that "Christmas and my birthday alone are unthinkable as I am a family man." He scribbled on the note: "my birthday is near – 28 -11." He died on that day. Cards and photos littered the scene.[212] It was not Robert Hewitt's own birthday that caused him to reassess his life, but that of his son David. To his estranged wife, Hewitt had written, "tomorrow is David's birthday and it will be the last of me. I do not wish to knock about the world by myself any longer."[213] When David Nelson's estranged wife refused to come to his birthday party, the abusive sullen man took his own life.[214]

There were undoubtedly innumerable private triggers, dates inaccessible to suicide researchers or clinicians, dates that prompted self-critical assessments. Exposure to the unalloyed happiness of others could initiate a damning self-review. A birthday party, an event that involved couples and children, reminded lonely Wayne Russell of "a few women problems."[215] After a bout of heavy drinking, struggling carpenter Pat O'Connell ranted unpleasantly about an award ceremony for his brother the following night.[216] Anniversaries of important life events such as marriage, divorce, and the death of a loved one appeared in statements only when a witness knew the deceased quite well and felt moved to mention the timing. At Daphne Horne's inquest, a close friend noted that the time of her death marked "the anniversary of a relationship she had with a man in Australia who died five years ago. She loved him very much and said that she wished she was with him."[217] The importance of private anniversaries raises once more the idea that vital personal thoughts lie beyond our ken, but they have meaning in someone's life. A researcher's presuppositions cannot discover, let alone imagine, all these private meaningful events.

CONCLUDING OBSERVATIONS

This chapter opened with a question. Discussion moved indecisively around it and will continue to do so in perpetuity since the question is unanswerable. Any list of risk factors provided by current or future sociological, biological, or psychological research will encounter the problem of false positives. Many individuals who will exhibit alleged risk factors will endure and not choose self-destruction. Theories will be negated by these invisible non-conforming individuals.

Decisions to act, as described in this chapter, can best be labelled situational. Men and women were in various states of sobriety, rationality, rage, passion, or hopelessness. On the one hand, there were irrational and impulsive acts. On the other hand, some acts were rational and deliberate. Self-euthanasia is an example. However, the terminally ill were not the only individuals to weigh their circumstances, the meaning of life, and the nature of death. Many individuals considered what death meant and believed in immortality; some thought about bravery and cowardice in relation to suicide and planned to use an aid to shore up their nerve.[218] People calculated the impact of the act on others. Occasionally, the desired impression was meant to be emotionally devastating and exact vengeance on family members, friends, neighbours, the police, or employers. One spouse left a note for her husband that well captures this idea: "I hope my spirit will haunt you to the end for the way you behaved to me."[219] Often in trouble with the law and recently having surrendered his license for driving under the influence of alcohol, trucker George Sutherland concluded his note sarcastically by "thanking the police."[220] Suicide could have a nasty intent but be semi-rational in the situation. At the other extreme, a few remarkable individuals wrote notes to console others.

An added complication with theorizing about suicide is that, if we accept the merits of the two-step model for investigating suicide that has been proposed in this book, then the situational feature evident in the first step must take into account the culture and economy of a jurisdiction. The troubles that overwhelmed people changed with the times and the demographic groups most affected shifted in accompaniment.

The advantages of a century-long historical inquiry include the opportunity to see swings in the age groups most vulnerable and movement in the related reasons for suicide. Thus the book reports that alcoholism was an astonishingly common debility in the early twentieth century; the welfare state eased the crises of economic setbacks after the 1930s; youth unemployment at century's end contributed to a distinct social problem. Unmarried pregnant girls early in the century were more likely to commit suicide out of shame than their late-century counterparts.[221] However, the sexual revolution was no bed of roses. A long-term and case-based approach also covers the impact of war on suicide rates by showing the lingering consequences of conflict for returned soldiers and a few civilians. Methods of suicide changed as the country became more urban, car-oriented, and drawn onto a pharmacological path; however, one change was the return of hanging, perhaps as the method of the economically marginalized. Suicides do not occur in a timeless present, and psychologists should consider this element of fluidity.

When trying to answer the basic question about suicide, psychologist Thomas Joiner highlights the idea of perception. A few individuals who thought of their pending suicide as a sacrifice, he indicates, were not necessarily a perpetual burden or even a temporary burden, but they perceived that they were. They were not necessarily dishonoured but perceived that they were. We can add that some people merged life and death into immortality and that this blending was also a perception. All such perceptions have a historical context. In this chapter, sensitivity to cultural trends over time helps to identify time-specific reasoning processes, and to identify the aids that were requisitioned by people to overcome hesitation. Judeo-Christian ideas of immortality and an omniscient God were prominent until mid-century. Youth nihilism, understandable in relation to the employment crises of the 1980s and early 1990s, was a significant new phenomenon that conditioned how and why many psychologists studied suicide. Clinical psychology and its supporting research branches had matured coincidental with the rise of youth suicide.

The idea of perception would put the study of suicide squarely into the field of psychology, but although the term "perception" is useful to a degree, it trips over the clutter of untidy realities. On occasion people *were* a burden and were made aware of how others felt about that burden. There were a number of suicides by elderly men and women whose relatives tried to keep them at home but found the circumstances a burden and in a moment of careless candour let slip their feelings or made moves to put them in a charity home or hospital.[222] The crucial factor here is surely not perception, but human interaction and situations. Often the objective reality of the burden should not be questioned and then downgraded to a perception, because there is the real conduct of those closest to the affected individual, as well as the quality of society's supports for the disabled and elderly. Psychology dwells on the mind of the affected individual, but realities impinge. Hopelessness is not always a matter of perception; for example, self-euthanasia can be a reaction to a real situation as well as a perceived situation.

Certain individuals did not merely perceive that they had thrown their lives away; they knew that they had, through drink, drugs, gambling, and crime. People confronted a reality, not a perception. However, on the face of it, other individuals who wrote that "my life is nothing but huge mistakes" really had not wasted their lives. Perception applies, but not universally. Sex offenders, the numerous wife beaters, and rogue fraudsters did not just perceive that they were shamed when the police knocked at the door. They *were* shamed. To take one of many possible examples, Richard Parsons was shamed when his daughter ran to a neighbour's house. "The [Parsons] girl came to my house," the neighbour testified, "and told me that her father was very drunk and was knocking her mother about and asked me if I would go over and try to quieten him."[223] People who handled mail or cash accounts had both aspirations for middle-class respectability and opportunities for theft. When matters "were in the hands of the police" they were overcome by shame.[224]

History spoils neatness and strengthens scepticism. Specialists in suicide studies will not want to forfeit aspirations to propose a theory of suicide; neither will they wish to abandon devising tests to confirm a theory. Striving professionals want to be taken seriously as scientists; they aspire to respect and authority in public life. However, abandonment of claims to have elucidated and verified theories is the right course to insist upon. The pseudo-scientists' aspirations for theory will always fall short. First, the organizing concepts for human conduct can never be sufficient for an intimate understanding of how individuals think about themselves unless we assume an impoverished sense of reality and human imagination. Compression inherent in theory surrenders too much and can marginalize or exclude important details, including historical circumstances. Second, pseudo-theories employ roomy words that permit manoeuvring. There is so much leeway for convenient interpretation that the words mean little in any operational sense. Something that can mean anything means nothing. Karl Popper expressed the matter bluntly when he recounted his search for the boundary between sciences and pseudo-sciences. "It is a typical soothsayer's trick to predict things so vaguely that their predictions can hardly fail; that they become irrefutable."[225] Fuzzy writing can conceal self-doubt or deception. It makes sense for "suicidologists" to accept and declare that they are engaging in an activity that is less than a science. When set in relation to actual lives that ended in suicide, certain insights from "suicidologists" are substantiated, modified, expanded, but found lacking.

Conclusion: History's Patterns and Prevention's Obstacles

Historical inquiry falls outside the therapy industry, whose practitioners routinely deal with front-line suicide prevention. Nevertheless, having claimed that historical research can contribute to knowledge about the difficult subject of suicide, we are obligated to comment on prevention. In this summation, we consider how historical patterns can contribute. As might be expected from strong hints throughout the book, the position taken on the healing professions and on suicide prevention more generally is agnostic. Grandiose claims and predictions are suspect; circumspection is appreciated. We believe that this call for openness reinforces scepticism about the effectiveness of suicide prevention, a term which can mean intervention to assist individuals, societal action to mitigate despair, and statutory measures to deter by controlling fatal means.

From historical accounts it is feasible to note possibilities, costs, and limitations in each of these ways of addressing suicide prevention. The numerous clinical reports read for this study leave no doubt as to the compassion and energy of the individuals who have staffed the therapy industry. Unquestionably, the majority cared for the individuals they tried to assist, although the health care system itself faltered during restructuring, and there were rifts among professionals and examples of human error. Where do these observations lead? To cite one of many probing evaluations of the efficacy of intervention practices, "there are more questions than answers."[1] That statement applies to societal action and deterrence as well.

Today suicide prevention is commonly thought of either as intervention in people's lives or as measures to deny access to lethal means. Practitioners deal with individuals currently in crisis. Or, more accurately phrased, they deal with individuals willing to come forward for counselling sessions or young people brought into therapy by parents or guardians. The wayward mobility of people, their reluctance to submit to help, and the enduring stigma of going for treatment were noted in the sections of chapter five that dealt with patients' reluctance to adhere to a regimen of psychiatric treatment. These challenges endure, and in recent times are evident in "therapeutic encounters" with psychologists.[2] Not everyone at risk can be or wants to be assisted.

Prevention in a deeper sense than immediate intervention or restricting the fatal means can mean working toward measures that recognize how crises originate over time. On several occasions we proposed that psychiatrists and psychologists overstated the frequency of mental illnesses among suicide cases. In their defence, what they saw were people in distress; training predisposed them to feel that emotional or mental states called for therapy. Our interests extended to people's immediate states too, hence the discussion of impulse and deliberation, and the reconstruction of the reasoning processes for setting aside the will to live. On several grounds, however, we part company with those who attribute almost all suicides to mental illness. The strangeness of some internal arguments to end one's life was worthy of an effort to understand them on the individuals' own terms. The mental illness label may pre-empt that inquiry by moving the discourse too quickly and directly to an end point, to a conclusion of illness or maladjustment.

Not every professional in the therapy industry worked exclusively near the end of the life-course. Family doctors for much of the century, and certainly before 1930, knew something of the individual's life circumstances. We should mention too that late in the century, adherents of psycho-dynamic therapy showed interest in individuals' life histories, and more than once we encountered specialists who mentioned that life experiences were important. To repeat a point to avoid misunderstanding, we found abundant cases of mental illness and, especially notable, a century-long effort to define and comprehend depression as a mental illness. But even when these depression cases, broadly defined, are incorporated into the category of mental illness motives, the estimates of psychiatrists and psychologists seem extreme and the categorization myopic. Additionally, the gathering-up of various modes of non-conformity as mental illnesses has at times in the past over-reached and blundered.

We felt it essential to go back into individuals' personal histories to gain an appreciation of what led them to see death as a solution. Whether they suffered from undiagnosed or diagnosed mental illnesses, many had experienced stresses. Some sources of stress were beyond their control: economic depressions, wars, accidents, and illnesses. When considering these troubles, we should keep in mind what we will call "deep prevention." A grieving father expressed matters eloquently when he wrote, "all a parent can do is provide support and a loving stable environment. What society must do is provide hope, employment opportunities and a sense of balance."[3] Amen!

Case-based evidence recommends deep-prevention measures that are long-term and pertain to health from cradle to grave, meaningful work, and far-reaching education. The broad concept of deep prevention is frankly utopian, because it emphasizes extensive social action to improve lives before they slump into despair about the future. It is also utopian because some measures would have to be administered by parents who need to take responsibility, although sometimes it can be their own rank irresponsibility that is a core issue. The involvement of family members in the suicide prevention of individuals under treatment for a mental illness is quite a delicate matter, because offsetting the many examples of dysfunctional families there were plenty of instances of articulate caring parents who expressed frustration with late-twentieth-century enforcement of privacy and confidentiality. One mother spoke for all such parents when she stated that "I do wish that mental health services could have talked to me more, because I am sure that maybe it would have given Charles a little more of a chance if they had."[4]

Education may be helpful. Government-sponsored publications in the 1990s and into the new millennium certainly presented sound information. The warning signs of suicide risk for pre-adolescents and adolescents listed in a manual circulated by the New Zealand Ministry of Education at the end of the century harmonize with our observations. However, in many depositions that we read, parents and teachers claimed not to have seen any of the leading risk factors, such as relationship troubles, poor body image, loss of expectations, low self-esteem, and a background of family abuse.[5] Awareness can be advanced by media reporting of well-considered facts. By the end of the century, coronial inquests attained high standards for the collection and assessment of information. Coroners' findings should be immediately available to the media and researchers; access can contribute to public awareness and education.

With incessant calls for more research, psychologists disclose that their methods may be utopian too; a close reading of forthright authors in the field produces lists of contradictory or bland general conclusions mixed with honest disclaimers. "The data are obviously controversial and open to interpretation and debate," stated one such report.[6] Despite considerable groping in the dark, the model of immediate intervention for dealing with suicide crises has political currency because it is linked with the unstoppable force of medical optimism and it implies life-saving now rather than years or decades away. Short-term and seemingly low-cost solutions appeal to governments which uniquely have the capacity to press a national agenda in a small unitary state such as New Zealand.

It is understandable that prevention in the shape of case-work intervention has an established position, albeit a fairly recent one, if one excludes the century-long first-response attention of general practitioners. Medical intervention by nature is immediate and analgesic. It answers to a politically led insistence that something be done, but its effectiveness is open to question since no one can estimate the number of suicides that would have transpired had there been no counselling, no public education, no instruction in the schools, no publication of booklets advising people of warning signs, and no post-suicide counselling. By the same token, it is impossible to credit intervention with downturns in overall national suicide rates, in age group suicide rates, or in gender-specific suicide rates without taking into account the economic, social, and cultural factors that could have mitigated rates independent of directed action. The drop in rates in the 1950s, for example, owed nothing to intervention, and another drop around 2000 may predate concerted efforts to address youth suicide.

In recent years, several reviews of research on specific modes of intervention, prepared for health authorities in several countries, have found little or no current evidence of effectiveness of the following: school education, behaviour-changing programs for youth at risk, crisis hotlines, and limits to media reporting.[7] Mental health interventions to promote self-esteem were believed to be of limited effectiveness. Proof positive of the effectiveness of any measure is unlikely to be achieved, because of a concatenation of variables.

In addition to clinical intervention and education, there is the other immediate measure that gets attention in suicide prevention discussions, namely restricting access to the means. In New Zealand, attention has been given to access, in particular the long-standing but inevitably porous regulation of poisons. There were gentle, then forceful, measures taken to control barbiturates in the 1970s. Control of long guns in rural areas everywhere in the world is problematic, but the prominence of the use of firearms as a method of suicide outside towns and cities is a concern; owners of weapons have an obligation to secure them and keep them for personal use. It is likely that fencing off high places from which people have leapt to their death is effective in reducing a few suicides, but these deaths have always been rare (1.3 to 3.4 percent of all New Zealand suicides per decade) and other techniques remain plentiful and simple. The shifts in methods charted in chapter one suggest that as soon as a prominent method was blocked or faded away by chance, another was discovered, or else there was a growth in an established technique. The straight razor vanished; barbiturates were more tightly controlled; catalytic converters reduced access to carbon monoxide. Hanging correspondingly increased. Our evidence finds that closing off particular methods is unlikely to reduce the suicide rate; rates can increase even when a major means is denied. Of course, neither we nor any other suicide researchers can make a reasonable guess at what the numbers of deaths would have been without prevention. In sum, the question of the efficacy of prevention by restricting methods is as intractable as any other question involving suicide.

The prominence of hanging – indeed its growth – poses an immense challenge for prevention strategies. Studies of methods report that hanging is a leading technique worldwide; it was prominent in New Zealand and increased with appalling speed among young people at century's end.[8] In the closely controlled environment of a police lock-up, remand centre, or prison, well-known measures to prevent hanging are feasible and have been implemented; however, outside these locales the method defies restriction. Individuals in custody are at high risk; they can be placed under intrusive surveillance and denied access to the means. But who is at such risk in the population at large that their rights can be suspended to restrict access to the means (close to impossible in a non-custodial environment) or their every move scrutinized to steer them away from a diffuse method?

Possibly adolescents "perceived to be at risk" can be managed more than other individuals, but supervision cannot be total. Drowning declined as soon as more reliable methods became available. However, as one man put it in 1950, "there is always the river."[9] The larger point stemming from this remark is that planned suicides will be exceedingly hard to prevent by attempting to control lethal means. Impulsive acts pose distinct and serious prevention problems too.

Deep prevention is a tricky approach since it does not focus energy on the dedicated professionals and well-mobilized interest groups of the therapy industry. On a grand scale it would also be costly, but on the cheap it could pursue open, ongoing, and unflinching debates about public health and parental responsibility, plus education about relationships, family violence, responsible alcohol consumption, and access to meaningful work. To reverse the perspective, we can say that a lot of suicides were indictments of culture, society, and the economy. Culture, society, and the economy evolve and spin off new variations on timeless sources of unhappiness and trauma, sorrow and rage. The medicalization or the therapy industry route to prevention is more politically palatable than deep prevention, not just due to the probable higher costs of the latter but on account of the prevalence of upbeat government chatter and avoidance in public life of expressions such as "intractable problem." Promises of effectiveness amount to a hostage to fortune; questions about effectiveness can and eventually will build into scepticism. Interestingly, when mental health clinicians faced claims that they had dropped the ball in particular deaths, they took the position that "there was nothing that could have prevented this [adolescent] suicide."[10] Can mental health professionals have it both ways, claiming utility and backing off when there are failures?

With the backing of some decent evidence, this book has argued that deep prevention has been evident and perhaps even successful in two areas. On account of a historical perspective, it has been possible to see the likely impact of social welfare. First, New Zealand social security and labour legislation addressed particular forms of troubles and the suicide rates of older men fell. Second, the treatment of the elderly improved, including palliative care. The lessons to be taken from *Sorrows of a Century* cannot be mapped in fine detail for the purposes of steering policy. The book's emphasis on changes in motives, methods, and rationales over the decades implies that wisdom is found in hindsight, predictions are ill-advised, and situations that affect lives are subject to circumstances that can change for better or worse. The types of years that we identified are testimony to that.

All is not lost in a chaos of micro-biographies and the unpredictability of changes over time. Rewarding work and employment security have been consistently important throughout the century, first for adult men, increasingly for women, and then, after the establishment of the welfare state, for many young people who by all accounts wanted a future and not simply welfare assistance. At its best, work provided a meaningful activity and developed relationships. Alcoholism and drug abuse have had multiple consequences for health, work, and relationships. Worries about work and the damage of substance abuse have contributed to mental illnesses. Of course, these are not the only sources of the mental illnesses which have had a presence among the motives for suicide.

We noticed and remarked on atavistic posturing by men. It was fairly persistent. It showed up in episodes of violence in the family and threats of self-harm to force a point. In these shocking circumstances, police intervention or court action occasionally pushed unstable men into rash deeds. More often, though, the men acted out their vengeance or controlling threats. Societal values about what is manly need addressing through education and example.[11] The prominence of physical ailments was a striking feature too. In many instances, physical decline was accelerated by lifestyle decisions contributing to high blood pressure, emphysema, congestive heart problems, liver disease, and obesity. Here again, prevention can benefit from long-term educational efforts that are now, thankfully, public health orthodoxy.

This book opened with a comment from the early-nineteenth-century British journalist William Hazlitt: "Our attachment to life depends on our interest in it." Deep prevention means the maintenance of an interest in life. Deep prevention is nothing more – but also nothing less – than putting into action a concern and respect for those around us.

Appendix One: Methodology

The abundance of case files required systematic selection to reduce note-taking. From the outset, we believed that qualitative evidence would be important and that there could never be too much information on people's situations. However, there could be limits to our stamina. We tested the limits on that count. To contain the research but secure a fine selection of cases for qualitative analysis, we decided to study half of all suicides. Rather than select a sample by random numbers, we read every case from even-numbered years. That eliminated a potential problem with a supposedly random selection. Some coroners forwarded their inquest files to the Ministry of Justice in batches, and thus the case-file numbers assigned when they arrived in Wellington do not represent a chronological sequence for the entire country but rather clusters of files from particular cities and regions. The implications of this feature were unclear to us. Moreover, by working with all cases in even years, we assumed we might encounter sets of related suicides from specific locales. That occurred. The pursuit of all instances of death by suicide for a calendar year led to a practical problem when we reached mid-century. By then, coroners demanded more extensive preparatory evidence; investigations took much longer. That led to delays in holding inquests. Quite a few inquests had to be postponed and some were conducted a year or even more after the date of death. Therefore, we had to review files deep into odd-numbered years to pick up the deferred inquests into deaths occurring in even-numbered years. Thoroughness was a costly watchword.

Delays in holding an inquest eventually affected government reporting. In recognition of the fact that accurate numbers of suicide deaths occurring in a calendar year could only be established by working through death certificates or inquest files several years down the road, the *New Zealand Official Yearbook* in 1985 abandoned reporting on suicide deaths for the calendar year and gave instead the number of suicide inquests held during that year. We adopted this latter expedient only for 2000, because Archives New Zealand currently holds inquests only through to the end of 2000. To complete the century in a consistent fashion, it would have been necessary to secure special consent to sort and view nearly 200 inquests held on site by Coronial Services, an awkward and costly effort since there would have been a retrieval fee. Some files of particular importance, especially in respect of psychiatric services, were made available by Coronial Services beyond 2000.

In addition to conventional note-taking, we assembled two data sets for analysis using SPSS (Statistical Package for the Social Sciences). The first data set contained information on all suicide deaths that occurred in the selected years (n = 11,000). The second set included all suicide inquests held in 2000 (n = 495). Two people working on and off for eight years completed the note-taking and coding of case-file information. Based in Wellington, Doug Munro conducted a large share of the post-1920 research. I examined the files from 1900 to 1920 and joined Doug for several months each year until we completed our work in July 2012.

Even working in tandem, two people can arrive at different judgements about details in some cases. Parts of several years were re-examined to see if there was great variation in our coding. There was, but only at the margins. In rare cases, we differed over whether a death was accidental or a suicide. Since it is possible to have conflicting philosophical outlooks on self-euthanasia, we established thresholds; self-euthanasia cases were defined as instances where an individual was mentally competent and had a terminal illness. However, we also included a few cases where there was a serious loss of quality of life and a clear expression of this circumstance by the individual. This point is mentioned to show the complexity of suicide as a category of action, and it indicates our collaboration on coding. When in doubt about the certainty of suicide or about the prime motive, we conferred.

By and large, the coding decisions were straightforward, although the heart of a matter sometimes came near the end of a witness' statement, doctor's report, or autopsy. Files had to be read carefully.

Coroners' summaries and findings often provided a fine outline of the case, but the supporting documents were the sources most relied upon for our judgements and note-taking. As much as possible, we wanted to cite the words of the parties. Of course, the authenticity of the witnesses' words can be questioned, because many depositions assembled responses to questions from a police officer or coroner. Yet credibility is advanced by the vernacular quality of replies, the free flow of numerous statements, and the amazing candour of some witnesses in respect to their own contributory conduct. More concerning was the incompleteness of some investigations; a few coroners discharged their responsibilities perfunctorily and wrote evasive findings. It was tempting to fill in the blanks by weighing every word for a hidden meaning. Our suspicions ultimately did not condition our coding; we used the designation "unknown" liberally.

A run of thin files could be worked through at the rate of twenty per researcher per seven-hour day; the rate for thick files was half that. When not working in tandem, we consulted by e-mail. Once the coding for a year was completed, I checked the data set for errors, and made corrections by re-reading the original files. When data sets were merged, I recoded the data in the master file to add new compressed variables.

Extraordinary luck enabled us to cover the century. Our original idea was less ambitious than a century-long study, but a chain of events enabled us to exceed our plan. The initial project compared Queensland and New Zealand from 1900 to 1950 and concluded with the publication of *A Sadly Troubled History: The Meanings of Suicide in the Modern Age*. Toward the end of the research for the New Zealand portion of that work, the Department of Justice transferred to Archives New Zealand all inquest files up to and including inquests held in 1988. We decided to press ahead with a new project covering 1950 to 1988. When we were nearing the completion of that work, the archives accessioned inquests held from the beginning of 1989 to the end of 2000. Each time we approached an apparent end of the road, more years became available until we could conceive of this century-long study. Original files for 1963 to 1975 were destroyed after microfilming; in some years the microfilm copies are disorganized and documents seem to be missing; most problems seemed to affect the records for 1974. Therefore, we excluded files from 1974 from the data set and notes. To access the microfilmed records, we needed approval from Coronial Services, because on strips of film there was no means of preventing our seeing restricted material: for example, disturbing police photographs, which we did not wish to see and which, in any event, were summarized in police testimony.

During the period of our research, all paper files for the century were open to researchers because sensitive material could be closed off; some files held sealed envelopes containing the disturbing photographs mentioned above, or suicide notes. Often the notes were placed in sealed envelopes because some were recriminatory, written with the intention of causing distress to acquaintances or relatives of the writer. Coronial Services granted us access to these notes; indeed, coroners urged us to access them because they knew from their experience that these statements were often powerful and important evidence. It is true that notes occasionally changed our attribution of motives and especially provided better insight into the deceased's mental state, their reasoning behind the suicide solution to a problem, and their attitude toward intimates. However, notes taken alone would not necessarily further an understanding of the suicide in question. Most were deeply personal communications and either employed private allusions or were short and anodyne; many of these latter brief notes provided no clues about motives or reasoning. The various documents are most revelatory when considered together.

In the midst of the case-file research, the key digital search facility (Archway) at Archives New Zealand replaced the traditional finding aids assembled in binders. Archway enabled us to locate important files scattered throughout many government departments on subjects such as mental hospitals, mental health interest groups, the control of barbiturates, the introduction of psychotropic drugs, social security, elements of youth subcultures, government suicide studies, censorship, self-euthanasia, and much more. Without Archway, for example, it is unlikely that we would have discovered the caches of records supporting chapter six.

Another stroke of good luck combined with government accommodation enabled us to be certain about individuals' ages. Inquest forms did not always require the person's age. Occupation and marital status were usually provided; however, age was not. Since age was bound to be an essential variable, we approached the office of the Registrar General of Births, Deaths, and Marriages for permission to see death certificates. This specific request was denied, but since the records were digitized, that office agreed to conduct searches for a reasonable fee. We submitted the names and dates on an Excel spreadsheet, and a staff member inserted the missing information and e-mailed back the Excel spreadsheet. In the final data set that included the added age information, we were missing ages for only one in twenty cases (5.4 percent). There were no missing ages after 1980, an important consideration because of the focus on youth suicides at the end of the century.

The initial data set assembled values for the following variables: name, date of death, gender, marital status, ethnicity, age, occupation, employment or financial status, recent emotional state, recent conduct of others toward the deceased, impact of war, evidence of emotional support, certainty of suicide, evidence of warnings or threats, primary motive for suicide, medical treatment, method of suicide, and information on the witnesses. After 1950, we recorded up to three motives in some cases, but usually additional motives were closely associated with the primary one.

We retained considerable detail in the initial coding scheme in keeping with a long-standing practice in quantitative historical research. Thus to cite some examples, for the variable on whether the deceased was affected by war, the number 2068 was the code for "wounded, WWI, shrapnel caused trouble, neurasthenia, depression since 1919, in pain." Several more examples will give an idea of the amount of detail that filled a codebook of over one hundred and fifty pages. Motive 30019 of the motives variable captured the details that the individual was "separated or divorced and the wife or de facto has custody of a child or was applying for custody." Medical treatment 4476 stood for the fact that the deceased had been on "Ward 12 of Invercargill Hospital with depression two years earlier." All of this information was retained in the codebook, which in itself became a useful set of notes. Subsequently many values for several important variables were recoded into new compressed variables. For some tables and statements in the book, the original values were useful; however, most tables and graphs express recoded values. Table 9.1 suggests the effort that went into recoding. During recoding, a few original coding errors were detected and corrected.

The spread between the number of raw values and the number of recoded values is a reminder of individuality. In order to relate fundamental human diversity, we relied in the book on qualitative evidence composed of quotes from witnesses' statements, doctors'

Table 9.1
Examples of the recoding of raw values into groups of values

Original variable name	*N of raw values for the variable*	*N of values accounting for half or more of cases*	*New variable name*	*N of values for the recoded variable*
Occupation	549	10 = 51.9%	Groups by work type and status	23
Marital status	30	2 = 68.3%	Marital status compressed	7
Employment situation	48	5 = 57.1%	Work and financial state	10
Motive	3,211	99 = 50.6%	Motive clusters	11
Emotional state noted	282	6 = 51.5%	Not recoded	
Action toward deceased	659	40.5% good care	Not recoded	
Medical treatment	2,374	190 = 50.0%	Type of illnesses	35
Affected by war	149	93.4% not affected	Types of impact	12
Method	445	4 = 56.3%	Types of methods	18
Exact location	218	5 = 52.6%	Not recoded	
Community name	1,489	51 = 50.0%	Type of community	11

reports, and suicide notes. The labour-intensive practice of typing up notes on most cases proved its worth when collating examples at the writing stage. We gave many notes thematic tags; recorded at the time of note-taking, these tags embodied our thinking when reading the evidence and assisted with recovering information at the writing stage. Photographing case files was reserved for something remarkable or visually significant, and not relied upon for the routine collection of information. Since our assumption was that this project would take an immense amount of time on-site, we did not feel constrained to photograph and digest material later. We believe there are advantages to thinking about and working with the material while taking notes.

Appendix Two: Writing Style

At one time, attempted suicide was a criminal offence. In New Zealand, it was rarely prosecuted in the twentieth century. The expression "to commit suicide" derived from the idea promoted by Christian churches that suicide was a sin; the individual who had "committed" the mortal sin could not be buried in consecrated ground. Pedantically speaking, people no longer "commit suicide"; however, the term remains in common usage and few people have the slightest idea of its correct origins. The term is thus retained in this book with today's vernacular understanding; our use of the expression conveys no critical judgement about the act.

Research for this book is the product of a fruitful partnership with Doug Munro. In addition to encoding thousands of cases in the data set and writing associated notes, Doug shared in the intellectual enterprise of developing questions and attempting answers; he was far more than a dedicated research assistant. Although his commitments as a South Pacific historian precluded his drafting sections on the topics that most interested him, his contributions are such that it has been impossible to discuss points in the first person singular. I have used "we" to capture our partnership.

Quotes from the documents retain the original spelling and use of upper case letters. In a few instances the punctuation was corrected to convey meaning more effectively. Quotations also retain New Zealand spelling. As mentioned in the introduction, almost all names have been fictionalized in ways that retain an individual's ethnic identity.

Due to government reorganizations, the Department of Health became the Ministry of Health in 1993, and in 1995 the Department of Justice became the Ministry of Justice. We have used "department" throughout.

Notes

INTRODUCTION

1 Archives New Zealand, Coroners' Inquests, ABVP, W5521 17298, 2000/1093. Henceforth files will be cited in an abbreviated form. For example, ABVP, 2000/1093.
2 See the account of games and sports in New Zealand in Belich, *Paradise Reforged*, 361–88.
3 ABVP, 2000/395.
4 ABVP, 2000/454.
5 ABVP, W5682 7410, Box 174, Legal, Interpretations, Rulings, Opinions, Coroners, LEG 12-3-1, Evidence and Verdict, Documents Produced during Inquest: Re: Picard, 13/7/83. ABVP, W5682 7410, Box 175, Coroners, LEG 12-5-9, Part 2. Coroners Handbook. New Zealand's Accident Compensation Commission, which started in 1972 to handle death benefits for the families, had a generous practice respecting suicides. No compensation would be paid in respect of a suicide. However, the wife or children might receive a payment if in need of assistance. ANZ, ACCT W2853 620 Box 40, Accident Compensation Act: Willfully Self-inflicted Injuries and Suicides. Case files suggest that ACC was generous. Coroners had no reason to render an open verdict to help a family with a claim. In the overwhelming number of cases in the late twentieth century, their findings were professional and based on common-law precedent and evidence. We disputed some findings where a coroner seemed to have unreasonably applied the common-law maxim that any doubt, however far-fetched, permitted an open finding.
6 Not every suicide note written has survived; on occasion individuals finding a body and a note secreted the note or destroyed it. We know for

certain that families wanted to retain them. This makes it impossible to estimate what proportion of suicides wrote notes or if notes disclosed any pattern. Once the police arrived, all physical evidence, including notes, was secured.

7 Mac Donald and Murphy, *Sleepless Souls*, 338–53; Anderson, *Suicide in Victorian and Edwardian England*, 191–259; Kushner, *Self-Destruction in the Promised Land*, 13–61.

8 Bailey, "*This Rash Act*," 7, 32–3, 94–5. Olive Anderson also covers this topic, *Suicide in Victorian and Edwardian England*, 41–103.

9 Weaver, *A Sadly Troubled History*.

10 Kushner, *Self-Destruction*, 89.

11 See for example a coroner's remark in 2000/477. He stated that suicide baffled the people who "treat the illness, and it is an illness."

12 Kitanaka, *Depression in Japan*, 200. See too a similar assertion in Lawlor, *From Melancholia to Prozac*, 195, 200.

13 We know that the set is essentially complete because the clerks maintaining the ledger abstract books assigned a number to each file as it arrived from outlying centres. During the microfilming of files from 1963 to 1975, some files were missed and all original files for this period were destroyed. Paper originals exist for all other years.

14 See the discussion of Norbert Elias in Mac Donald and Murphy, *Sleepless Souls*, 275.

15 Joiner, *Why People Die by Suicide*, 136.

16 Joiner, *Myths about Suicide*, 272.

17 Bailey, "*This Rash Act*," 7, 32–3, 94–5.

CHAPTER ONE

1 J46, 1930/77; 1930/966.

2 J46, 1960/982; 1976/335; 1976/572.

3 See for example these cases from one year: J46, 1964/722; 1964/1168; 1964/1216.

4 ABVP, 1992/989.

5 J46, 1954/569.

6 J46, 1976/311.

7 J46, 1961/186.

8 ABVP, 2000/846.

9 ABVP, 2000/1004.

10 J46, 1950/872.

11 ABVP, 1995/397.

12 J46, 1960/973.
13 For an articulation of the modern coroner's position, see ABVP, 2000/614, and Coroners Court, Wellington, New Zealand, Decision 75/2006. A good example of a lawyer's efforts to raise doubt about a suicide appears in ABVP, 2000/828.
14 J46, 1961/533–5.
15 We could have normalized suicide rates by one of several tables employed in epidemiological studies to adjust for variations in the age distributions among countries. No advantage is gained by taking this step, since we are not comparing New Zealand rates to those of another jurisdiction. Comparison is the fundamental reason for normalizing rates and, because we are sceptical about the quality of rates from many other countries, there is no reason to venture beyond simple rates. While the official rates and our inquest-derived rates form separate series, both moved in parallel over the years.
16 A royal commission in 1967 recommended a comprehensive no-fault insurance scheme. It was established in 1972 and adopted the principle that accident compensation was a community responsibility. AATD W3294 6136, Royal Commission on Social Policy. Original Submissions, Box 8, Submission 767, Review of the Accident Compensation Scheme.
17 ABVP, W5682 7410, Box 174, Legal, Interpretations, Rulings, Opinions, Coroners, LEG 12-3-1, N.R.A. Netherclift, Solicitor, Accident Compensation Commission, to Chief Advisory Officer, Legal Section, Department of Justice, 18 April 1977 (att: Mr Sisarich).
18 Brooking, "Economic Transformations," 226–49.
19 Belich, *Paradise Reforged*, 315.
20 J46, 1906/672.
21 Comparisons with the general population on the matter of marital status are impossible, because inquests often were forthright in describing the states of relationships that were not captured in the census. De facto status was first reported in the 1981 census. Also, couples living apart might report their status as married for the census, but police investigations for the inquests turned up the actual status. On the reporting of de facto status see *Yearbook 2000*, 123.
22 Abbott, "Overview of the Symposium," 6.
23 Recent surveys conducted in Britain indicate that happiness dips in the thirties and forties on account of loneliness and work-life balance. This is the period when relationships disintegrate. *The Economist*, 18 August 2012, 53.

24 The calculation of a rate of suicides for farmers in each era would be a simple way of making comparisons. The problem is that occupations are not consistently defined in the New Zealand census.

25 The easiest way to access official statistics is to access the annual reports on suicide (2003 to 2010) from the New Zealand Ministry of Health: http://www.health.govt.nz/nz-health-statistics/health-statistics-and-data-sets/suicide-data-and-stats, accessed 1 March 2013.

26 Private communication from Alison Ainsworth, Business Support Officer, Births, Deaths, and Marriages, 5 December 2012. See http://www.bdmonline.dia.govt.nz/NonHistoricrecords/DataCollection#deathmaoriregisters, accessed 1 March 2013.

27 J46, 1900/733; 1908/264; 1910/274; 1912/299; 1914/1076;1916/58; 1916/854; 1916/993; 1922/794; 1922/1135; 1922/1219; 1924/961; 1924/1200; 1926/912; 1926/1051; 1928/1474; 1929/2; 1936/400; 1936/763; 1936/869; 1936/994; 1936/1244; 1940/1302; 1942/337; 1968/1386.

28 J46, 1902/952; 1904/373; 1904/616; 1904/1047; 1908/87; 1908/216; 1910/223; 1910/306; 1910/325; 1912/127; 1914/278; 1914/300; 1914/921; 1914/1438; 1922/447; 1922/1226; 1924/792; 1926/157; 1926/314; 1926/350; 1928/233; 1928/743; 1928/998; 1930/605; 1930/785; 1934/1278; 1934/1384; 1936/849; 1936/1083; 1936/1464; 1936/1471; 1936/1528; 1938/126; 1938/1942; 1940/417; 1949/307; 1952/691; 1954/554; 1958/724; 1961/173; 1964/791; 1964/1168.

29 See Ministry of Social Development, http://socialreport.msd.govt.nz/introduction/index.html (note the section on ethnic differences), accessed 1 March 2013.

30 ABQU W4452 632 Box 2, Accidents – Statistics on Accidental Drowning and Submersion, 1948 to 1971; Box 275, National Health Statistics – National Health Statistics Centre – Drowning, 1983 to 1991.

31 ABVP, 2000/1181.

32 See for example the correspondence from 1961 to 1970 in AAFB W2788 632 Box 73, Poisons – Substances – Nicotine. On antidotes see ABQU W4452 632 Box 936, Poisons – Substances – Nicotine, J.B. Hammond, Division of Public Health, to W.E. Pierson, Pierson's Livestock Remedies, 4 July 1975. Atropine was an antidote for nicotine-based pesticides.

33 ABVP, 2000/700.

34 "Not deep enough," said one slowly dying individual to a constable. J46, 1904/138. Also see J46, 1930/360.

35 J46, 1912/312; 1916/988.

36 ABQU W4452 632 Box 943, Poisons – Substances – Carbon Monoxide, 1926–1987, World Health Organization, *Environmental Health Criteria for Carbon Monoxide* [1978].

37 ABGX W5189 16127, Box 147, TR 4/1/1/9, Transport Committee – Catalytic Converters. Dave Brash, Manager, Pollution and Risk Management for Secretary for the Environment, to Hon. Rob Story, Chairman, Transportation Select Committee, 24 August 1995.

38 J46, 1950/409.

39 AADB W3463 632 Box 46 – Poison Prescription – Barbiturates, Remarks by R.A. Barker, Conference on Barbiturates, February 1977.

40 AADB W3463 632 Box 46 – Poison Prescription – Barbiturates, F.S. Maclean, Director, Division of Public Hygiene, to Minister of Health, 1 February 1952; Duncan Cook, Director, Division of Clinical Services, to Minister, 4 September 1952; warning circular to medical practitioners, 24 April 1961; clipping, *Sunday News*, 8 February 1976; A.A. Fraser, President, Pharmaceutical Society of New Zealand, to Minister of Health, 5 October 1976; Barbiturates: Background Paper [1977]; Barbiturates Conference, 4 February 1977.

41 AADB W3463 632 Box 46 – Poison Prescription – Barbiturates, Recommendations of the Conference of 23 February 1977.

42 AADB W 3463 632 Box 46 – Poison Prescription – Barbiturates, Harold D. Law, Visiting Medical Practitioner, Department of Health, District Office, Auckland, to Dr A.A. Andrews, Director of Clinical Services, Department of Health, 7 February 1977.

43 AADB W 3463 632 Box 46 – Poison Prescription – Barbiturates, A.A. Fraser, President, Pharmaceutical Society of New Zealand, to Minister of Health, 5 October 1976.

44 AADB W 2788 632 Box 168, Narcotics – Methadone, Memorandum of Discussion – Dr G. Blake-Palmer, Assistant Commissioner of Police, Mr Austing and Sergeant Stewart of the Auckland Drug Squad, 18 January 1972. Also see Police Report by Detective Sergeant B.J. Stewart, Drug Squad, 26 January 1972; N.T. Barnett, Medical Officer of Health, "Prescribing by General Practitioners, Auckland Health District – Methadone and Amphetamines" [February 1972]. These reports were critical of an Auckland doctor whom police believed had made methadone available too freely. The doctor was severely dealt with at an inquest. See ABVP, 1972/1483.

45 AADB W 3463 632 Box 46 – Poison Prescription – Barbiturates, Clipping from *New Zealand Herald*, 1 August [1974]. A similar assessment

that over-the-counter medications consumed with alcohol were at least as effective as an overdose of prescription drugs was offered by a coroner. ABVP, 2000/821.

46 Consider these cases from 1930: J46, 1930/435; 1930/960; 1930/971; 1930/1336.

47 J46, 1930/430; 1930/486; 1930/677.

CHAPTER TWO

1 ABVP, 2000/1247.

2 ABVP, 1998/974.

3 Joiner, *Myths about Suicide*, 42.

4 J46, 1961/47.

5 J46, 1961/176.

6 J46, 1930/1537.

7 J46, 1936/1083.

8 J46, 1938/1317.

9 ABVP, 1988/104.

10 J46, 1936/101.

11 J46, 1928/790.

12 J46, 1934/1380.

13 J46, 1912/33.

14 J46, 1934/1016.

15 J46, 1900/813.

16 J46, 1952/577.

17 J46, 1936/101.

18 ABVP, 1988/1208.

19 J46, 1908/1091.

20 J46, 1925/509.

21 J46, 1946/597.

22 J46, 1976/1518.

23 J46, 1952/1272.

24 The quote is from J46, 1912/58.

25 J46, 1968/681. Appearances troubled a few young men who felt they would never find a girl. J46, 1942/637.

26 ABVP, 2000/1178. See ABVP, 2000/1200. A woman tried to turn an affair back to friendship.

27 J46, 1912/459.

28 J46, 1908/364.

29 J46, 1906/244.
30 J46, 1936/1395.
31 J46, 1936/339.
32 ABVP, 2000/1181.
33 J46, 1936/1395.
34 J46, 1946/239.
35 J46, 1912/94.
36 J46, 1914/390.
37 ABVP, 2000/869.
38 J46, 1946/1364.
39 J46, 1972/74.
40 ABVP, 2000/1100.
41 ABVP, 1998/938.
42 J46, 1912/587.
43 ABVP, 2000/512.
44 ABVP, 1986/1547.
45 J46, 1902/292.
46 J46, 1926/1264.
47 ABVP, 2000/789.
48 J46, 1904/658.
49 J46, 1910/1176.
50 J46, 1916/1038.
51 J46, 1900/262; 1904/520.
52 J46, 1924/624.
53 For more on this subject see Richards and Weaver, "'I may as well die'," 304–27.
54 J46, 1904/373.
55 J46, 1916/1409 and 1410.
56 J46, 1964/389.
57 J46, 1934/1286.
58 J46, 1934/1354.
59 J46, 1912/1273.
60 ABVP, 1982/338; 1984/621.
61 J46, 1918/1187.
62 J46, 1976/825.
63 J46, 1922/58.
64 J46, 1922/656 and 657.
65 ABVP, 2000/1312.
66 J46, 1925/37 and 38.

67 ABVP, 1999/29 and 30.
68 For double cases that may have simply have involved close male friends who were in legal trouble see ABVP, 1998/639 and 715. Two patients at a mental hospital had planned a double suicide. See J46, 1908/446. For another where the motive is uncertain, see ABVP, 1994/620 and 621.
69 ABVP, 1989/216.
70 J46, 1922/289.
71 J46, 1930/696.
72 J46, 1959/697.
73 J46, 1928/431.
74 J46, 1904/119.
75 J46, 1926/1442.
76 J46, 1900/757.
77 J46, 1922/229.
78 J46, 1924/677.
79 ABVP, 1988/1226; 2000/374.
80 J46, 1918/368.
81 J46, 1954/380.
82 J46, 1904/600.
83 J46, 1940/1427.
84 J46, 1976/914.
85 ABVP, 1997/181.
86 J46, 1942/1262.
87 J46, 1976/1687.
88 J46, 1936/805.
89 J46, 1940/296.
90 J46, 1900/554.
91 J46, 1902/202.
92 J46, 1902/658.
93 ABVP, 1991/381.
94 J46, 1928/377.
95 J46, 1960/1097.
96 J46, 1976/469.
97 ABVP, 1998/864.
98 ABVP, 1998/913.
99 For more on the idea of a gender script and suicide see Canetto and Sakinofsky, "The Gender Paradox in Suicide," 19.
100 ABVP, 2000/1292.
101 On the history of these shelters see AATD W3294 6192, Box 1, Royal Commission on Social Policy: Research Papers Included in Submissions

Database: Family Violence DSW [Department of Social Welfare]. Neale, "Family Violence," 13–14. On police policy see Neale, 21.

102 ABVP, 2000/1057.
103 ABVP, 2000/896.
104 J46, 1908/837.
105 J46, 1906/1028.
106 J46, 1908/50.
107 J46, 1912/190.
108 J46, 1920/1009.
109 J46, 1928/1344.
110 J46, 1918/385.
111 ABVP, 2000/851.
112 ABVP, 2000/1212.
113 J46, 1936/278.
114 J46, 1942/1252.
115 J46, 1942/341.
116 J46, 1972/249.
117 ABVP, 1989/236.
118 J46, 1910/773.
119 J46, 1916/344.
120 J46, 1924/344.
121 J46, 1924/1213.
122 J46, 1926/1287.
123 J46, 1972/1518.
124 J46, 1976/338.
125 J46, 1914/300.
126 J46, 1976/749.
127 J46, 1952/1153.
128 J46, 1960/977.
129 J46, 1940/794.
130 J46, 1900/554; 1906/452.
131 J46, 1936/426.
132 J46, 1936/435.
133 J46, 1942/849.
134 J46, 1961/84.
135 J46, 1976/423.
136 J46, 1920/229.
137 J46, 1972/1224; 1976/441.
138 J46, 1914/278.
139 J46, 1936/1464.

140 J46, 1925/1442.
141 J46, 1928/640.
142 J46, 1916/1409.
143 J46, 1960/1062.
144 J46, 1976/499.
145 J46, 1924/1014.
146 J46, 1924/1291.
147 J46, 1900/380; 1902/968; 1904/852; 1906/28; 1908/924.
148 ABVP, 1988/1355.
149 J46, 1908/973.
150 ABVP, 1998/925.
151 ABVP, 1994/562.
152 J46, 1912/127.
153 J46, 1949/307.
154 J46, 1926/1473.
155 For example see inquests held in 1998: ABVP, 1998/821; 1998/901; 1998/888.
156 J46, 1920/585.
157 J46, 1964/389.
158 J46, 1990/830 and 850.
159 J46, 1934/1493.
160 J46, 1939/1356.
161 J46, 1954/141; for a similar case see 1960/1065.
162 ABVP, 1994/1007.
163 J46, 1980/1184.
164 J46, 1922/1013.
165 J46, 1902/712.
166 J46, 1908/824.
167 J46, 1931/66.
168 J46, 1919/202.
169 J46, 1924/1253.
170 J46, 1956/1128.
171 ABVP, 1987/218.
172 J46, 1960/823.
173 ABVP, 2000/1059.
174 J46, 1960/928.
175 This observation has abundant support from other studies. Canetto, "Gender Roles," 611; Norstrom, "The Impact of Alcohol," 310.
176 J46, 1908/882; ABVP, 1986/507; ABVP, 1998/852.
177 Roy and Linnoila, "Alcoholism and Suicide," 162–6.

178 J46, 1914/892.
179 J46, 1924/74.
180 Stearns, *Be a Man*, 5–72.
181 Canetto, "Gender Roles," 611.
182 Entry for 13 December 1935, Diary of Peter Carter Lovell-Smith, MSX-5461, Alexander Turnbull Library, National Library of New Zealand.
183 Hamer and Copeland, *Living with Our Genes*, 133–4.
184 J46, 1904/492.
185 For an explanation that relies on neurochemistry, see Ashton, "Delirium and Hallucinations," 185–6.
186 Brådvik and Berglund, "A Suicide Peak," 189–90.
187 J46, 1922/122.
188 J46, 1914/443.
189 J46, 1914/116.
190 J46, 1914/1245.
191 J46, 1916/628.
192 J46, 1916/843.
193 J46, 1902/176.
194 J46, 1910/689.
195 J46, 1912/504.
196 J46, 1914/968.
197 J46, 1914/358.
198 J46, 1914/1001.
199 J46, 1914/1215.
200 J46, 1916/302.
201 J46, 1916/734.
202 J46, 1916/1388.
203 J46, 1917/58.
204 J46, 1914/1058.
205 J46, 1914/36.
206 J46, 1914/843.
207 J46, 1914/183.
208 J46, 1914/206.
209 J46, 1916/210.
210 J46, 1916/1148.
211 J46, 1922/127.
212 J46, 1922/19.
213 J46, 1912/437.
214 J46, 1938/1393.
215 J46, 1942/341.

216 J46, 1950/80.
217 J46, 1918/274.
218 J46, 1914/174.
219 J46, 1912/1290.
220 J46, 1906/163; 1906/848.
221 J46, 1916/59.
222 J46, 1914/1175.
223 J46, 1926/914.
224 J46, 1910/295.
225 J46, 1914/955.
226 J46, 1910/186.
227 J46, 1940/1474.
228 J46, 1906/1015.
229 J46, 1916/728.
230 J46, 1942/138.
231 J46, 1912/684.
232 J46, 1914/372.
233 J46, 1914/469.
234 J46, 1914/183.
235 J46, 1914/1076.
236 J46, 1914/1347.
237 J46, 1915/36.
238 J46, 1914/1001.
239 J46, 1922/61.
240 J46, 1922/811.
241 J46, 1916/327.
242 J46, 1912/425.
243 J46, 1914/501.
244 J46, 1914/879.
245 For a brief discussion of a study that found a high rate of suicides among hotel occupants, see Zarkowski and Avery, "Hotel Room Suicide," 580.
246 ABVP, 1998/761.
247 ABVP, 2000/1120.
248 AAYE W5048 7433, Box 127, B&P 6-6-1, Part 2. Benefits and Pensions – Invalids Benefit Correspondence. Senior Executive Office, Policy and Legislation Unit, to Wellington Regional Training and Support Officer, 4 November 1980. The benefit was means-tested.
249 AAYE W5048 7433 Boxes 226 and 227, Organisation and Departments – Drug and Alcohol Rehabilitation Centres – Alcohol Substance Abuse Programme – New Funding Assistance. Assorted files from 1985 to 1987.

250 ABQZ 6802, Box 4, Substance Abuse, Clipping Files, *The Star* (Christchurch), 31 May 1990. Believing cannabis harmless, a few adults passed joints to children. *Wanganui Chronicle*, 31 March 1990. For one of many examples, see ABVP 1998/820.

251 ABQZ 6802, Box 14, *The Evening Post*, 22 August 1995 and 2 August 1996.

252 J46, 1976/959.

253 AATD W3294 6192, Box 1, Royal Commission on Social Policy: Research Papers Included in Submissions Database: Family Violence DSW [Department of Social Welfare]. Neale, "Family Violence," 7. New Zealand public and private agencies were well aware of the problems and remedies, but had to work with restricted funding and volunteer "burn-out." Neale, 8.

CHAPTER THREE

1 For a discussion of some New Zealand studies on unemployment and incidents of self-harm see AATD W3294 6136, Royal Commission on Social Policy. Original Submissions, Box 61, Submission 5371, Mental Health Foundation of New Zealand, Keith Macky and Hilary Haines, "The Psychological Effects of Unemployment: A Review of the Literature," 4–6.

2 Brooking, *History of New Zealand*, 89.

3 Ibid., 89–90. In a prior study of suicide that compared New Zealand and Queensland up to 1950, we argued that New Zealand's lower suicide rate during the early twentieth century was partly due to its early initiatives in welfare legislation. Compared to those in Queensland, the destitute New Zealand elderly were treated better. See Weaver, *A Sadly Troubled History*, 109–37.

4 Belich, *Paradise Reforged*, 261–4.

5 Brooking, "Economic Transformations," 226.

6 J46, 1906/777.

7 Belich, *Paradise Reforged*, 142–4.

8 J46, 1912/947.

9 J46, 1914/1000.

10 Belich, *Paradise Reforged*, 145.

11 J46, 1914/318.

12 J46, 1916/988.

13 J46, 1906/271.

14 J46, 1916/404.

15 J46, 1912/1279.

16 J46, 1914/200.

17 J46, 1904/423.

18 J46, 1904/36.
19 J46, 1900/135.
20 J46, 1906/404.
21 J46, 1908/646.
22 J46, 1914/1456.
23 J46, 1914/1073.
24 J46, 1912/1237.
25 J46, 1926/166. The coroner's complaints to the Department of Justice are enclosed in the file.
26 J46, 1924/1121.
27 J46, 1900/129.
28 J46, 1980/933.
29 J46, 1902/81.
30 J46, 1918/57.
31 J46, 1912/1275.
32 J46, 1912/814.
33 J46, 1910/1232.
34 J46, 1904/1045; 1908/837.
35 J46, 1904/537.
36 J46, 1902/173.
37 J46, 1902/1086.
38 J46, 1912/808.
39 J46, 1914/638.
40 J46, 1912/712.
41 J46, 1914/1344.
42 J46, 1914/1234.
43 J46, 1914/1381.
44 J46, 1914/825.
45 J46, 1902/81; 1904/230; 1930/1464.
46 J46, 1922/122.
47 J46, 1922/385.
48 J46, 1930/1451.
49 J46, 1930/1062.
50 J46, 1904/524; 1906/712; 1920/481; 1934/1494; 1938/1789; 1958/1182; ABQZ 6802, Box 4, Substance Abuse, Clipping Files, *The Dominion*, 3 July 1989.
51 J46, 1930/966.
52 J46, 1930/1057.
53 J46, 1906/163.

54 J46, 1912/12; 1912/13.
55 J46, 1922/251.
56 J46, 1902/401.
57 J46, 1902/96.
58 J46, 1918/134.
59 J46, 1900/62.
60 J46, 1914/197.
61 J46, 1922/172.
62 J46, 1914/648.
63 J46, 1904/16; 1908/881.
64 J46, 1920/299.
65 J46, 1916/406.
66 J46, 1924/170.
67 J46, 1920/1336.
68 J46, 1910/1057.
69 J46, 1920/1311.
70 J46, 1904/209.
71 J46, 1920/1324.
72 J46, 1930/1326.
73 J46, 1916/930.
74 J46, 1920/66.
75 J46, 1920/286.
76 J46, 1920/618.
77 J46, 1914/1263.
78 J46, 1930/1025.
79 J46, 1900/154.
80 Ibid.
81 J46, 1910/1034.
82 J46, 1912/655.
83 J46, 1912/777.
84 Belich, *Paradise Reforged*, 255–6.
85 For a description and assessment of the economy of the 1920s, see Brooking, *History of New Zealand*, 107–10.
86 LS36, Box 24, File on Discharged Soldiers Settlement Account: Report for the Year Ended 30th June 1935, 1.
87 J46, 1916/262.
88 Macdonald and Thomson, "Mortgage Relief," 228–50; Belshaw, Williams, and Stephens, "Farming Industries," 786–806; Philpott, *A History of the New Zealand Dairy Industry*, 202–3, 255–60.

89 LS1, File 22/4476, John Mee, Supervising Field Inspector, Department of Lands and Surveys, to The Undersecretary for Lands, Memorandum on Farm Labour, 11 January 1939.
90 J46, 1938/233.
91 McAloon, *No Idle Rich*, 118.
92 J46, 1934/1307.
93 J46, 1934/1126.
94 J46, 1936/1533.
95 J46, 1936/278.
96 J46, 1936/819.
97 J46, 1936/583.
98 National Efficiency Board, Box 15, File 679, Thomas Moss, Wellington District Commissioner, Report on Farms in Taranaki, 1 November 1917.
99 J46, 1930/636.
100 J46, 1930/385.
101 J46, 1938/594.
102 J46, 1936/1394; 1938/192.
103 J46, 1936/421.
104 J46, 1938/1714; 1938/2021.
105 J46, 1938/1044; 1938/1246; 1938/1843.
106 J46, 1926/556.
107 J46, 1940/584.
108 J46, 1930/166.
109 J46, 1934/1354.
110 J46, 1934/1353.
111 J46, 1938/1514.
112 LS 36, File on Discharged Soldier Settlement Account, Report for the Year Ended 30th June 1935, 3.
113 J46, 1932/309.
114 J46, 1934/318.
115 J46, 1928/553.
116 J46, 1930/1325.
117 J46, 1937/206.
118 J46, 1936/798.
119 J46, 1938/937.
120 J46, 1936/1284.
121 J46, 1936/974.
122 J46, 1938/330.
123 J46, 1938/1270.

124 J46, 1938/1044.
125 J46, 1936/1409.
126 J46, 1934/1322.
127 J46, 1934/1409.
128 J46, 1930/253.
129 J46, 1932/848.
130 J46, 1936/344; 1938/768.
131 J46, 1936/258.
132 J46, 1938/1795.
133 Dalley, "The Golden Weather," 321.
134 Brooking, *History of New Zealand*, 137.
135 Hensley, *Beyond the Battlefield*, 243–9.
136 J46, 1954/329.
137 J46, 1940/265.
138 Gustafson, *Kiwi Keith*, 51.
139 J46, 1944/492.
140 J46, 1950/676.
141 J46, 1950/1214.
142 Brooking, *History of New Zealand*, 137–8.
143 J46, 1958/815.
144 J46, 1960/339.
145 J46, 1958/1069.
146 J46, 1960/604.
147 J46, 1961/313.
148 J46, 1960/145.
149 J46,1954/789.
150 J46, 1955/1; 1954/1283; 1955/145.
151 J46, 1952/1215; 1954/1283; 1955/145.
152 J46, 1964/114.
153 J46, 1952/985.
154 J46, 1972/779.
155 J46, 1952/1362. Also see 1968/645; 1968/648.
156 J46, 1960/690; 1961/105; 1973/186.
157 J46, 1958/931.
158 J46, 1968/1262.
159 J46, 1976/1800.
160 J46, 1952/1321.
161 J46, 1973/115.
162 ABVP, 2000/1118.

CHAPTER FOUR

1 J46, 1928/1104.
2 J46, 1968/780.
3 ABVP, 1980/467.
4 J46, 1904/248.
5 J46, 1902/968.
6 J46, 1946/1419; ABVP, 1980/811; 2000/1173.
7 J46, 1930/135.
8 J46, 1944/467.
9 J46, 1965/85.
10 ABVP, 1995/924.
11 J46, 1942/1383.
12 ABVP, 1980/790.
13 J46, 1942/807.
14 J46/1902/704; 1904/815; 1908/501; 1912/117; 1912/388; 1914/630; 1914/879; ABVP, 1999/448.
15 J46, 1941/197.
16 ABVP, 2000/612.
17 Research staff, *Voluntary Euthanasia*, 3–4. http://www.life.org.nz/euthanasia/abouteuthanasia/nzeuthanasiahistory3/Default.htm, accessed 1 March 2013.
18 Dowbiggin, *A Concise History of Euthanasia*, 112.
19 These were articles recommended by euthanasia publications. ABVP, 1997/1129; 1998/733.
20 For a history of debates over expanding euthanasia beyond the terminally ill see Dowbiggin, *A Concise History of Euthanasia*, 123–6.
21 ABVP, 1991/324.
22 ABVP, 1999/339.
23 "Over My Dead Body," *The Economist* (20 October 2012), 55.
24 ABVP, 1991/389.
25 ABVP, 1999/30.
26 ABVP, 1973/224.
27 ABVP, 1988/1304.
28 ABVP, 1997/1129.
29 ABVP, 1988/1280.
30 ABVP, 1980/1181.
31 ABVP, 1968/821.
32 ABVP, 1996/913.
33 ABVP, 1998/1026.

34 ABVP, 1998/843.
35 ABVP, 1980/790.
36 ABVP, 1996/350.
37 On the global growth of euthanasia groups between the 1960s and 1990s, see Dowbiggin, *A Concise History of Euthanasia*, 123–6.
38 ABVP, 1998/1387.
39 ABVP, 1985/385.
40 ABVP, 1982/318; 1998/733.
41 ABVP, 1997/609.
42 ABVP, 1997/272.
43 ABVP, 1985/385; 1988/723.
44 ABVP, 1990/1225; 1992/452; 1992/461; 1992/1088; 1998/1026; 1999/29.
45 ABVP, 1995/693.
46 ABVP, 1996/693.
47 ABVP, 1980/733.
48 AAFB W2788 632 Box 58, Tuberculosis Act, World Health Organization, "Twenty-Years Against Tuberculosis, 1948–1968" (1968), 3–5.
49 J46, 1904/760.
50 J46, 1908/1172.
51 J46, 1920/389.
52 J46, 1922/856.
53 J46, 1912/251.
54 J46, 1902/822.
55 J46, 1904/16.
56 J46, 1908/679.
57 J46, 1920/1336.
58 J46, 1926/1087.
59 ABVP, 2000/886.
60 J46, 1912/851.
61 ABVP, 1988/1343.
62 J46, 1902/913.
63 J46, 1904/45.
64 J46, 1904/658; 1904/827; 1916/1384.
65 J46, 1912/155.
66 J46, 1930/1134.
67 J46, 1924/1111.
68 J46, 1926/1157.
69 J46, 1930/756.
70 J46/1930/822.
71 J46, 1924/628.

72 J46, 1903/9.
73 J46, 1908/218.
74 J46, 1912/597.
75 J46, 1916/993.
76 J46, 1918/146.
77 J46, 1926/1286; 1928/214; 1934/1487.
78 J46, 1924/1294.
79 J46, 1926/725.
80 J46, 1960/919.
81 J46, 1936/287.
82 J46, 1916/1289.
83 J46, 1922/822.
84 J46, 1916/1232.
85 J46, 1925/152.
86 J46, 1940/1082.
87 J46, 1925/90.
88 J46, 1934/1443.
89 J46, 1918/127.
90 J46, 1918/1253.
91 J46, 1918/1372.
92 J46, 1922/759.
93 J46, 1902/11.
94 J46, 1904/375.
95 J46; 1910/1141.
96 J46, 1910/839.
97 J46, 1900/518.
98 J46, 1904/459; 699/1908; 1233/1910.
99 Osler, *The Principles and Practices of Medicine*, 118.
100 J46, 1943/18.
101 ABVP, 1986/912; 1997/11. Also see 1989/770.
102 Barry, *The Great Influenza*, 379–81.
103 J46, 1914/818.
104 ABVP, 1994/0336; 1995/207.
105 J46, 1942/1383.
106 J46, 1928/495.
107 J46, 1912/1105.
108 J46, 1928/392.
109 J46, 1940/974.
110 J46, 1954/533.

111 J46, 1952/923; ABVP, 1976/181; 1980/1758; 1984/1505; 1986/682; 1986/1226; 1986/1630; 1991/388.
112 J46, 1977/826; ABVP, 1980/831.
113 Dwyer, "Neurological Patients," 47.
114 J46, 1908/111.
115 J46, 1924/798.
116 ABVP, 1994/893.
117 ABVP, 1998/1143.
118 ABVP, 1988/1280.
119 J46, 1942/560.
120 J46, 1924/1192; 1934/1132.
121 J46, 1936/159.
122 J46, 1976/1097.
123 J46, 1914/471.
124 J46, 1942/995; 1942/995; 1943/4; 1943/18.
125 J46, 1929/62.
126 J46, 1924/248; 1936/1447; 1940/121.
127 J46, 1924/1296; 1942/1326.
128 J46, 1928/824.
129 J46, 1938/569.
130 J46, 1938/680.
131 J46, 1926/1269.
132 J46, 1940/420.
133 J46, 1924/918.
134 J46, 1936/1409.
135 J46, 1944/585; ABVP, 1980/1812; 1981/11; 1989/716; 1990/444; 1992/711; 1992/1018; 1994/503; 1996/599; 1996/633; 1996/521.
136 J46, 1902/650.
137 J46, 1928/1171.
138 J46, 1940/1493.
139 J46, 1940/1664.
140 ABVP, 2000/237.
141 ABVP, 2000/1298.
142 ABVP, 1994/996.
143 ABVP, 1980/549.
144 J46, 1964/530.
145 ABVP, 1989/142.
146 ABVP, 2000/1000.
147 J46, 1938/594.

148 AVBP, 1997/557.
149 ABVP, 1996/1024.
150 ABVP, 2000/1173.
151 J46, 1906/1072.
152 J46, 1934/1548.
153 J46, 1976/580.
154 J46, 1930/836.
155 J46, 1936/1463.
156 J46, 1942/1103.
157 J46, 1961/29.
158 J46, 1938/874.
159 J46, 1926/1224..
160 J46, 1908/232.
161 J46, 1928/124; 1934/1224.
162 J46, 1976/1685.
163 The number cited here is double the number of cases in the data set, which was based on files from just the even-numbered years.
164 J46, 1938/613.
165 J46, 1976/1304.
166 J46, 1940/595.
167 J46, 1942/354.
168 J46, 1914/644.
169 J46, 1936/1325.
170 J46, 1928/1293.
171 J46, 1922/788; ABVP, 1980/664.
172 J46, 1922/692.
173 J46, 1924/1095.
174 J46, 1902/390; 1904/65.
175 J46, 1906/580; 1908/869; 1914/1408; 1916/841; 1916/1064; 1918/85; 1928/1484; 1934/1221; 1946/567; 1954/399; 1954/433.
176 J46, 1922/924.
177 J46, 1931/129.
178 J46, 1926/1405.
179 J46, 1954/399.
180 J46, 1972/1275.
181 ABVP, 1980/1075.
182 J46, 1940/86.
183 J46, 1924/183.
184 J46, 1936/1239.
185 J46, 1926/912.

186 J46, 1904/505.
187 J46, 1929/87.
188 J46, 1942/1575.
189 J46, 1976/276.
190 J46, 1908/817.
191 J46, 1916/1382.
192 J46, 1914/638.
193 J46, 1946/1273.
194 ABVP, 1989/219.
195 J46, 1942/540.
196 ABVP, 1998/396.
197 J46, 1908/998.
198 J46, 1924/961.
199 ABVP, 2000/748.
200 J46, 1902/232.
201 J46, 1920/166.
202 J46, 1904/567.
203 J46, 1902/477.
204 J46, 1938/579.
205 J46, 1914/307.
206 J46, 1942/25.
207 J46, 1927/39.
208 J46, 1938/193.
209 J46, 1928/550.
210 J46, 1922/911.
211 J46, 1908/253.
212 J46, 1930/820.
213 J46, 1908/1083.
214 J46, 1930/1930.
215 J46, 1954/437.
216 J46, 1960/751.
217 J46, 1902/633.
218 J46, 1916/949.
219 SS7 W2756, Box 17, Accounts, Miscellaneous Publicity and Returns – Returned Servicemen – Miscellaneous Statistics, Annual Returns on Pensions, 1936–56.
220 Ibid.
221 J46, 1926/1445.
222 J46, 1928/716.
223 J46, 1926/685; 1926/1343; 1929/62.

224 J46, 1924/1294.
225 J46, 1928/319.
226 J46, 1918/257.
227 J46, 1918/567; 1918/602; 1922/1101; 1954/174.
228 J46, 1924/512.
229 J46, 1922/146.
230 J46, 1922/773.
231 J46, 1924/568.
232 J46, 1918/1000; 1926/1326; 1926/263; AABK 18805, W555, Box 102, 0124688.
233 J46, 1922/861.
234 J46, 1922/959.
235 J46, 1924/530.
236 J46, 1930/1262.
237 J46, 1924/706.
238 J46, 1928/1051; 1928/1068; 1928/1355.
239 J46, 1928/930.
240 J46, 1928/1295.
241 J46, 1944/478; 1944/558; 1944/625; 1944/742; 1946/1306.
242 J46, 1952/1276.
243 J46, 1954/67.
244 J46, 1920/265.
245 J46, 1922/332.
246 J46, 1924/186.
247 J46, 1925/550; AABK 18805, W555, Box 102, 0124688.
248 J46, 1922/805; 1922/1046.
249 J46, 1924/70.
250 J46, 1922/335; 1922/935; 1924/648; 1923/87 and for this case also see Military Records, AABK 18805, W5539, Box 70, 0049430.
251 J46, 1918/1244.
252 SS7 W2756, Box 17, Accounts, Miscellaneous Publicity and Returns – Returned Servicemen – Miscellaneous Statistics, Annual Returns on Pensions, 1936–56, Memorandum for Minister of Pensions, 11 August 1936.
253 J46, 1922/262; 1924/946; 1924/1111.
254 J46, 1918/882.
255 J46, 1922/292.
256 J46, 1924/661.
257 J46, 1918/707.
258 J46, 1918/402.
259 J46, 1918/1121; 1922/321.

260 J46, 1918/625.
261 J46, 1955/103.
262 J46, 1950/1157; 1957/64; 1957/169.
263 J46, 1956/1316.
264 J46, 1954/1263.
265 J46, 1956/470.
266 J46, 1956/1282.
267 J46, 1947/250.
268 J46, 1956/1009.
269 J46, 1952/206.
270 IA1, Department of Internal Affairs, Patriotic Funds – Rehabilitation – Psychosis Cases – Treatment, 1942–43.
271 Joiner, *Why People Die By Suicide*, 128.
272 J46, 1918/167; 1918/610; 1918/914.
273 J46, 1916/981.
274 J46, 1918/987.
275 J46, 1924/367.
276 J46, 1946/234.
277 J46, 1956/1245.

CHAPTER FIVE

1 Porter, *A Social History*, 223. See the list of case histories indexed in Gay, *Freud*, 790.
2 Paterson, *A Mad People's History*; Porter, *A Social History*. Porter alleged that hundreds of autobiographical accounts "by (allegedly) mad people" existed in English.
3 Porter, *A Social History*, 232.
4 Porter has recently been criticized for an obsolete appeal for studies on patients and for helping to deflect attention from the study of the patient as a concept or category of modernism. Cooter, "Neuropatients in Historyland," 215–17. Reaume discusses first-person accounts in *Remembrance of Patients Past*, 266. The self-reflections by an eminent medical researcher appear in Campbell, *Not Always on the Level*, 177–92, 217–44. Afflicted with a bi-polar disorder, the author felt that medication was no help and that talk therapy was useful as it provided him with insights into his condition and coping techniques. He was suicidal.
5 Moran, *Committed to the State Asylum*, 3–12, 170–2. At private asylums, circumstances were different for they had "to grant a greater voice … to [their] paying patients." Warsh, *Moments of Unreason*, 171.

6 Porter alleged that he did not want "to add the big guns of history to the anti-psychiatric broadside," but he and the asylum historians sniped at "the true fantasists ... who have claimed to hold the master key to madness." Porter, *A Social History*, 232.
7 For a discussion of the law governing the finding of suicide, see ABVP, 2000/532. A well-to-do family secured legal representation to assist with raising doubt about suicide, although the physical evidence pointed to suicide. The noose used in the hanging was not of a quick-release type associated with sexual misadventure.
8 For an outstanding example of a doctor's engagement with a patient's problems, see J46, 1976/1694. A leading professor of psychological medicine at the University of Otago emphasized that mental health was associated with environment: marriage, recreation, work, housing, and the law. COM 12, Royal Commission on Hospital and Related Services, 1972–1974. Submission 74, Personal Submission of Basil James.
9 Lawlor, *From Melancholia to Prozac*, 136–202.
10 For a cautious and professional critique of experts who display confidence about causes and treatments, see Dawes, *House of Cards*, 283–93.
11 J46, 1969/140.
12 See the shifting categories in the annual reports for the mental health branch of the Department of Health entitled *Medical Statistics Report: Part II – Mental Health Data*.
13 Shorter, *A History of Psychiatry*, 291.
14 J46, 1960/920.
15 *The Economist*, 11 March 1972, 60.
16 For an introduction to psychiatrists' efforts to define the essence of depression or, alternately, to subdivide it and define the categories, see Shorter, *A Historical Dictionary*, 78–89.
17 J46, 1906/399.
18 J46, 1906/297.
19 J46, 1906/300.
20 J46, 1976/713.
21 For explanations of the remarkable increase in diagnoses of depression see Dowbiggin, *The Quest for Mental Health*, 169–72.
22 For a good summary of the controversy see Dowbiggin, *The Quest for Mental Health*, 170–1. On the profit motive, see Whitaker, *Mad in America*, 147–50.
23 Deleuze and Guattari, *Anti-Oedipus*, 341.
24 COM 12, 6, Royal Commission on Hospital and Related Services, Submission 24, Campaign against Psychiatric Atrocities.

25 Szasz, *Law, Liberty, and Psychiatry*; *The Manufacture of Madness*; *The Myth of Mental Illness*; *The Therapeutic State*.
26 Hirshbein, *American Melancholy*, 28–9.
27 Ibid., 28–37.
28 Ibid., 42, 53.
29 COM 12, 6, Royal Commission on Hospital and Related Services, Submission 35, The Medical Association of New Zealand, 29.
30 J46, 1976/535.
31 These aspects of a patient's history appeared in a fair number of late century reports. For good examples, see J46, 1976/959; 1981/50.
32 AAAC W4946 6015 Box 60, Application for Lottery Funds, J.S. Werry, Biochemical Correlates of Schizophrenia. For a background discussion on a trend toward statistical analysis see Lawlor, *From Melancholia to Prozac*, 160–4.
33 Kramer, *Against Depression*, 51.
34 J46, 1906/271.
35 J46, 1918/331.
36 J46, 1976/1241.
37 J46, 1977/653.
38 J46, 1976/612.
39 ABVP, 1986/1495.
40 J46, 1954/466.
41 J46, 1976/1294.
42 Kramer, *Against Depression*, 115–49.
43 J46, 1914/1069.
44 J46, 1908/471.
45 J46, 1912/16.
46 J46, 1918/356.
47 J46, 1906/314.
48 J46, 1918/547.
49 For early references see J46, 1904/305; 1906/821. For late century see J46, 1976/665.
50 J46, 1906/193.
51 J46, 1906/1001.
52 J46, 1912/712.
53 J46, 1920/343.
54 J46, 1940/1181.
55 J46, 1942/1350.
56 J46, 1918/873.
57 J46, 1906/1001.

58 J46, 1902/733; 1904/925; 1906/193; 1906/1110; 1912/686.
59 J46, 1906/1110.
60 J46, 1904/853.
61 J46, 1904/564.
62 J46, 1912/1116.
63 J46, 1904/853; 1906/1110.
64 J46, 1920/605.
65 J46, 1918/331.
66 J46, 1940/129.
67 J46, 1930/562.
68 Lawlor, *From Melancholia to Prozac*, 153–4.
69 J46, 1904/869; 1906/619; 1910/259; 1914/1069; 1918/651; 1920/1392; 1920/1397.
70 J46, 1920/1342.
71 J46, 1910/689.
72 J46, 1916/688.
73 For the longevity of chloral hydrate's use see Dowbiggin, *The Quest for Mental Health*, 147.
74 J46, 1900/664.
75 J46, 1902/932.
76 J46, 1912/496.
77 J46, 1902/733.
78 J46, 1920/13.
79 J46, 1964/584.
80 Stone, "Shell Shock," 242–71.
81 For histories of shell shock as the precursor to PTSD, see, inter alia: Bill Rawling, "Providing the Gift of Life," 7–20; Mersky, "Post-Traumatic Stress Disorder," 490–500; and Merskey, "After Shell Shock," 89–118. For more critical examinations of the social construction of shell shock, see Brown, "Post-Traumatic Stress Disorder," 500–8.
82 AD 1, 49/301 (49 refers to a sub-series and 301 to a subject file; the archives retained the army file numbering system), Mental Patients, Memorandum, Federation of New Zealand Patriotic War Relief Societies to James Allen, Minister of Defence, 28 August 1917.
83 AD 1, 49/301, Mental Patients, Secretary, Rotoroa Returned Soldiers' Association, to Acting Director Medical Services (henceforth ADMS), Wellington, 2 December 1918; James Allen, Minister of Defence, to Miss Holland, Secretary, Victoria League of Auckland, 4 February 1919; F.S. Emmett to James Allen, 19 December 1919, 25 January 1920. AD 49/301/1, Mental Health Patients, NZEF (New Zealand Expeditionary

Force), General File, William Power, Taranaki Provincial War Relief Association, to Minister of Defence, 16 June 1920.

84 AD 1, 49/301, Mental Patients, Secretary, Auckland Returned Soldiers' Association, to James Allen, Minister of Defence, 26 September 1919.

85 AD 78, 15/28, Mental Patients, Director of Base Records, to the Officer in Charge, New Zealand Record Office, London, 14 December 1917.

86 The argument here parallels that of Roper in *The Secret Battle*. Roper stressed that soldiers relied on families for support.

87 These two terms were related; they were used for supposedly light mental illness cases. The former largely meant somatic illnesses, or those believed to be caused by brain lesions, while the latter was reserved for emotional trauma. At times, however, shell shock was the label applied to both concepts.

88 AD 1, 49/284/3, Neurasthenia Cases, Minute Sheet for Minister of Defence, 22 November 1918. The sheet mentioned studies and treatments.

89 AD 1, 39/319, Hospitals – England, Report on Hospitals by [illegible signature] to General Officer Commanding, 14 August 1917.

90 AD 1, 49/301, Mental Patients, Director of Military Hospitals to DGMS, 21 April 1916.

91 AD 1, 49/301, Mental Patients, Director of Military Hospitals to DGMS, 4 May 1916.

92 AD 1, 49/301, Mental Patients, Inspector General, Mental Hospitals, Department Memorandum, to Col. Valintine, 28 April 1916.

93 AD 78, 15/28, Mental Patients, Truby King to Inspector General, Mental Hospitals, 29 May 1916.

94 AD 78, 15/28 Mental Patients, Truby King to Col. Valintine and Dr Frank Hay, 3 June 1916.

95 AD 1, 49/921, Neurasthenia, DGMS, Memorandum, Transfer of Patients, 30 October 1919.

96 ABVP, 2000/1120. For a glimpse of the collaboration among the Salvation Army, the courts, and the government, see J Series 8 (JJ8), 1/13, Reformatory Institutions, Inebriates Homes, Rotoroa Island, Advisory Board Minutes, 1957–1967; AAQB, W3950 889, Box 648, Prisons, Inebriates Home, Rotoroa Island, 1945–1979.

97 AD 1, 49/301, Mental Patients, Secretary, Auckland Returned Soldiers' Association, to James Allen, Minister of Defence, 26 September 1919.

98 Department of Justice (JU), Series 9, Circular Memos, Item 16, Memo to Stipendiary Magistrates, 4 December 1918.

99 Many reports for Hanmer survive from 23 October 1916 to 21 March 1920. They show average weekly admission rates of (1916) four, (1917)

nine, (1918) six, and (1919) six; multiplying these by the number of weeks (15 weekly reports were missing) gives an estimate of 1,000. A separate report mentioned 481 admissions in 1920 and 368 in 1921, bringing the estimate to around 1,850 admissions from October 1916 to the end of 1921. These included a few patients receiving treatment for joint and chest problems. An inspection of Hanmer on 29–30 September 1917 showed that of 82 patients, 60 required massage treatment, so perhaps 20 percent of patients were there for shell shock. In late March 1919, Hanmer became the designated army centre for shell shock and neurasthenia. The army's anxiety over the mounting numbers of cases in 1920 and 1921 suggests a rising proportion. If functional mental illness cases were around 20 percent through 1916, 1917, and 1918, 50 percent in 1919, and close to 100 percent in 1920 and 1921, then perhaps 1,150 men had been treated for mental illness at Hanmer.

Another estimate can be made for soldiers in civilian mental hospitals. The Minister of Defence required reports to answer critics. These documents provided cross-sectional glimpses. The following are the dates and number of soldier patients in all mental hospitals presented in scattered reports: 1914 (3), 1915 (23), 1916 (36), October 1920 (186), March 1921 (108), April 1921 (139), October 1921 (117), December 1921 (104), April 1922 (106). Seacliff held about a quarter to a third of the total number. A single report gave the total number of returned soldiers that Seacliff held from March 1915 to January 1920 as 94. Thus, for Seacliff a total flow-through estimate of 130 to 150 soldier patients from March 1915 to January 1922 is reasonable. With about a quarter of all soldier patients in mental hospitals at Seacliff, it is possible that 400 men were in hospitals during that period. From the start of the war until August 1919, returned soldiers at Avondale numbered 42, and a few more may have entered between August 1919 and January 1922. Several cross-sectional reports put the proportion of all soldier cases here at about one-sixth; an estimate based on Avondale would be roughly 300 soldiers in mental hospitals. Perhaps 1,500 men were institutionalized for assorted mental ailments, about 1,150 at Hanmer and 300 to 400 in mental hospitals. See AD 1, 40/301, Mental Patients, Nominal Rolls of Military Patients at Mental Hospitals, 1921; McGavin to Secretary, National War Funds Council, 29 November, 1921; AD 1, 49/301/1, Mental Patients, Return of Soldiers Received into Seacliff Mental Hospital from March 1915 to January 1920, 17 January 1920; R. Heaton Rhodes to Secretary, Returned Soldiers' Association, Dunedin, 11 October 1920; DGMS to Dr. W.E. Collins, 18 April 1921; AD 1, 64/30, Mental Cases in NZEF 1918, Ending 31 January 1919; AD 78,

15/28, List of Patients in Mental Hospitals [no date, but probably October 1920]; Return of Returned Soldiers, Mental Patients [no date, but probably March 1921].

100 AD 1, 49/284/3, Neurasthenia Cases, Minute Sheet for Minister of Defence, 22 November 1918.

101 AD 1, 49/922, Training of Medical Officers in Psychotherapy.

102 AD 1, 49/922, Training of Medical Officers in Psychotherapy, minute on cable of 17 February 1919.

103 AD 1, 49/921, Neurasthenia, HQ (Medical), Canterbury Medical District, Memorandum for the DGMS, 27 March 1919.

104 AD 1, 49/921, Neurasthenia, Director, Division of Hospitals, to All Medical Practitioners, 10 February 1921.

105 H11 11/1/1, Queen Mary Hospital, Lieutenant Colonel P. Chisholm to D.S. Wylie, 12 October 1921.

106 There were Hanmer cases among the inquest files. J46, 1926/1064; 1938/590. For a request to remove a patient see J46, 1930/295.

107 J46, 1938/590.

108 See for example these cases that mentioned Hanmer from 1996: ABVP, 1996/1113; 1996/1281; 1997/30; 1997/93; 1997/110.

109 J46, 1930/1145.

110 J46, 1928/283.

111 J46, 1928/357.

112 J46, 1928/427.

113 J46, 1930/455.

114 Brunton, "To imitate."

115 Fennell, "Psychiatry in New Zealand," 146–7.

116 AAFB W4452 2788, Box 118, Hospitals – Private Hospitals – "Selwyn," G. Blake-Palmer to Dr. P. Kennedy, 12 May 1960.

117 AAFB W4914 632 Box 35, Private Hospitals – Private Psychiatric Hospitals – "Piki-te-ora," Wellington.

118 ABQU W4452 632, Box 82, Hospitals – Private Hospitals – "Selwyn," Report on Selwyn Hospital, 16 June 1990. ECT was administered in the patients' bedrooms. More about psychiatric care appeared in Nurse Inspector's Report on Licensed Private Hospital, 16 December 1977, 11 November 1976, 22 June 1973. Earlier reports documenting the growth in psychiatric out-patients are found in AAFB W4452 2788, Box 118, Hospitals – Private Hospitals – "Selwyn." See for example Report on Licensed Private Hospital 5 August 1971, 8 December 1964; W.S. Barber to Dr Miller, 3 September 1965; J.R. Kennedy to Medical Officer of Health, Auckland, 3 June 1964.

119 AAFB W4452 2788, Box 118, Hospitals – Private Hospitals – "Selwyn," Duncan Cook to Dr Russell, 30 March 1949; W.S. Barber to the Minister of Health, 22 March 1960.
120 Archives New Zealand, COM, 12, 1, Campaign Against Psychiatric Atrocities, Submission number 24. This submission was thin and superficial. For a history of ECT that strongly supports it as an effective therapy in some circumstances, see Shorter and Healy, *Shock Therapy*.
121 ABVP, 1992/1366.
122 For positive reports, see J46, 1976/963; 1980/907.
123 J46, 1989/271.
124 J46, 1950/1280; 1954/507.
125 J46, 1976/1226.
126 J46, 1954/86.
127 J46, 1954/507.
128 J46, 1964/584.
129 J46, 1976/196.
130 J46, 1976/695.
131 J46, 1976/1126.
132 ABVP, 2000/838; 2000/1072.
133 *The Economist*, 11 March 1972, 60.
134 J46, 1964/738.
135 J46, 1964/235.
136 J46, 1960/1091.
137 J46, 1976/612.
138 ABVP, 1980/1752.
139 ABVP, 1980/1661.
140 J46, 1964/590; 1964/648; 1964/665.
141 ABVP, 1989/171.
142 AATD W3294 6136, Royal Commission on Social Policy. Original Submissions, Box 42, Submission 4256, New Zealand Association of Psychotherapists and Counsellors [December 1987], 2. The association was also critical of the loss of valuable social and health facilities with de-institutionalization.
143 AATD W3294 6136, Royal Commission on Social Policy. Original Submissions, Box 61, Submission 5371, Mental Health Foundation of New Zealand; Box 62, Submission 5378, Mental Health Foundation of New Zealand.
144 ABVP, 1990/525.
145 ABVP, 2000/982.
146 ABVP, 1990/1080; 1985/420; 1981/449; 1982/646.

147 J46, 1980/1771; ABVP, 1989/524.

148 Lawlor, *From Melancholia to Prozac*, 159–160.

149 ABVP, 1982/629. For a discussion of the differences between American and British psychiatrists on the matter of endogenous and reactive depression, see Hirshbein, *American Melancholy*, 35–6.

150 ABVP, 1988/1219.

151 ABVP, 1986/832.

152 ABVP, 2000/946.

153 ABVP, 2000/219.

154 ABVP, 2000/1082.

155 ABVP, 2000/1020.

156 ABVP, 2000/949. In 2000 a Whakatane coroner who had recently conducted five suicide inquests wrote in the finding of one of these deaths that the common factors were all social in origin: alcohol abuse, broken relationships, and unemployment. For his report see ABVP, 2000/1208.

157 ABVP, 2000/206.

158 ABVP, 2000/982.

159 ABVP, 2000/1009.

160 ABVP, 2000/118.

161 ABVP, 2000/206.

162 J46, 1924/119.

163 ABVP, 2000/872.

164 J46, 1968/1650.

165 For a report that raised the possibility of a genetic predisposition by mentioning a "strong family history of Schizophrenia," see ABVP, 2000/1242.

166 AAFB 632 W3463/49, Mental Health, Committed Patients, Review, Sunnyside Hospital, Report on Patient MT.

167 J46, 1972/158.

168 ABVP, 1982/164.

169 ABVP, 1988/1397; 1996/735.

170 See two widely separated cases: J46, 1918/733; ABVP, 1992/587. They were not unusual.

171 ABVP, 1988/302.

172 For a survey of harm see a report based on 558 heavy drinker case files held by seventeen social agencies. SS W2363 30, 34/11/6, Research on Social Problems – New Zealand Population – Survey on Alcoholism. Robb, McCreary, and Morton, "Survey of Social Agency Involvement," 1–56. Also note AATD W3294 6136, Royal Commission on Social Policy. Original Submissions, Box 5, Submission 369, Auckland Council on Alcohol and Drugs.

173 ABQZ W5328 16364, Box 6, Health – Substance Abuse. Meredith, *Report to the Commonwealth Drugs Conference*, 1.

174 AAFB 632 W3463/49, Mental Health, Committed Patients, Review, Sunnyside Hospital, Report on Patients DD, YH, and TF. See also ABVP, 1981/89; 1997/195.

175 J46, 1916/814; ABVP, 1980/1516; 1988/302; 1996/1242; 2000/988. Archives New Zealand, AAFB 632 W3463/49, Mental Health, Committed Patients, Review, Sunnyside Hospital, Report on Patients BB, TF, AR, YH, and BA.

176 ABVP, 1980/745.

177 ABVP, 1988/1397.

178 ABVP, 1989/12, 1989/33; 2000/598.

179 ABVP, 2000/678.

180 ABVP, 1989/623.

181 ABVP, 1980/1047.

182 See for example AAAC W4946 6015 Box 86 Application for Lottery Funds – Schizophrenia Fellowship of New Zealand Inc., Christchurch, Undated statement from the fellowship [1978].

183 ABVP, 1994/912.

184 ABVP, 1989/623. AATD W3294 6136, Royal Commission on Social Policy. Original Submissions, Box 19, Submission 2603, The Royal Australian and New Zealand College of Psychiatrists. In this brief the college focused on schizophrenia.

185 ABVP, 1989/342.

186 For a discussion of the complexities of depression among schizophrenia patients see DeLisi, *Depression in Schizophrenia*, 27–36.

187 ABVP, 2000/398.

188 Lawlor, *From Melancholia to Prozac*, 169.

189 ABVP, 1980/1382.

190 De-institutionalization was international. During and immediately afterward, there were criticisms of its pace and the economizing that reduced community elements. See Brown, *The Transfer of Care*; Cohen, *Psychiatry Takes to the Streets*.

191 ABVP, 1980/1516.

192 ABVP, 1988/876.

193 ABVP, 1988/1391.

194 ABVP, 1987/3.

195 Dowbiggin, *The Quest for Mental Health*, 146–7. Swazey, *Chlorpromazine in Psychiatry*, 8; Grob, *From Asylum to Community*, 150–4; Healey, *The Creation of Psychopharmacology*, 130.

196 AAFB W4914 632 Box 123, Supplies – Drugs – Chlorpromazine, S.W.P. Mirams, N. Callow, Notes on Quantities of Chlorpromazine Hydrochloride Consumed in New Zealand, 9 February 1968.
197 Ibid.
198 Ibid.
199 AAFB W4914 632 Box 123, Supplies – Drugs – Chlorpromazine, S.W.P. Mirams, Director, Division of Mental Health, Memo, 17 January 1968
200 AAFB W4914 632 Box 123, Supplies – Drugs – Chlorpromazine, S.W.P. Mirams, Director, Division of Mental Health, to the Solicitor-General, 12 May 1966. ABVP, 2000/855.
201 ABVP, 1980/926.
202 ABVP, 1986/1008; J46, 1976/294.
203 ABVP, 1986/1008; 1992/645.
204 ADHS W5502 18913, Box 1, Store – Electro Convulsive Therapy Machines. This file contains letters on topics other than ECT. S.W.P. Mirams, Circular Memorandum No. M.H. 1961/153.
205 ABVP, 1982/284.
206 ABVP, 1982/361.
207 ABVP, 1992/1393.
208 ABVP, 2000/398.
209 ABVP, 1980/885.
210 ABVP, 1992/979.
211 ABVP, 1988/1402.
212 DeLisi, ed., *Depression in Schizophrenia*, 55.
213 COM 12, 6, Royal Commission on Hospital and Related Services, Submission 35, The Medical Association of New Zealand, 3–4.
214 On fear see ABVP, 1980/1371.
215 ABVP, 1990/423.
216 On transfers see J46, 1961/81. On male nurses see COM 12, Royal Commission on Hospital and Related Services, 1972–1974. Submission 4, Hospital Boards' Association of New Zealand, 2.
217 ABVP, 2000/953. On the scale of operations and staff see ABQU W4452 632, Box 1353. Social Security – Hospital Benefits – Ashburn Hall, B.D. Smaill, Mental Health Branch, to Basil James, Ashburn Hall, 19 November 1981. Ashburn was privately owned but received subsidies and collected patients' benefits. For a financial statement see "Summary of Results, 1970–1977" and Memo on "Ashburn Hall Hospital Benefit" in Box 1353.
218 *New Zealand Official Yearbook 1980*, 143.
219 *New Zealand Official Yearbook 2000*, 194.

220 AAAC W4946 6015, Box 86, Application for Lottery Funds – Schizophrenia Fellowship of New Zealand Inc., Christchurch, Undated statement from the fellowship [1978].

221 ABVP, 1981/449.

222 For the expansion at the hospitals see AAFD W2347 811, Box 99, Health – Mental Hospitals, 1950–1957.

223 ABVP, 1982/406.

224 ABVP, 1982/629.

225 J46, 1976/634.

226 For references to several facilities, see ABVP, 1998/741; 1998/825; 1998/859; 1998/990.

227 ABVP, 1988/1063.

228 ABVP, 2000/1023.

229 *New Zealand Official Yearbook 1988–9*, 303; *New Zealand Official Yearbook 1996*, 159. Also see AATD W3294 6136, Royal Commission on Social Policy. Original Submissions, Box 61, Submission 5371, Mental Health Foundation of New Zealand. This was a long and well-conceived submission. Note pages 14–26.

230 The expression comes from Castel, Castel, and Lovell, *La société psychiatrique avancée*. See Porter and Micale, "Introduction," 13.

231 For an example of the team approach see ABVP, 1997/171. Also see AATD W3294 6136, Royal Commission on Social Policy. Original Submissions, Box 61, Submission 5371, Mental Health Foundation of New Zealand, "Mental Health Foundation National Report on Community Mental Health Services for Psychiatric Patients," 7–16.

232 COM 12, Royal Commission on Hospital and Related Services, 1972–1974. Submission 7. L.M. Franklin, Director, Department of Psychiatry, Southland Hospital [no date], 2–3. Franklin articulated the new openness and anti-authoritarianism.

233 COM 12, Royal Commission on Hospital and Related Services, 1972–1974. Submission 6. L.I. Sullivan, Charge Tutor, Oakley Hospital [June 1972], 3.

234 Numerous cases illustrate this point. Some family members came forward to cross-examine or denounce medical witnesses. See for example these cases from late in the century after coroners had long been exposing the problems: ABVP, 2000/628; 2000/678; 2000/705.

235 AAAC W4946 6015, Box 86, Application for Lottery Funds, Schizophrenia Fellowship of New Zealand Inc., Christchurch, Schizophrenia Fellowship Newsletter, NZ (no. 6, vol. 1; November 1979), 9.

236 AATD W3294 6136, Royal Commission on Social Policy. Original Submissions, Box 36, Submission 3869, Schizophrenia Fellowship; Box 57, Submission 5128, Schizophrenia Fellowship, Wanganui Branch.
237 AATD W3294 6136, Royal Commission on Social Policy. Original Submissions, Box 32, Submission 3547, Auckland Mental Health Interest Group on Housing [October 1987]. This submission is packed with criticism of the way de-institutionalization was carried out. See Box 4, Submission 236, The Mental Health Foundation of New Zealand. This submission was cautious and supported institutionalization only for the chronically ill. For more critical statements see Box 5, Submission 367, Task Force for Mental Health Law Reform; Box 6, Submission 519, The Schizophrenia Fellowship.
238 ABVP, 1996/918.
239 ABVP, 2000/1138.
240 There was an explosion of inquests with critical remarks. Note these from 2000. ABVP, 2000/65: The patient "had the feeling that his health team are abandoning him." ABVP, 2000/884: The patient was denied admission to a psychiatric ward and left his assessment session agitated. ABVP, 2000/114: Mental Health and Alcohol and Addiction Services were not coordinated. ABVP, 2000/968: The deceased had complained about the lack of continuity in care. ABVP, 2000/1094: The family complained about "gapping holes" in health services. ABVP, 2000/1065: A husband complains about the release of his suicidal wife. ABVP, 2000/1151: A husband worried that release from hospital could endanger the children. ABVP, 2000/1178: the coroner remarks that medical personnel should have considered the state of the custodial parent. Also ABVP, 2000/821; 2000/1253.
241 ABVP, 2000/953.
242 J46, 1980/1480.
243 ABVP, 1980/1480.
244 ABVP, 1986/1495.
245 ABVP, 1987/100.
246 ABVP, 1988/115.
247 ABVP, 1996/483.
248 ABVP, 2000/762.
249 ABVP, 1989/320.
250 J46, 1964/590.
251 ABVP, 2000/798.
252 ABGX W5188 16127, Box 75, Social Services Committee – Correspondence: *Report of the Controller and Auditor General on Community Care*

for People with Mental Illness [1993], 19–24, 32–5. Based on a study of two regions where the psychiatric hospitals had been closed, the report concluded that many care staff believed patients were released too soon and without a proper assessment of needs.

253 ABVP, 1988/1063; 1984/1518; 1996/1077; 1997/324; 2000/454.
254 ABVP, 1992/1442.
255 J46, 1976/639; ABVP, 1980/954; 1980/168; 2000/65.
256 Records of the Coroners' Court, Wellington, New Zealand: Decision 22/2004; 77/2004; 64/2010; 90/2010; 93/2010; 131/2010; 132/2010; 133/2010.
257 ABVP, 1988/1389.
258 ABVP, 2000/1025.
259 ABVP, 2000/855.
260 ABVP, 1996/535.
261 ABVP, 1996/852.
262 J46, 1976/1693; 1980/1300; ABVP, 2000/1000.
263 J46, 1980/1271.
264 J46, 1968/1174.
265 Wendy Hunter Williams, *Out of Sight Out of Mind: The Story of Porirua Hospital* (Wellington: Porirua Hospital, 1987), 41–139.
266 ABVP, 1996/416; 2000/990.
267 ABVP, 1999/943; 2000/993.
268 ABVP, 1980/1751. Also see the use of the term "drug psychosis" in *New Zealand Official Yearbook, 1983*, 166.
269 ABVP, 1992/291; 1997/217; 2000/762.
270 ABVP, 1996/1083.
271 Recently created area health boards had to manage a Health Department imposition of a 9.5% staff cut. AAFH W5510 6790, Box 310, Social Impact Unit – Administration – Regional Managers Meeting. Regional Report: Gisborne – Wairoa – East Cape [March 1988].
272 Kavanagh, "Cherry Farm," 182. On a number of occasions, family members at inquests held in the years after de-institutionalization wished that their loved one could have been committed. ABVP, 2000/678.
273 ABVP, 2000/993.

CHAPTER SIX

1 ABQZ 6802, Box 4, Substance Abuse, Clipping Files, *The Evening Post*, 28 February 1991.

2 ABQZ W5328 16363, Box 17, Parts 1–3, Youth Affairs – Youth Issues – Youth Suicide, Clipping Files, 1988–1996. *New Zealand Herald*, 29 November 1988. Henceforth, the source for clippings will be cited only as ABQZ.
3 ABQZ, *Auckland Star*, 22 September 1988.
4 COM 12, 6, Royal Commission on Hospital and Related Services, Submission 16, Cherry Farm Group of Hospitals [June 1972]; Submission 63, Department of Justice [November 1972].
5 COM 12, 6, Royal Commission on Hospital and Related Services, Submission 35, The Medical Association of New Zealand [October 1972], 35; Submission 57, Hospital Boards' Association of New Zealand Incorporated [October 1972], 15–16.
6 *Report of the Committee of Inquiry into Procedures Used in Certain Psychiatric Hospitals in Relation to Admission, Discharge or Release on Leave of Certain Classes of Patients* (August 1988), 66.
7 *Report of the Committee of Inquiry*, 34.
8 ABQZ, *The Christchurch Press*, 23 December 1995.
9 ABQZ, *Otago Daily Times*, 19 November 1988.
10 ABQZ, Waimea College guidance counsellor Jim Scott quoted in *Nelson Evening Mail*, 10 February 1996.
11 ABQZ, *Evening Post*, 26 September 1988.
12 ABQZ, *The Dominion*, June 1996
13 ABQZ, *Sunday Star*, 15 November 1987. The clipping files held some material from before 1988.
14 ABQZ, *The Dominion*, 16 July 1996.
15 See for example the claim made by Carolyn Coggan who wrote a PhD thesis on youth suicide. *New Zealand Herald*, 14 August 1996.
16 ABQZ, *New Zealand Herald*, 25 Oct 1988.
17 A youth affairs portfolio had been created in November 1987. By an Order-in-Council a ministry was formally established effective 1 July 1989. In 2003, its activities were taken on by the Ministry of Youth Development. See AAAC, Box 45, Youth Affairs – Policy – Joint Papers, A Ministry of Youth: A Report to Hon. P.B. Goff MP, Minister of Youth Affairs by The Youth Affairs Establishment Unit, 14 November 1988.
18 ABQZ, *Daily News* (New Plymouth), 21 August 1996.
19 ABQZ, *New Zealand Herald*, 5 March 1988.
20 ABQZ, *Dominion Sunday Times*, 11 June 1989.
21 ABQZ, *Dominion Sunday Times*, 11 June 1989.
22 See for example ABVP, 1976/185.

23 ABQU, Ministry of Health, Child Health, Youth Suicide, vol. 3, Barbara Disley to Simon Upton, 29 May 1992.

24 ABQZ, *The Press* (Christchurch), 28 November 1988.

25 ABQZ, *The Press* (Christchurch), 25 May 1989. Barry Taylor returned to the virus analogy on later occasions. See ABQZ, *The Dominion*, 26 April 1993.

26 ABQZ, *Otago Daily Times*, 19 November 1988. Also see *New Zealand Herald*, 28 November 1988.

27 For an insightful assessment of youth culture and drunkenness see ABQZ W5328 16364, Box 6, Health – Substance Abuse. Taylor, "Drinking, Drunkenness."

28 ABQZ, *Dominion Sunday Times*, 19 February 1989.

29 ABQZ, *New Zealand Herald*, 5 March 1988.

30 ABQZ, *Dominion Sunday Times*, 19 February 1989.

31 ABQU, *Youth Suicide Prevention Project: Workshop Report and Literature Review* (Unpublished), 22.

32 ABQZ, *New Zealand Herald*, 2 February 1989.

33 For insights into clinical psychologists practices and ambitions, see COM 12, 6, Royal Commission on Hospital and Related Services, Submission 46, B.S. Parsonson and P.N. Priest [October 1972], 1–17.

34 COM 12, 6, Royal Commission on Hospital and Related Services, Submission by The New Zealand Psychological Society [October 1972], 3–8.

35 See for example COM 12, 6, Royal Commission on Hospital and Related Services, Submission 66, Professor A.J.W. Taylor, submission 65 [November 1972].

36 For an interesting articulation of this position, see COM 12, 6, Royal Commission on Hospital and Related Services, Phase Two: Psychiatric Services, New Zealand Medical Association, Submission No. 1, submission number 69 [undated].

37 See the list of articles provided as background by the General Assembly Library Reference Section, 11 December 1987: *Otago Daily Times*, 18 March 1985; 16 September 1986; *Auckland Star*, 20 May 1986; *Evening Post*, 24 November 1986; *Sunday Star*, 15 November 1987. ABQZ, 1988–1989.

38 ABVP, 1988/997. The correct name is used in this case and the next because of the ample newspaper reporting.

39 ABVP, 1988/1289.

40 ABVP, 1988/1298.

41 ABQZ, 1988–1989, *Auckland Star*, 23 September 1988.

42 ABQZ, *Auckland Star*, 23 September 1988.

43 ABVP, 1988/1298.

44 ABQZ, *Dominion Sunday Times*, 11 June 1989.
45 ABQZ, *The Star* (Christchurch), 23 May 1989.
46 ABQZ, *The Press* (Christchurch), 24 May 1989.
47 ABQZ, *The Star* (Christchurch), 25 May 1989.
48 ABQZ, *Dominion Sunday Times*, 29 May 1989.
49 ABQZ, *Christchurch Press*, 24 May 1989.
50 Hirshbein, *American Melancholy*, 69.
51 ABQZ, *The Press* (Christchurch), 25 May 1989.
52 ABQZ, Box 18: YA 1/9/3 Part 1 Youth Affairs – Youth Issues – Unemployment, *New Zealand Herald*, 25 Oct 1988.
53 See for example, ABQZ, 1990–1993, *The Evening* Post, 28 April 1993; ABQZ, 1995–1996, *Manawatu Standard*, 30 October 1996.
54 ABKH, Women Supporting Women: Suicide Grief Counsellors Conference, File on Grant Application to Women's Suffrage Trust.
55 ABQZ, *The Press* (Christchurch), 24 May 1989.
56 ABQZ, *The Dominion* (Wellington), 25 May 1989.
57 ABQZ, *The Star* (Christchurch), 23 May 1989.
58 Ibid.
59 ABQZ, 29 November 1988.
60 ABVP, 1988/1205, Thomas Tender. See also ABQZ, *The Star* (Christchurch), 23 September 1988.
61 ABVP, 1988/1289, Marc Hitchcock.
62 ABQZ, *Auckland Star*, 23 September 1988.
63 ABVP, 1994/775; 1994/911.
64 ABVP, 1988/1289.
65 See for example, ABVP, 1988/1289; 1988/997.
66 ABVP, 1992/861.
67 ABVP, 1993/172.
68 ABVP, 1992/1242.
69 ABVP, 1993/128.
70 ABQZ, *The Dominion*, 23 September 1988.
71 ABQZ, *Dominion Sunday Times*, 25 September 1988.
72 ABVP, 1988/1289.
73 ABQZ, *New Zealand Herald*, 5 May 1992.
74 ABVP, 1998/226.
75 ABVP, 1999/338.
76 ABQZ, *Auckland Star*, 9 October 1988.
77 ABVP, 2000/765.
78 ABQZ, *Evening Standard*, 24 February 1989; Otago *Daily Times*, 13 May 1989.

79 Note the high quality of the reports in AATD W3294 6136, Royal Commission on Social Policy. Original Submissions, Box 61, Submission 5371, Mental Health Foundation of New Zealand.
80 ABQZ, *New Zealand Herald*, 15 July 1988.
81 ABQZ, *New Zealand Herald*, 3 March 1992.
82 *Report of the Suicide Prevention Review Group: Review of Suicide Prevention in Prisons* (Wellington: Department of Justice, 1995), 40–53. ABVP, 1991/267.
83 ABQZ, *New Zealand Herald*, 16 May 1992; *The Dominion*, 15 May 1992.
84 ABQU, vol. 3, Velma McClellan to Lindsay Morgan of the *Evening Post*, 14 May 1992.
85 ABQU, vol. 3, Kaye Saville Smith, Manager, Women and Younger People Health Policy to Velma McClellan, Policy Analyst, 20 May 1992.
86 ABQU, vol. 3, Kaye Saville Smith to Katherine O'Regan, 29 May 1992.
87 This lodge was the site of various government conferences on economic restructuring in the 1980s and 1990s. AAFH W5510 6790, Box 310, Social Impact Unit – Administration – Regional Managers Meeting. National Transition Managers Seminar [November 1987].
88 ABQU, vol. 3, Helena Barwick, "Introduction," *Youth Suicide Prevention Project Workshop Report and Literature Review* (unpublished and confidential report, November 1992), 4.
89 ABQU, vol. 3, Helena Barwick to Velma McClellan, 10 November 1992.
90 ABQZ, 1990–1993, *The Press* (Christchurch), 12 February 1993.
91 ABQU, vol. 3, Helena Barwick, "Introduction," *Youth Suicide Prevention Project Workshop Report and Literature Review* (unpublished and confidential report, November 1992), 56.
92 ABQZ, 1990–1993, *The Press* (Christchurch), 12 February 1993.
93 Ibid.
94 ABQZ, 1990–1993, *Otago Daily Times* 12 February 1993.
95 ABQZ, *The Press* (Christchurch), 15 February 1993.
96 ABQZ, *The Dominion*, 13 February 1993.
97 ABQZ, *The Evening Post,* 26 September 1988.
98 ABQZ, *The Dominion*, 28 April 1996. For Bulls see ABVP, 1997/345; 1997/388; 1997/599.
99 ABQZ, *The Dominion*, 30 September 1996.
100 ABQZ, *Greymouth Evening Star*, 23 March 1996.
101 ABQZ, *New Zealand Herald*, 27 August 1996.
102 ABQZ, *The Evening Post*, 26 August 1996.
103 See the discussion of under-counting of Māori deaths by cause in *New Zealand Official Yearbook 1947–9*, 86.

104 ABVP, Box 175, Coroners, LEG 12-5-9, Part 2. Coroners, Coroners Handbook. Memo on Publication of Suicide Details: Prepared by New Zealand Press Council, 2 Feb 1982, 1.

105 ABQZ, *The Press* (Christchurch), 15 February 1993.

106 ABQZ, *The Dominion Sunday Times*, 14 February 1993.

107 ABQZ, *The Dominion*, 16 July 1996.

108 ABVP, Box 175, Coroners, LEG 12-5-9, Part 2. Coroners Handbook. Memo on Publication of Suicide Details: Prepared by New Zealand Press Council, 2 Feb 1982, 1. Out of seven hundred complaints over nine years, only four concerned suicides.

109 ABQZ, *The Evening Post*, 13 February 1993.

110 ABQZ, *The Evening Post*, 13 February 1993.

111 ABQZ, *Greymouth Evening Star*, 23 March 1996.

112 ABVP, 1994/666.

113 ABVP, 1995/1181.

114 ABVP, 1996/440.

115 ABQZ, *Waikato Times*, 23 October 1996; *The Press* (Christchurch), 23 October 1996.

116 ABQZ, *The Press* (Christchurch) 21 October 1996.

117 ABQZ, *The Press* [Christchurch], 24 July 1996.

118 COM 12, 1, Royal Commission on Hospital and Related Services, Submission 30, Bay of Plenty Hospital Board [October 1972], 2; Submission 40, Psychology Department, Sunnyside Hospital [October 1972], 2. For a psychologist's views on professional tensions and the growth of psychology, see Taylor, *Cockney Kid*, 269–92.

119 Jim Anderton had written movingly and intelligently about his daughter's suicide, but could not get press attention for his party's mental-health-focused policy on youth suicide. ABQZ, Letter to the Editor, *Evening Post*, 2 November 1996.

120 ABQZ, Summary of Report Written by A.J.W. Taylor, Victoria University, and M.D. Cummings, Chief Superintendent, New Zealand Police [1987]. For the report itself see *A National Cohort of Suicides* (Auckland: Mental Health Foundation of New Zealand, 1985).

CHAPTER SEVEN

1 ABQU W4452 632, Box 248, Child Health – Adolescent Health – Youth Suicide, volume 3, Barwick, "Introduction," 4.

2 ABQZ W5328 16363, Box 17, Youth Affairs – Youth Issues – Mental Health, *The Dominion*, 2 November 1988.

3 ABVP, 2000/1096.
4 Lesage et al., "Suicide and Mental Disorders," 1065.
5 ABVP, 2000/793.
6 ABVP, 2000/964.
7 ABVP, 1998/844.
8 ABVP, 2000/1228.
9 ABVP, 1994/177.
10 For examples from earlier decades, see J46, 1912/667; 1912/1239; 1924/271; 1936/83.
11 Joiner, *Why People Die By Suicide*, 111.
12 A.L. Beautrais, "Child and Young Adolescent Suicide," 651–2. Beautrais used inquest files for the 1990s. She had sixty-one cases. For the same even-numbered years that we used, she had thirty-three cases. We had thirty-one. For the year of death, we used the year in which death occurred, but starting in 1985 deaths were officially reported by the year in which the inquest was held. In many cases that was one or two years after death on account of delays in holding inquests. See *New Zealand Official Yearbook*, 1985, 146. Beautrais may have used files according to the date of registration. Our findings are consistent with hers, but we supplement data with qualitative information.
13 J46, 1910/898.
14 J46, 1912/295.
15 J46, 1946/1323.
16 For an instance of theft and parental discipline see J46, 1973/180.
17 J46, 1976/769.
18 ABVP, 1980/347.
19 ABVP, 1997/54.
20 ABVP, 2000/347.
21 ABVP, 1991/64.
22 ABVP, 1998/245.
23 ABVP, 1984/1359.
24 ABVP, 1999/902.
25 ABVP, 2000/923.
26 ABVP, 1997/251.
27 ABVP, 1990/474.
28 ABVP, 1988/997.
29 ABVP, 1988/1289.
30 ABVP, 1996/1239.
31 ABVP, 1988/1330.
32 Trovato, "A Durkheimian Analysis," 425.

33 J46, 1936/83.
34 ABVP, 1976/518.
35 ABVP, [Number omitted for anonymity]. Also see the case of a fifteen-year-old juvenile delinquent: ABVP, 2000/57.
36 Massey, *New Zealand*, 7, 108–9, 113.
37 Dalley, "The Golden Weather," 321. Tom Brooking labels the period from 1951 to 1967 "the last good years." Brooking, *The History of New Zealand*, 137.
38 Massey, *New Zealand*, 8–9, 13–15.
39 AAFH W4160, Box 27, Social Impact Unit – Rural Package. Re-establishment of Farming Families [May 1986].
40 AAFH W5510 6790, Box 310, Social Impact Unit – Administration – Regional Managers Meeting. National Transition Managers Seminar [November 1987].
41 All data for the suicide graphs come from the data set and Census and Statistics Department, *Monthly Abstract of Statistics* (1972 to 1989); *Key Statistics* (1989 to 1997). AAFH W5510 6790, Box 312, Social Impact Unit – State Owned Enterprises – Forestry Corporation. Surplus NZ Forestry Service Wage Workers [February 1987].
42 Social Impact Unit, *Regional Social Impact Review: East Cape* (Mimeographed, March 1987), section 1.1; Social Impact Unit, *Regional Social Impact Review: Rotorua* (Mimeographed, March 1987), 56; Social Impact Unit, *Regional Social Impact Review: South Auckland* (Mimeographed, March 1987), 38–40.
43 AAFH W5510 6790, Box 314, Social Impact Unit – Social Issues – Social Impact Advice to Government. Short Guide to the Job Creation and Training Programmes Administered by the Department of Labour [November 1981].
44 There was a brief commodity price boom in the early 1970s. Dalziel and Lattimore, *The New Zealand Macroeconomy*, 14–15.
45 AANK, Box 606, Ministry of Labour, Employment Division – Client Files – National Youth Council, Jim Brown, President, National Youth Council, to J.B. [Jim] Bolger, 16 April 1982.
46 AANK, Box 606, Ministry of Labour, Employment Division – Client Files – National Youth Council, *Out of Work* (Wellington: National Youth Council, 1981). The government's annoyance is documented in the file. See J.B. Bolger, Minister of Labour, to National Secretary, National Youth Council, 23 December 1981.
47 "All Blacks in the Red," *Economist*, 25 May 1996, 80; Martin Wolf, "Lessons from the Antipodes," *Financial Times*, 12 March 1996, 20. For a

collection of economic data from 1960 to 1995, see Dalziel and Lattimore, *The New Zealand Macroeconomy*, 115–26.

48 Easton, *The Commercialisation of New Zealand*. He used the expression "blitzkrieg" on page 243. Dalziel and Lattimore provide a defense in *The New Zealand Macroeconomy*. They concede that recovery was long and unemployment levels shocking. See page x.

49 For a chronology, see Massey, *New Zealand*, 205–16.

50 ABQZ, Box 18, Youth Affairs – Youth Issues – Unemployment, *Otago Daily Times*, 15 September 1988; *The Dominion*, 7 September 1988; *The Evening Post,* 14 and 24 November 1988; *The Dominion,* 6 December 1989. Chapple, Harris, and Silverstone, "Unemployment," 156. On the policy of full employment, labour assignment practices, and regional unemployment see AATD W3294 6198, Box 10. Royal Commission on Social Policy. Drafts of Papers. Deborah Mabbett, "Restructuring, Full Employment and Regional Policy" [September 1987], 1–21. On the social services full-employment practices of government departments see AAFH W4160, Box 24, Social Impact Unit – State Owned Enterprises – Social Costs. Clipping from *Sunday Star*, 21 September 1986.

51 AAQB W5108 7842, Box 170, Background Papers – Corporatisation. Memo on Impact of Restructuring on Ministry of Works and Development [May 1987]. AAFH W5510 6790, Box 401, State Owned Enterprises – Targeted Organisations: Post-Office – Mason Morris Report. AAFH W5510 6790, Box 401, State Owned Enterprises – Targeted Organisations: Post-Office – Mason Morris Report.

52 AAFH W5510 6790, Box 314, Social Impact Unit – Regional Representatives – Huntly and Waikato. Role of SIU in Waikato [June 1988].

53 AAFH W5510 6790, Box 312, Social Impact Unit – State Owned Enterprises – Forestry Corporation. Forestry Corporatisation: Northland [Report, February 1987].

54 Civil servants aware of local employment needs appealed for continuing or alternate funding. AAFH W5510 6790, Box 310, Social Impact Unit – Administration – Regional Managers Meeting. Notes from Discussion on Work Development and Community Development Funding Schemes [March 1988]. Recognizing that the government had a responsibility as an employer to assist redundant workers who would not relocate, Cabinet in October 1986 approved a "contingency fund" to provide seed money to explore or initiate new businesses. AATJ W3566 7428, Box 101, Regional Development – Contingency Fund Committees. Memo on Uses of Contingency Fund, 28 November 1986.

55 Easton, "Income Distribution," 130, 169; AATD W3294 6136, Royal Commission on Social Policy. Original Submissions, Box 5, Submission 362, Submission of the Umbrella Group of Auckland Unemployed and Beneficiaries [1986].
56 ABQU, *Youth Suicide Prevention Project: Workshop Report and Literature Review* (Unpublished), 22.
57 Stephens, "Social Services," 459.
58 Weaver and Munro, "Country Living," 933–61.
59 AAFH W4160, Box 27, Social Impact Unit – Rural Package. Re-establishment of Farming Families [May 1986]. ABHR W3847, Box 8, Correspondence – Government Departments – State Services Commission – Social Impact of Corporatisation – Unit. Memo on Establishment of Social Impact Unit, 26 September 1986.
60 ABQZ, Box 17, Youth Affairs – Youth Issues – Mental Health, quoted in *Bay of Plenty Times*, 22 Oct 1988. For a comparable assessment based on submissions to the Royal Commission on Social Policy see AATD W3294 6198, Box 10. Royal Commission on Social Policy. Drafts of Papers. "Work: An Overview Paper" [March 1988], 12–21.
61 ABQZ, Box 18, Youth Affairs – Youth Issues – Unemployment, *New Zealand Herald Weekend Magazine*, 22 October 1988.
62 ABQZ, Box 18, Youth Affairs – Youth Issues – Unemployment, *The Evening Post*, 24 November 1988. The three-hundred-member organization representing guidance counsellors felt that employment was essential to self-esteem and socializaion. AATD W3294 6136, Royal Commission on Social Policy. Original Submissions, Box 57, Submission 5148, New Zealand Counselling and Guidance Association.
63 ABVP, 1996/460.
64 ABQU, Child Health – Adolescent Health – Youth Suicide, volume 3, Barwick, "Introduction," 4.
65 J1 W2304 82, Record Number 18/12, Part 1. Legislation – Miscellaneous – Divorce and Matrimonial Act – General. Report on the increase in divorces [May 1970].
66 ABVR W5063 7763, Box 10, Courts, CRTS 2-6-4, Part 1. Activities, Family Courts, Counselling, Anger Management. Maxwell, *Changing Family Structures*, 10–14; Maxwell, *Marriage and Divorce Trends*, 3–4.
67 ABVP, 1990/603.
68 ABVP, 1994/953.
69 ABVP, 2000/1009. The medical report for the inquest went back to 1992.
70 On girlfriends see ABVP, 2000/1012.

71 ABVP, 1992/1242.
72 ABVP, 1994/1057.
73 ABVP, 1997/330. The young girl's diary was filled with entries on her relationship with her mother. Also see the extended report on a youth's troubled life after her father left. ABVP, 1997/388. Evidence of parental disinterest is common in the files from 1980 to 2000. ABVP, 2000/949; 2000/950; 2000/1027.
74 ABVP, 1996/1251.
75 ABVP, 1990/1150; 1991/80.
76 ABVP, 2000/1060.
77 ABVP, 2000/110.
78 ABVP, 1986/1550; 1987/168; 1987/175; 1987/1126; 1988/268; 1988/405; 1988/589; 1988/590; 1988/616; 1990/470; 1990/730; 1990/737; 1990/865; 1991/402.
79 ABVP, 1988/1208.
80 ABVP, 1988/104; 2000/909.
81 ABVP, 1988/384; 1988/745; 1991/467; 1994/209; 2000/893.
82 ABVP, 1985/470.
83 ABVP, 1991/554.
84 ABVP, 1982/205, 1988/384, 1990/730, 1990/1105, 1991/554, 1992/432, 1994/144, 1994/209, 1994/536, 1996/1010, 1996/383; 2000/986.
85 J46, 1976/1193; ABVP, 1998/1075.
86 J46, 1976/1278; ABVP, 1990/801; ABQZ, Box 7, Health – Young Women's Health – Liking Your Body. For a well-documented case, see ABVP, 1998/848.
87 ABVP, 1991/48.
88 ABVP, 2000/948.
89 ABVP, 2000/1111.
90 ABVP, 1990/865.
91 ABVP, 2000/1021.
92 ABVP, 1994/1058.
93 ABVP, 1997/330.
94 ABVP, 1988/276.
95 ABVP, 1997/209.
96 That was the opinion of church organizations in Northland. See AATD W3294 6136, Royal Commission on Social Policy. Original Submissions, Box 19, Submission 732, Northland Churches Submission. There were conflicting research findings on sexual abuse among Māori children. ABJZ W4644 7019, Box 21, Policy and Research – Welfare – Family Violence,

1989–1990. Clipping, *New Zealand Herald*, 5 October 1989. Also see the report *The Cultural Facilitators of Family Violence: A Maori Perspective.*

97 For an example of a prisoner mentioning how the time he had on his hands led to critical self-reflection, see ABVP, 1999/127.

98 ABVP, 1990/405.

99 ABVP, 1990/1135.

100 ABVP, 1991/140.

101 ABVP, 1987/168.

102 ABVP, 1986/1550.

103 ABVP, 1990/1201.

104 *Report of the Suicide Prevention Review Group: Review of Suicide Prevention in Prisons* (Wellington: Department of Justice, 1995), 43–9, 66–8.

105 ABVP, 1989/174.

106 ABVP, 1985/48.

107 ABVP, 1980/1138.

108 ABVP, 1986/1109.

109 ABVP, 2000/1247.

110 ABVP, 1990/924.

111 ABVP, 1990/405.

112 ABVP, 1980/945.

113 ABQU, *Youth Suicide Prevention Project: Workshop Report and Literature Review* (unpublished), 22.

114 For an introduction to psychiatrists' efforts to define the essence of depression or, alternately, to subdivide it and define the categories, see Edward Shorter, *A Historical Dictionary of Psychiatry* (Oxford, UK: Oxford University Press, 2005), 78–89.

115 ABVP, 1990/1083.

116 ABVP, 2000/229.

117 ABVP, 1980/1480; 1986/1495; 1986/1495; 1987/100; 1988/115; 1996/483.

118 ABVP, 1994/211.

119 ABQZ W5328 16364, Box 6, Health – Substance Abuse. "Perspectives for Change: Conference on Alcohol, Tobacco, and Drugs" [Keynote Address, 1991], 4. On drug abuse prevention initiatives see in the same file John Hannifan, "Drug Education in New Zealand: There Must be a Better Way" [Paper Prepared for National Drug Educators' Workshop, 1989], 1–15.

120 ABVP, 2000/968. On the debate over legalization, see the correspondence in ABVP W5682 7407, Box 584, Policy and Research – Offending – Substance Abuse and Related Offending – Cannabis Offences.

121 J46, 1976/683. A concern that cannabis was erroneously accepted as harmless was expressed in a series of newspaper reports in 1991. ABQZ 6802, Box 4, Substance Abuse. *New Zealand Herald*, 17 October 1991; *Sunday News*, 3 November 1991. A recently published study indicates that regular use of cannabis, defined as four times a week, can lead to memory loss and a lower IQ. The study was led by Madeline Meier of Duke University. See Madeline H. Meier, Avshalom Caspi, Antony Ambler, Hona Lee Harrington, Renate Houts, Richard S.E. Keefe, Kay McDonald, Aimee Ward, Richie Poulton, and Terrie E. Moffitt, "Persistent Cannabis Users Show Neuropsychological Decline from Childhood to Midlife," PNAS Plus (Proceedings of the National Academy of the Sciences of the United States of America, Social Sciences – Psychological and Cognitive Sciences) 2012; published ahead of print 27 August 2012.

122 ABVP, 1996/735; 1996/941; 1997/342; 1997/482; 1998/999; 2000/720; 2000/1106; 2000/1209; 2000/1211.

123 ABGX, Box 125, Health Committee, House of Representative – Inquiry into Mental Health Effects of Cannabis. Information Package [17 December 1998], 2.

124 For example, see cannabis references in 1996 youth suicides. ABVP, 1996/483; 1996/735; 1996/941; 1996/1096; 1996/1113; 1997/255; 1997/342; 1997/361; 1997/682. For a report on high consumption see ABQZ 6802, Box 4, Substance Abuse. Newspaper clipping files for 1991. *Dominion Sunday Times*, 1 September 1991.

125 ABVP, 1989/484.

126 ABVP, 1997/162.

127 ABVP, 1980/1033.

128 ABVP, 1998/831. Also see 1998/1110.

129 ABVP, 1987/94.

130 ABVP, 1984/1049.

131 ABVP, 2000/427.

132 ABVP, 1988/400; 1988/1005; 1988/1171.

133 ABVP, 1980/531.

134 ABQZ 6802, Box 4, Substance Abuse, Clipping Files, *The Dominion*, 31 August and 24 September 1990, 19 March 1991. For a well-documented case, see ABVP, 1998/909.

135 AAFB, Box 168, Narcotics – Methadone, Notes on Preventive and Social Medicine, J.S. Roxburgh, Nelson District Health Officer, 11 April 1972; clippings, *New Zealand Herald*, 30 November 1972 and 22 February 1973; W2788 632 Box 168, Narcotics – Methadone, Memo on Inquests, A.R. Matheson, Chief Inspector of Police, 2 November 1972; Memo

on Methadone Deaths, S.L. Pugmire, Medical Superintendent, Lake Alice Hospital, 2 November 1972; J46, 1972/1483; 1973/198; ABVP, 1980/1271.

136 ABVP, 1989/177.

137 J46, 1968/1460.

138 J46, 1973/48.

139 ABVP, 1997/335.

140 ABVP, 1996/964.

141 ABVP, 1996/987.

142 On poverty in the Lower Hutt Valley see AATD W3294 6136, Royal Commission on Social Policy. Original Submissions, Box 62, Submission 5373, "Hard Times: The Breadline Study: A Study on Poverty and Its Effects on the Physical, Mental, and Emotional/Spiritual Well-Being of Lower Hutt Valley Residents" [January 1988].

143 ABQZ W5328 16363, Box 8, Youth Affairs – Income – Benefit Reform. Appendix II, Statistical Profile of Client Groups, 6 [Early 1991]. See also Social Impact of Proposed Reforms on Youth, 2–3.

144 On mental depression after a romantic break up, see ABVP, 1990/546; 1990/823; 1991/140; 1991/338.

145 ABVP, 1994/1406.

146 ABQZ W5328 16363, Box 8, Youth Affairs – Income – Benefit Reform. Preliminary Analysis of Impact of Task Force Proposal for Youth Benefits [1990].

147 A government briefing paper on social assistance reform asked for discussion on the social impact of reducing benefits. Stress, encounters with the law, substance abuse, and suicide were mentioned. ABQZ W5328 16363, Box 8, Youth Affairs – Income – Benefit Reform. Briefing Paper for Liaison Section on Youth Benefit Changes [January 1992]; April Welfare Changes: An Update [August 1991], 4. Officials in the Ministry of Youth were concerned about the consequences of reductions of benefits and a removal of the unemployment entitlement for 16–17-year-olds. Briefing Paper for the Liaison Section on Youth Benefit Changes [December 1991].

148 ABVP, 1991/1444.

149 ABVP, 1991/132.

150 ABVP, 1994/636.

151 ABVP, 1990/743.

152 ABVP, 1994/81.

153 ABVP, 1996/392.

154 ABVP, 1996/446.

155 ABVP, 1994/636.

156 ABVP, 1981/209.
157 ABVP, 1986/1653.
158 ABVP, 1996/802.
159 ABVP, 1996/859.
160 J46, 1976/937.
161 There were also a few women. ABVP, 1992/1065.
162 ABVP, 1990/947.
163 ABVP, 1988/484.
164 ABVP, 1997/469.
165 ABVP, 1997/113.
166 ABVP, 1990/212.
167 ABVP, 1996/950.
168 ABVP, 1998/226.
169 ABVP, 1990/843.
170 ABVP, 1996/1251.
171 ABVP, 1998/1354.
172 ABVP, 1987/109; 1987/112; 1997/10; 1997/162.
173 ABVP, 1996/1128.
174 New Zealand Ministry of Health, *New Zealand Suicide Prevention Action Plan, 2008–2012: The Evidence for Action* (Wellington: Ministry of Health, 2008), 4, Figure 1.
175 ABVP, 2000/951.
176 ABVP, 2000/269.
177 ABVP, 2000/1025.

CHAPTER EIGHT

1 Douglas, *The Social Meanings of Suicide*, 339. This book is brilliant, difficult, and inspiring.
2 Douglas, *The Social Meanings of Suicide*, 340.
3 In *Myths about Suicide*, Joiner sets up false propositions to knock over; thus he attacks the "myth" that suicide is the result of impulsive action. This is true; however, his demolition work leaves the impression that impulse rarely if ever plays a role, when in some cases it does. He considers people who stress impulse as pernicious because they challenge the idea that suicide is tractable. *Myths about Suicide*, 84.
4 J46, 1922/1224.
5 J46, 1922/729.
6 Joiner, *Why People Die by Suicide*, 136.

7 This section follows the line of critical search for the boundary between science and pseudo-science pioneered by Karl Popper. He articulated his insights in many places, but for a brief account see Popper, *The Growth of Scientific Knowledge*. A more tendentious and acerbic commentary on the claims of the social sciences and psychology is found in Andreski, *Social Sciences as Sorcery*. Andreski thought that many social science propositions were "nebulous, untestable, pseudo-theoretical meanderings" (107).
8 Weaver, *A Sadly Troubled History*, 19–61.
9 Trovato, "The Relationship between Marital Dissolution and Suicide," 346–7.
10 Stack, "The Impact of Divorce on Suicide in Norway," 230.
11 Berman, Jobes, and Silverman, *Adolescent Suicide*, 29.
12 Meehl, "Theoretical Risks," 811.
13 So-called findings from the more honest of these studies are strewn with warnings about their shaky quality. See Johnson, Krug, and Potter, "Suicide among Adolescents," 80.
14 Berman et al., *Adolescent Suicide*, 42.
15 Ibid., 108.
16 Ibid., 160.
17 Ibid., 116–17.
18 J46, 1922/656.
19 J46, 1950/1280.
20 ABVP, 2000/1100.
21 J46, 1910/327.
22 J46, 1910/1083.
23 J46, 1930/877.
24 J46, 1930/1539.
25 J46, 1908/120.
26 J46, 1914/540.
27 J46, 1930/805.
28 J46, 1910/839; 1910/854.
29 J46, 1916/542; 1968/1650.
30 J46, 1916/58; 1922/61.
31 J46, 1914/1245.
32 J46, 1908/264; 1912/968; 1914/1215.
33 J46, 1902/176.
34 J46, 1908/121; 1916/31.
35 J46, 1900/565.
36 J46, 1906/221.

37 J46, 1908/882.
38 J46, 1968/1650; 1968/1386.
39 J46, 1912/721.
40 J46, 1914/66.
41 J46, 1914/879.
42 J46, 1900/933; 1924/1114.
43 J46, 1950/1296.
44 J46, 1925/20.
45 J46, 1906/169.
46 J46, 1930/542.
47 J46, 1910/59.
48 J46, 1926/157.
49 ABVP, 2000/525. The deceased put the barrel of the gun in her mouth. It is possible that as she made a threat to get attention during the argument, the gun went off accidentally.
50 J46, 1902/64.
51 J46, 1910/1076.
52 J46, 1930/1336.
53 J46, 1930/140.
54 J46, 1914/921.
55 J46, 1954/554.
56 J46, 1900/856; 1904/243; 1926/503; 1968/1375; ABVP, 1988/1226.
57 ABVP, 2000/1138.
58 J46, 1930/605.
59 J46, 1906/996.
60 J46, 1912/312.
61 J46, 1924/1218.
62 J46, 1908/154.
63 J46, 1912/396.
64 J46, 1950/59.
65 J46/1981/261.
66 J46, 1941/62.
67 J46, 1946/1364.
68 ABVP, 2000/1059.
69 ABVP, 1998/914.
70 ABVP, 1989/708.
71 J46, 1976/1706.
72 ABVP, 1976/913.
73 ABVP, 1997/242.
74 ABVP, 1989/283.

75 ABVP, 1989/309.
76 ABVP, 1988/1381.
77 ABVP, 1997/171.
78 ABVP, 1997/242.
79 ABVP, 1996/934.
80 Douglas, *The Social Meanings of Suicide*, 286–300.
81 J46, 1900/703.
82 J46, 1924/795.
83 J46, 1926/848.
84 J46, 1930/1026.
85 J46, 1931/7.
86 J46, 1942/1136.
87 J46, 1949/307.
88 J46, 1951/471.
89 J46, 1950/862.
90 J46, 1906/1062.
91 J46, 1964/749.
92 ABVP, 2000/221.
93 J46, 1940/265.
94 J46, 1960/923.
95 J46, 1951/232.
96 J46, 1976/276. TAB is the abbreviation for the Totalisator Agency Board. Created in 1950, it operates off-track betting shops.
97 ABVP, 1997/177.
98 ABVP, 1994/400.
99 ABVP, 2000/1228.
100 ABVP, 2000/940.
101 J46, 1976/238.
102 ABVP, 2000/1238.
103 ABVP, 1976/325.
104 ABVP, 1996/631.
105 J46, 1931/121.
106 J46, 1946/1364.
107 ABVP, 1997/599.
108 J46, 1950/914.
109 J46, 1972/1284.
110 J46, 1976/937.
111 J46, 1968/1453.
112 ABVP, 1992/1065.
113 ABVP, 1994/1189.

114 ABVP, 1994/985.
115 ABVP, 1996/684.
116 ABVP, 2000/1007. Matt may have suffered from schizophrenia, although there was no report on treatment in the file. However, he was living rough on the streets of Auckland. His mode of death, jumping from the Grafton Viaduct, was consistent with schizophrenia.
117 ABVP, 1994/1189.
118 Joiner, *Why People Die By Suicide*, 120.
119 J46, 1953/716.
120 J46, 1976/548.
121 ABVP, 1984/533.
122 ABVP, 1995/1294.
123 ABVP, 1985/425.
124 J46, 1926/124.
125 ABVP, 1995/840.
126 ABVP, 1986/640.
127 ABVP, 1996/559.
128 J46, 1914/702.
129 J46, 1940/1301.
130 ABVP, 1996/890.
131 J46, 1946/1364.
132 J46, 1924/344.
133 J46, 1968/1514.
134 J46, 1928/854.
135 ABVP, 1994/953.
136 J46, 1902/826.
137 J46, 1926/355.
138 J46, 1928/1051.
139 ABVP, 1985/103.
140 J46, 1951/697.
141 J46, 1968/1449.
142 ABVP, 1986/53.
143 J46, 1976/325.
144 The phenomenon had an international aspect. A study of teenagers in Seattle and Washington, DC with tattoos claimed that the youths were more likely to suffer from low self-esteem, delinquency, and drug abuse. ABQZ 6802, Box 4, Substance Abuse, Clipping Files, bundle for 1989 to 1991. *The Star* (Christchurch), 20 February 1991.
145 ABVP, 1980/1098; 1980/1271; 1990/605; 1990/613; 1992/771; 1992/98; 1992/1053; 1993/60; 1996/749.

146 ABVP, 1997/239.
147 ABVP, 1984/1292.
148 ABVP, 1984/1505.
149 ABVP, 1991/578.
150 ABVP, 1987/358.
151 ABVP, 1986/855.
152 ABVP, 1997/177.
153 ABVP, 1997/560.
154 ABVP, 1997/79.
155 ABVP, 1992/1352; 1993/1151a.
156 ABVP, 1990/1153.
157 ABVP, 1992/1072.
158 ABVP, 1993/3.
159 ABVP, 1996/1024.
160 ABVP, 2000/889.
161 ABVP, 2000/1110.
162 ABVP, 1994/282.
163 ABVP, 1997/380.
164 ABVP, 1990/666.
165 ABVP, 2000/850.
166 J46, 1908/498.
167 J46, 1914/1365.
168 J46, 1916/1141.
169 J46, 1906/260.
170 J46, 1942/704.
171 J46, 1920/1079.
172 J46, 1922/427.
173 J46, 1916/919.
174 J46, 1924/918.
175 ABVP, 2000/450; 2000/678.
176 See cases for 2000. ABVP, 2000/109; 2000/873; 2000/1111; 2000/1302.
177 J46, 1924/303.
178 Joiner, *Why People Die By Suicide*, 97.
179 J46, 1912/152.
180 J46, 1930/837.
181 J46, 1976/376.
182 J46, 1946/515.
183 J46, 1960/721.
184 ABVP, 2000/1024.
185 J46, 1960/920.

186 J46, 1969/147.
187 J46, 1976/1313.
188 J46, 1976/665; 1980/595; 1980/624.
189 J46, 1968/1531.
190 J46, 1972/256.
191 ABVP, 1982/440.
192 ABVP, 2000/1177.
193 J46, 1914/405.
194 J46, 1946/1314.
195 J46, 1912/1148.
196 J46, 1968/1389; 1969/498.
197 J46, 1916/823.
198 J46, 1914/966.
199 J46, 1926/457.
200 J46, 1950/1151.
201 ABVP, 1994/628.
202 ABVP, 1998/871.
203 J46, 1922/729.
204 J46, 1930/1529.
205 J46, 1918/72.
206 J46, 1943/206.
207 J46, 1911/75.
208 J46, 1930/154.
209 J46, 1954/355.
210 ABVP, 1997/114.
211 ABVP, 2000/904.
212 ABVP, 2000/581.
213 J46, 1904/119.
214 ABVP, 2000/886.
215 ABVP, 2000/1080.
216 ABVP, 2000/1160.
217 ABVP, 2000/939.
218 J46, 1930/1464.
219 J46, 1924/323.
220 J46, 1964/682.
221 J46, 1900/262; 1904/520; 1910/325; 1912/384; 1916/1410; 1922/195.
222 J46, 1900/62; 1924/1012.
223 J46, 1924/74.
224 J46, 1924/191.
225 Popper, *Conjectures and Refutations*, 37.

CONCLUSION

1 Philip Crowley, Jean Kilroe, and Sara Burke in conjunction with the Health Development Agency on behalf of the UK and Ireland Public Health Evidence Group, *Youth Suicide Prevention: Evidence Briefing* (Health Development Agency, 2004), 45.
2 Berman et al., *Adolescent Suicide*, 211–21.
3 ABVP, 2000/1240.
4 ABVP, 2000/756.
5 ABVP, 2000/925.
6 Ibid., 84.
7 Crowley et al., *Youth Suicide Prevention*, 40–5.
8 Ibid., 34–5.
9 J46, 1950/34.
10 ABVP, 2000/1178.
11 Conner et al., "Violence, Alcohol, and Completed Suicide," 1704; Lawlor, *From Melancholia to Prozac*, 195.

Bibliography

1. GOVERNMENT RECORDS: ARCHIVES NEW ZEALAND, TE RUA MAHARA O TE KĀWANATANGA

The Wellington repository of Archives New Zealand offers a cornucopia for social historians. Due to the digital revolution, researchers can more readily than ever discover files on a topical basis. "Archway," the search mechanism for all collections held in Wellington, Auckland, Christchurch, and Dunedin, facilitated research immeasurably. Knowledgeable archivists have written helpful descriptions of the records and the government branches that created them. While much has been done to assist research, the official citations for records accessioned in recent decades offer no clues as to the department that originated them.

Citations for earlier records are more readily understood. Files or boxes often bear original government labels. Archivists added record group and series designations to these original references. For example, the Army Department was designated AD, Justice J, Health H, Internal Affairs AI, and Land Department L. Within these record groups, archivists next established particular series. Coroners' inquests from 1900 to 1974 were designated as Series 46 of the Justice Department record group; they were cited simply as J46. Within J46, each file was numbered sequentially as it arrived at the Justice Department during the course of a year. For example, J46, 1928/315 identified the 315th inquest file received in Wellington during 1928. To cite another example, AD Series 1, 49/301, refers to a sub-series 49 in the Army Department records and 301 to a subject file; the archives retained the army file numbering system. In this case the file was labeled Mental Patients, Memorandum, The Federation of New Zealand Patriotic War Relief Societies. For older collections, these original archives designations are retained in this bibliography and endnotes. These older designations can still be used to access records through "Archway."

Bland archival citations were introduced for records accessioned around 1990 and later. They have no relationship to the title of the government unit that created them. For example, coroners' inquests covering 1978 to 1988 were designated as ABVP W5450 17298; the file numbers still incorporate the order of arrival and the year, as in the case of 1992/1235. For the sake of brevity, an endnote citing that file will read ABVP, 1992/1235. Many record groups accessed for this book were transferred from government agencies to the archives after the adoption of this system. To show why certain files were consulted, this bibliography provides short descriptions copied from the original cover sheets of the government files. For example, the citation 'AAFB W4914 632, Box 123, Supplies – Drugs – Chlorpromazine' establishes that this Health Department file contains material on the early psychotropic drug chlorpromazine.

The remarkable scope of government involvement in the lives of New Zealanders has created immense paper legacies awaiting social history inquiry. So far, professional archivists as well as some civil servants have supported openness, although access varies by department, record type, and year. There are balances to be struck between the desirability of investigation and the right to privacy. During our research on post-1960 files, we were aware of intermittent discussions between archivists and government records managers over the period of time that some records should normally remain closed. Reasonableness and trust prevailed when we sought access to closed items. Where restrictions applied, privacy officers in government departments usually responded favourably to requests for access. Senior personnel at Coronial Services commendably supported the principle that all inquest records ought to be available to *bona fide* researchers, because the files were prepared for public proceedings partly with an objective to amend practices and save lives. We honoured privacy by adopting fictitious names for individuals, although strictly speaking this measure of privacy was not required. Case citations, however, are not disguised. The conventions of scholarship require that other investigators must be able to follow our steps. We cannot forecast if they will enjoy the level of accommodation accorded to us. We hope that our findings will justify the support we have had from the advocates of openness. Perhaps recognition of the value of inquests will lead to the discovery of similar materials in other jurisdictions and to their being opened to researchers.

Diverse files created in assorted departments contributed to our descriptions of mental health care, social welfare, substance abuse, and economic crises. They added to the narratives and arguments in chapters five, six, and seven. Several government departments maintained files of newspaper clippings as well as research papers on suicide or topics associated with motives for suicide.

For a description of the contents of the inquest case files that constitute the core resource for this book, see Appendix One which explains research methodology.

Army Department

AD 1, 40/301, Mental Patients, Nominal Rolls of Military Patients at Mental Hospitals, 1921.

AD 1, 49/301/1, Mental Health Patients, New Zealand Expeditionary Force, General File.

AD 1, 49/284/3, Neurasthenia Cases, Minute Sheet for Minister of Defence, 22 November 1918.

AD 1, 49/922, Training of Medical Officers in Psychotherapy.

AD 1, 49/921, Neurasthenia, HQ (Medical), Canterbury Medical District, Memorandum.

AD 1, 49/791, Alcoholism among Returned Soldiers.

AD 1, 64/30, Mental Cases in New Zealand Expeditionary Force.

AD 78, 12/12/2, Lists of Deceased Soldiers Including Suicides, Featherston Camp, New Zealand, 1916–1922.

AD 78, 15/28, Patients in Mental Hospitals.

Commissions of Inquiry and Royal Commissions

AATD W3294 6136, Various Boxes, Royal Commission on Social Policy. Original Submissions.

AATD W3294 6192, Box 1, Royal Commission on Social Policy: Research Papers Included in Submissions Database: Family Violence DSW [Department of Social Welfare].

AATD W3294 6198, Box 10, Royal Commission on Social Policy. Drafts of Papers.

COM 12, Royal Commission on Hospital and Related Services, 1972–1974. Various Submissions.

Department of Agriculture

ARNZ W5657 22499, Box 15, National Efficiency Board, File 679, Thomas Moss, Wellington District Commissioner, Report on Farms in Taranaki.

Department of Health

AADB W3463 632, Box 46 – Poison Prescription – Barbiturates.

AAFB W2788 632, Box 58, Tuberculosis Act.

AAFB W2788 632, Box 73, Poisons – Substances – Nicotine.

AAFB W2788 632, Box 168, Narcotics – Methadone.

AAFB W3463/49 632, Mental Health, Review of Committals at Sunnyside, 1970–2.

AAFB W4914 632, Box 35, Private Psychiatric Hospitals – "Piki-te-ora," Wellington.

AAFB W4914 632, Box 123, Supplies – Drugs – Chlorpromazine.

AAFB W4452 2788, Box 118, Hospitals – Private Hospitals – "Selwyn."

ABGX W5189 16127, Box 147, TR 4/1/1/9, Transport Committee – Catalytic Converters.

ABQU W4452 632, Box 2, Accidents – Statistics on Accidental Drowning, 1948 to 1971.

ABQU W4452 632, Box 82, Hospitals – Private Hospitals – "Selwyn."

ABQU W4452 632, Box 248, Parts 1–3, Child Health – Adolescent Health – Youth Suicide.

ABQU W4452 632, Box 275, National Health Statistics – National Health Statistics Centre – Drowning, 1983 to 1991.

ABQU W4452 632, Box 936, Poisons – Substances – Nicotine.

ABQU W4452 632, Box 943, Poisons – Substances – Carbon Monoxide, 1926–1987.

ABQU W4452 632, Box 1353, Social Security – Hospital Benefits – Ashburn Hall.

ABQZ W5328 16363, Box 17, Youth Affairs – Youth Issues – Health – Sex and Sexuality.

ABQZ W5328 16363, Box 17, Youth Affairs – Youth Issues – Mental Health.

ABQZ W5328 16363, Box 17, Youth Issues – Health – Solvent Abuse.

ABQZ W5328 16363, Box 7, Health – Young Women's Health – Liking Your Body.

ADHS W5502 18913, Box 1, Store – Electro Convulsive Therapy Machines.

Department of Internal Affairs

AAAC W5333 7536, Box 45, Youth Affairs – Policy – Joint Papers.

IA1, Department of Internal Affairs, Patriotic Funds – Rehabilitation – Psychosis Cases – Treatment, 1942–43.

Department of Justice and Courts

AAAP W3038 17298, Boxes 1 to 50, Coroners Inquest Case Files, 1975 to 1978.

AAAP W3475 17298, Boxes 1 to 22, Coroners Inquest Case Files, 1978.

AAAR W3605 500, Box 18, Allowances – Miscellaneous – Visiting Committees to Inebriates Institutions, 1933 to 1969.

AAQB W3950 889, Box 648, Prisons, Inebriates Home, Rotoroa Island, 1945–1979.

ABVP W5450 17298, Boxes 1 to 305, Coroners Inquest Case Files, 1978 to 1988.

ABVP W5521 17298, Boxes 1 to 419, Coroners Inquest Case Files, 1988 to 2000.

ABVP W5682 7407, Box 584, Policy and Research – Offending – Substance Abuse and Related Offending – Cannabis Offences.

ABVP W5682 7410, Box 174, Legal, Interpretations, Rulings, Opinions, Coroners, LEG 12-3-1, Evidence and Verdict, Documents Produced during Inquest: Re: Picard, 13/7/83.

ABVP W5682 7410, Box 175, Coroners, LEG 12-5-9, Part 2. Coroners' Handbook.

ABVR W5063 7763, Box 10, Courts, CRTS 2-6-4, Part 1. Activities, Family Courts, Counselling, Anger Management.

J Series 1 (J1) W2304 82, Record Number 18/12, Part 1. Legislation – Miscellaneous – Divorce and Matrimonial Act – General.

J Series 8 (J8) 1/13, Reformatory Institutions, Inebriates Homes, Rotoroa Island, Advisory Board Minutes, 1957–1967.

J Series 46 (J46), Coroners Inquest Case Files, 1900 to 1974. Microfilm reels U5426 to U5591.

JU Series 9 (JU9), Circular Memos to Magistrates, Boxes 5 to 8, 1901 to 1940.

Department of Labour

AANK W3574 947, Box 96, Social Research, Unemployment Survey – Study of Unemployed Youth in Christchurch, March 1979.

AANK W3574 947, Box 606, Employment Division – Client Files – National Youth Council.

AANK W4397, Box 369, Unemployment Benefit Return from Social Welfare, 1986.

Department of Social Welfare

AAYE W5048 7433, Box 127, B&P 6-6-1, Part 1. Benefits and Pensions – Invalids Benefit – Reform – Liaison Committee.

AAYE W5048 7433, Box 127, B&P 6-6-1, Part 2. Benefits and Pensions – Invalids Benefit Correspondence.

Department of Public Works

AAQB W5108 7842, Box 170, Background Papers – Corporatisation [Restructuring the Ministry of Works and Development].

Department of Youth Affairs

ABQZ 6802, Box 4, Substance Abuse, Clipping Files, 1989 to 1991; 1995 to 1996.

ABQZ W5328 16363, Box 8, Youth Affairs – Income – Benefit Reform.

ABQZ W5328 16363, Box 17, Parts 1–3, Youth Affairs – Youth Issues – Youth Suicide, Clipping Files, 1988–1996.

ABQZ W5328 16363, Box 17, Youth Affairs – Youth Issues – Mental Health.

ABQZ W5328 16363, Box 18, Youth Affairs – Youth Issues – Unemployment.

ABQZ W5328 16364, Box 6, Health – Substance Abuse.

Lands Department

LS Series 36, Records of the Lands Department, Series 36, File on Discharged Soldier Settlement Account, Report for the Year Ended 30th June 1935.

Lottery Commission

AAAC W4946 6015, Box 60, Application for Lottery Funds, J.S. Werry, Biochemical Correlates of Schizophrenia.

AAAC W4946 6015, Box 86, Application for Lottery Funds – Schizophrenia Fellowship of New Zealand Inc., Christchurch, Undated statement from the fellowship [1978].

Māori Affairs

ABJZ W4644 7019, Box 21, Policy and Research – Welfare – Family Violence, 1989–1990.

Military Service Records

AABK W5539 180805, Various Boxes, Assorted Service Files.

Ministry of Economic Development

AATJ W3566 7428, Box 101, Regional Development – Contingency Fund Committees, 1986–7.

Office of the Postmaster-General

AAFH W5510 6790, Box 401, State Owned Enterprises – Targeted Organisations: Post-Office –Mason Morris Report.

Parliament

ABGX W5188 16127, Box 75, Social Services Committee – Correspondence: Report of the Controller and Auditor General on Community Care for People with Mental Illness [1993].

ABGX W5188 16127, Box 125, Health Committee, House of Representatives – Inquiry into Mental Health Effects of Cannabis [1998].

Prime Minister's Department

AAFD W2347 811, Box 40, CAB 79/3/12, Social Welfare Home for Inebriates, 1952 to 1954.

AAFD W2347 811, Box 99, Health – Mental Hospitals, 1950–1957.

AAFD W3738 811, Box 911, CAB 79/3/12, Social Affairs – Hostels – Homes for Inebriates, 1958.

State Services Commission, Social Impact Unit

AAFH W4160, Box 24, Social Impact Unit – State Owned Enterprises – Social Costs.

AAFH W4160, Box 27, Social Impact Unit – Rural Package.
AAFH W5510, Box 305, Social Impact – Contingencies and Minutes.
AAFH W5510 6790, Box 310, Social Impact Unit – Administration – Regional Managers Meeting.
AAFH W5510 6790, Box 312, Social Impact Unit – State Owned Enterprises – Forestry Corporation.
AAFH W5510 6790, Box 314, Social Impact Unit – Regional Representatives – Huntly and Waikato.
AAFH W5510 6790, Box 314, Social Impact Unit – Social Issues – Social Impact Advice to Government.
AAFH W5510 6790, Box 316, Social Impact Unit – Regional Representatives – Wellington.
ABHR W3847, Box 8, Correspondence – Government Departments – State Services Commission – Social Impact of Corporatisation – Unit.

Social Security [Welfare] Department

AAYE W5048 7433, Boxes 226 and 227, Organisation and Departments – Drug and Alcohol Rehabilitation Centres – Alcohol Substance Abuse Programme – New Funding Assistance.
SS W2363 30, 34/11/6, Research on Social Problems – New Zealand Population – Survey on Alcoholism.

War Service Statistics

SS7 W2756, Box 17, Accounts, Miscellaneous Publicity and Returns – Returned Servicemen - Miscellaneous Statistics, Annual Returns on Pensions, 1936–56.

Other Government Bodies

ABKH W4788, Women Supporting Women: Suicide Grief Counsellors Conference, File on Grant Application to Women's Suffrage Trust.

2. GOVERNMENT RECORDS NOT IN NATIONAL ARCHIVES

Death Certificates (for missing ages), Registrar General, Internal Affairs, Wellington.
Records of the Coroners' Court, Wellington, New Zealand, Assorted Case Files, 2004–2010.

3. MANUSCRIPT COLLECTIONS: ALEXANDER TURNBULL LIBRARY, NATIONAL LIBRARY OF NEW ZEALAND

Diary of Peter Carter Lovell-Smith, MSX-5461.

4. GOVERNMENT PUBLICATIONS

Alcohol Liquor Advisory Council, *Directory of Addiction Services in New Zealand* (Wellington, various editions 1982 to 1986).

Committee of Inquiry into Procedures Used in Certain Psychiatric Hospitals, *Report of the Committee of Inquiry into Procedures Used in Certain Psychiatric Hospitals in Relation to Admission, Discharge or Release on Leave of Certain Classes of Patients* (August 1988).

Department of Health, Mental Health Division, *Annual Reports: Appendix to the Journals of the House of Representatives* (various titles), 1900 to 1960.

Department of Health, *Medical Statistics Report: Part II – Mental Health Data* (various years).

Monthly Abstract of Statistics (1950 to 1987). In 1988, the name changed to *Key Statistics* (1988–2000).

New Zealand Official Yearbook (1900 to 2005).

Research staff, Parliamentary Library, *Voluntary Euthanasia and New Zealand* (Wellington: Background Note, 2003).

Social Impact Unit, *Regional Social Impact Review: East Cape* (Mimeographed, March 1987).

Social Impact Unit, *Regional Social Impact Review: Rotorua* (Mimeographed, March 1987).

Social Impact Unit, *Regional Social Impact Review: South Auckland* (Mimeographed, March 1987).

Social Impact Unit, *Regional Social Impact Review: Southland* (Mimeographed, March 1987).

Suicide Prevention Review Group, *Report of the Suicide Prevention Review Group: Review of Suicide Prevention in Prisons* (Wellington: Department of Justice, 1995).

5. BOOKS AND ARTICLES: NEW ZEALAND GENERAL HISTORY AND NEW ZEALAND MEDICAL HISTORY

Abbott, Max, "Overview of the Symposium," in *Mental Health Foundation of New Zealand – New Zealand Z Psychological Society*

Symposium on Unemployment: Papers and Reports, edited by Max Abbott (Auckland: Mental Health Foundation of New Zealand, 1982).

Belich, James, *Paradise Reforged: A History of New Zealanders from the 1880s to the Year 2000* (Honolulu: University of Hawai'i Press, 2001).

Brooking, Tom, *The History of New Zealand* (Westport, CT: Greenwood Press, 2004).

– "Economic Transformations," in *The Oxford History of New Zealand*, edited by W.H. Oliver and B.R. Williams (Wellington: Oxford University Press, 1981).

Brunton, Warwick, "Out of the Shadows: Some Historical Underpinnings of Mental Health Policy," in *Past Judgment: Social Policy in New Zealand History*, edited by B. Dalley and M. Tennant (Dunedin: University of Otago Press, 2004).

– "The Origins of Deinstitutionalisation in New Zealand," *Health and History* 5 (2003).

– "'To imitate, if not to rival, in their arrangement, the asylums of the home country': The Scottish Influence on New Zealand Psychiatry before World War II," paper presented at the Annual Conference of the New Zealand Historical Association, 27–30 November 2003.

– "Mental Health: The Case of Deinstitutionalization," in *Health and Public Policy in New Zealand*, edited by P. Davis and T. Ashton (Auckland: Oxford University Press, 2001).

Dalley, Bronwyn, "The Golden Weather, 1949–1965," in *Frontier of Dreams: The Story of New Zealand*, edited by Bronwyn Dalley and Gavin McLean (Auckland: Hodder Moa, 2005).

Dalziel, Paul, and Ralph Lattimore, *The New Zealand Macroeconomy: A Briefing on the Reforms* (Melbourne: Oxford University Press, 1991).

Easton, Brian, *The Commercialisation of New Zealand* (Auckland: Auckland University Press, 1997).

– "Income Distribution," in *A Study of Economic Reform: The Case of New Zealand*, edited by Brian Silverstone, Alan Bollard, and Ralph Lattimore (Amsterdam: Elsevier, 1996).

– *An Introduction to the New Zealand Economy* (St Lucia: University of Queensland Press, 1982).

– ed., *The Making of Rogernomics* (Auckland: Auckland University Press, 1989).

Fennell, Susan, "Psychiatry in New Zealand, 1912–1948," in *'Unfortunate Folk': Essays on Mental Health Treatment, 1863–1992*, edited by Barbara Brookes and Jane Thomson (Dunedin: University of Otago Press, 2001).

Gould, John, *The Rake's Progress: The New Zealand Economy since 1945* (Auckland: Hodder and Stoughton, 1982).
Gustafson, Barry, *Kiwi Keith: A Biography of Keith Holyoake* (Auckland: Auckland University Press, 2007).
Hensley, Gerald, *Beyond the Battlefield: New Zealand and Its Allies, 1939–45* (Auckland: Penguin/Viking Press, 2009).
Kavanagh, Jeff, "Cherry Farm, 1952–1992: Social and Economic Forces in the Evolution of Mental Health Care in New Zealand," in Brookes and Thomson, *'Unfortunate Folk': Essays on Mental Health Treatment, 1863–1992* (Dunedin: University of Otago Press, 2001).
Lange, Raeburn, *May the People Live: A History of Maori Health Development, 1900–1920* (Auckland: University of Auckland Press, 1999).
Macdonald, Barrie, and David Thomson, "Mortgage Relief, Farm Finance, and Rural Depression in New Zealand in the 1930s," *New Zealand Journal of History* 21, no. 2 (1987).
McAloon, Jim, *No Idle Rich: The Wealthy in Canterbury and Otago, 1840–1914* (Dunedin: University of Otago Press, 2002).
Massey, Patrick, *New Zealand: Market Liberalization in a Developed Economy* (London: St Martin's Press, 1995).
Philpott, H.G., *A History of the New Zealand Dairy Industry* (Wellington: Government Printer, 1937).
Williams, Wendy Hunter, *Out of Sight Out of Mind: The Story of Porirua Hospital* (Wellington: Porirua Hospital, 1987).

6. BOOKS AND ARTICLES ON NEW ZEALAND: POPULATION AND SUICIDE STUDIES

Antonidis, Nicholas, *Suicide Risk and Prevention: A Study of Coroners' Files (1981)* (Wellington: Health Services Research and Development Unit, 1988).
Beautrais, A.L, "Child and Young Adolescent Suicide in New Zealand," *Australian and New Zealand Journal of Psychiatry* 35 (2001).
– "Risk Factors for Suicide and Attempted Suicide among Young People," *Australian and New Zealand Journal of Psychiatry* 34 (2000).
– "Cannabis Abuse and Serious Suicide Attempts," *Addiction* 94 (1999).
– "Unemployment and Serious Suicide Attempts," *Psychological Medicine* 28 (1998).
Beautrais, A.L., S.C.D. Collings, P. Ehrhardt, et al., *Suicide Prevention: A Review of Evidence of Risk and Protective Factors, and Points of Effective Intervention* (Wellington: Department of Health, 2005).

Crampton, Peter, Clare Salmond, and Russell Kirkpatrick, *Degrees of Deprivation in New Zealand: An Atlas of Socioeconomic Difference*, 2nd edition (Auckland: David Bateman, 2000).

New Zealand, *Suicide Trends in New Zealand, 1974–94* (Department of Health, 1997).

Pool, Ian, Arunachalam Dharmalingam, and Janet Sceats, *The New Zealand Family from 1840: A Demographic History* (Auckland: University of Auckland Press, 2007).

Soper, Margaret, *Coroners* (Wellington: Butterworths, 1996).

Taylor, A.J.W. (Tony), *Cockney Kid: The Making of an Unconventional Psychologist* (Paekakariki: Silver Owl Press, 2009).

Taylor, A.J.W. (Tony), Victoria University, and M.D. Cummings, *Cohort of Suicides* (Auckland: Mental Health Foundation of New Zealand, 1985).

7. BOOKS AND ARTICLES ON SUICIDE, MENTAL ILLNESS, MEDICINE, AND SCIENCE: HISTORICAL AND CONTEMPORARY

Anderson, J. Maxwell, *Discovering Suicide: Studies in the Social Organization of Sudden Death* (London: Macmillan, 1978).

Anderson, Olive, *Suicide in Victorian and Edwardian England* (Oxford, UK: Clarendon Press, 1987).

Andreski, Stanislav, *Social Sciences as Sorcery* (New York: St Martin's Press, 1972).

Andriessen, Karl, "On 'Intention' in the Definition of Suicide," *Suicide and Life-Threatening Behavior* 36 (October 2006).

Ashton, Heather, "Delirium and Hallucinations," in *Neurochemistry of Consciousness: Neurotransmitters in Mind,* edited by Elaine Perry, Heather Ashton, and Allan Young (Amsterdam/Philadelphia: John Benjamins Publishing Co., 2002).

Bailey, Victor, *"This Rash Act": Suicide across the Life Cycle in the Victorian City* (Stanford, CA: Stanford University Press, 1998).

Barber, James G., "Relative Misery in Youth Suicide," *Australian and New Zealand Journal of Psychiatry* 35 (2000).

Barham, Peter, *Forgotten Lunatics of the Great War* (New Haven, CT: Yale University Press, 2004).

Barry, John M., *The Great Influenza: The Story of the Deadliest Pandemic in History*, revised edition (New York: Penguin, 2009).

Belshaw, H., D.O. Williams, and F.B. Stephens, "Farming Industries during the World Crisis," in *Agricultural Organization in New Zealand*, edited by H. Belshaw et al. (Melbourne: Melbourne University Press in association with Oxford University Press, 1936).

Bennewith, Olive, et al., "The Usefulness of Coroners' Data on Suicides for Providing Information Relevant to Prevention," *Suicide and Life-Threatening Behavior* 35 (December 2005).

Berman, Alan L., David A. Jobes, and Morton M. Silverman, *Adolescent Suicide: Assessment and Intervention* (Washington, DC: American Psychological Association, 2006).

Brådvik, Louise, and Mats Berglund, "A Suicide Peak after Weekends and Holidays in Patients with Alcohol Dependence," *Suicide and Life-Threatening Behavior* 33 (Summer 2003).

Brown, Edward, "Post-Traumatic Stress Disorder and Shell Shock – Social Section," in *A History of Clinical Psychiatry: The Origin and History of Psychiatric Disorders*, edited by German Berrios and Roy Porter (London: The Athlone Press, 1995).

Brown, Phil, *The Transfer of Care: Psychiatric Deinstitutionalization and Its Aftermath* (London: Routledge and Kegan Paul, 1985).

Brugha, Traolac, and Dermot Walsh, "Suicide Past and Present – The Temporal Constancy of Under-Reporting," *British Journal of Psychiatry* 132 (1978).

Campbell, E.J. Moran, *Not Always on the Level* (Cambridge: British Medical Journal, 1988).

Canetto, Silvia, "Gender Roles, Suicide Attempts, and Substance Abuse," *The Journal of Psychology* 125 (1992).

Canetto, Silvia, and Isaac Sakinofsky, "The Gender Paradox in Suicide," *Suicide and Life Threatening Behavior* 28 (1998).

Cantor, C., P. McTaggart, and D. De Leo, "Misclassification of Suicide: The Contribution of Opiates," *Psychopathology* 34 (2001).

Castel, Robert, Françoise Castel, and Anne Lovell, *La société psychiatrique avancée* (Paris: Grasset, 1979).

Cohen, Neil, ed., *Psychiatry Takes to the Streets: Outreach and Crisis Intervention for the Mentally Ill* (New York: The Guilford Press, 1990).

Conner, Kenneth R., C. Cox, P.R. Duberstein, L.L. Tian, P.A. Nisbet, and Y. Conwell, "Violence, Alcohol, and Completed Suicide: A Case-Control Study," *American Journal of Psychiatry* 158 (October 2001).

Cooke, Simon, *Secret Sorrows: A Social History of Suicide in Victoria, 1841–1921* (PhD thesis: The University of Melbourne, 1998).

– "Terminal Old Age: Ageing and Suicide in Victoria, 1841–1921," *Australian Cultural History* 14 (1995).

Cooter, Roger, "Neuropatients in Historyland," in *The Neurological Patient in History*, edited by L. Stephen Jacyna and Stephen T. Casper (Rochester, NY: University of Rochester Press, 2012).

Crawford, M.J., and M. Prince, "Increasing Rates of Suicide in Young Men in England during the 1980s: The Importance of the Social Context," *Social Science and Medicine* 49 (1999).

Crowley, Philip, Jean Kilroe, and Sara Burke in conjunction with the Health Development Agency on behalf of the UK and Ireland Public Health Evidence Group, *Youth Suicide Prevention: Evidence Briefing* (Health Development Agency, 2004).

Cutright, Phillip, and Robert Fernquist, "Firearms and Suicide: The American Experience, 1926–1996," *Death Studies* 24 (2000).

Dawes, Robyn M., *House of Cards: Psychology and Psychotherapy Built on Myth* (New York: The Free Press, 1994).

De Leo, Diego, "Century of Suicide in Italy: A Comparison between the Young and the Old," *Suicide and Life-Threatening Behavior* 27 (Fall 1997).

Deikstra, R.F.W., and W. Gulbinat, "The Epidemiology of Suicidal Behaviour: A Review of Three Continents," *World Health Statistics Quarterly* 46 (1993).

Delgado, Pedro, "Common Pathways of Depression and Pain," *The Journal of Clinical Psychiatry* 65 (2004).

Deleuze, Gilles, and Félix Guattari, *Anti-Oedipus: Capitalism and Schizophrenia*, translated by Robert Hurley, Mark Seem, and Helen R. Lane (New York: Penguin Books, 2009).

DeLisi, Lynne E., ed., *Depression in Schizophrenia* (Washington, DC: American Psychiatric Press, 1990).

Denning, Diane, Yeates Conwell, Deborah King, and Chris Cox, "Method Choice, Intent, and Gender in Completed Suicide, *Suicide and Life-Threatening Behavior* 30 (2000).

Dineen, Tana, *Manufacturing Victims: What the Psychology Industry Is Doing to People* (Montreal: Studio 9/Robert Davies, 1996).

Douglas, Jack D., *The Social Meanings of Suicide* (Princeton, NJ: Princeton University Press, 1967).

Dowbiggin, Ian, *The Quest for Mental Health: A Tale of Science, Medicine, Scandal, Sorrow, and Mass Society* (Cambridge: Cambridge University Press, 2011).

– *A Concise History of Euthanasia: Life, Death, God, and Medicine* (Lanham, MD: Rowman and Littlefield, 2005).

Durkheim, Émile, *Suicide*, translated by John A. Spaulding and George Simpson (Glencoe, IL: The Free Press, 1951).

Dwyer, Ellen, "Neurological Patients as Experimental Subjects: Epilepsy Studies in the United States," in *The Neurological Patient in History*, edited by L. Stephen Jacyna and Stephen T. Casper (Rochester, NY: University of Rochester Press, 2012).

Firth, Christopher, and Eve Johnstone, *Schizophrenia: A Very Short Introduction* (Oxford, UK: Oxford University Press, 2003).

Gay, Peter, *Freud: A Life for Our Time* (New York: W.W. Norton, 1988).

Gibbs, Jack P., and Walter T. Martin, *Status Integration and Suicide: A Sociological Study* (Eugene, OR: University of Oregon Books, 1964).

Gove, Walter R, "Sex, Marital Status, and Mortality," *American Journal of Sociology* 79.

Grob, Gerald N., *From Asylum to Community: Mental Health Policy in Modern America* (Princeton, NJ: Princeton University Press, 1991).

Halbwachs, Maurice, *The Causes of Suicide*, translated by Harold Goldblatt (London: Routledge & Kegan Paul, 1978).

Hamer, Dean, and Peter Copeland, *Living with Our Genes: Why They Matter More than You Think* (New York: Doubleday, 1998).

Hassan, Riaz, *Suicide Explained: The Australian Experience* (Melbourne: University of Melbourne Press, 1995).

Hassan, Riaz, *A Way of Dying: Suicide in Singapore* (Kuala Lumpur, Malaysia: Oxford University Press, 1983).

Healey, David, *The Creation of Psychopharmacology* (Cambridge, MA: Harvard University Press, 2002).

Hirshbein, Laura, *American Melancholy: Constructions of Depression in the Twentieth Century* (New Brunswick, NJ: Rutgers University Press, 2009).

Jackson, Stanley W., *Melancholia and Depression from Hippocratic Times to Modern Times* (New Haven, CT: Yale University Press, 1986).

Johnson, Ann Braden, *Out of Bedlam: The Truth about Deinstitutionalization* (New York: Basic Books, 1990).

Johnson, G.R., E.G. Krug, and L.B. Potter, "Suicide among Adolescents and Young Adults: A Cross-National Comparison of 34 Countries," *Suicide and Life-Threatening Behavior* 30, no. 1 (Spring 2000).

Joiner, Thomas, *Myths about Suicide* (Cambridge, MA: Harvard University Press, 2010).

– *Why People Die by Suicide* (Cambridge, MA: Harvard University Press, 2005).

Kitanaka, Junko, *Depression in Japan: Psychiatric Cures for a Society in Distress* (Princeton, NJ: Princeton University Press, 2012).

Kramer, Peter D., *Against Depression* (New York: Penguin Books, 2005).

Kushner, Howard, "Taking Biology Seriously: The Next Task for Historians of Addiction?" *Bulletin of the History of Medicine* 80 (Spring 2006).

– *Self-Destruction in the Promised Land* (New Brunswick, NJ: Rutgers University Press, 1989).

Lal, Brij V., "Veil of Dishonour: Sexual Jealousy and Suicide on Fiji Plantations," *Journal of Pacific History* 20, no. 3 (1985).

Roger Lane, *Violent Death in the City: Suicide, Accident, and Murder in Nineteenth-Century Philadelphia* (Cambridge, MA: Harvard University Press, 1979).

Lawlor, Clark, *From Melancholia to Prozac: A History of Depression* (Oxford, UK: Oxford University Press, 2012).

Leenaars, Antoon, David Lester, and B. Yang, "The Effects of Domestic and Economic Stress on Suicide Rates in Canada and the United States," *Journal of Clinical Psychology* 49 (1993).

Leenaars, Antoon, et al., "Suicide Notes of Adolescents: A Life-Span Comparison," *Canadian Journal of Behavioural Science* 33 (2001).

Leenaars, Antoon, and Susanne Wenckstern, "Sylvia Plath: A Protocol Analysis of Her Last Poems," *Death Studies* 22 (1998).

Lesage, Alain, et al., "Suicide and Mental Disorders: A Case-Control Study of Young Men," *American Journal of Psychiatry* 151 (July 1994).

Lester, D., "The Sex Distribution of Suicides by Age in the Nations of the World," *Social Psychiatry and Psychiatric Epidemiology* 25 (1990).

– "Benefits of Marriage for Reducing Risk of Violent Death from Suicide and Homicide for White and Non-White Persons: Generalizing Gove's Finding," *Psychological Reports* 61 (1987).

Leys, R., *Trauma: A Genealogy* (Chicago: University of Chicago Press, 2000).

Lukes, Steven, *Emile Durkheim: His Life and Work: A Historical and Critical Study* (New York: Harper & Row, 1972).

Mac Donald, Michael, and Terence R. Murphy, *Sleepless Souls: Suicide in Early Modern England* (Oxford, UK: Clarendon Press, 1990).

Maris, Ronald E., "The Adolescent Suicide Problem," *Suicide and Life-Threatening Behavior* 15 (Summer 1985).

– *Pathways to Suicide: A Study of Self-Destructive Behaviors* (Baltimore, MD: The Johns Hopkins University Press, 1981).

Meehl, Paul, "Theoretical Risks and Tabular Asterisks: Sir Karl, Sir Ronald, and the Slow Progress of Soft Psychology," *Journal of Consulting and Clinical Psychology* 46 (1978).

Merskey, Harold, "After Shell Shock: Aspects of Hysteria since 1922," in *150 Years of British Psychiatry: Vol. II: The Aftermath*, edited by Hugh Freeman and German Berrios (London: The Athlone Press, 1996).
– "Post-Traumatic Stress Disorder and Shell Shock – Clinical Section," in *A History of Clinical Psychiatry: The Origin and History of Psychiatric Disorders*, edited by German Berrios and Roy Porter (London: The Athlone Press, 1995).
Micale, M., and P. Lerner, ed., *Traumatic Pasts: History, Psychiatry, and Trauma in the Modern Age, 1870–1930*, (Cambridge: Cambridge University Press, 2001).
Minois, Georges, *History of Suicide: Voluntary Death in Western Culture*, translated by Lydia A. Cochrane (Baltimore, MD: The Johns Hopkins University Press, 1999).
Moran, James E., *Committed to the State Asylum: Insanity and Society in Nineteenth-Century Quebec and Ontario* (Montreal and Kingston: McGill-Queen's University Press, 2000)
Morrissey, Susan K., *Suicide and the Body Politic in Imperial Russia* (Cambridge: Cambridge University Press, 2006).
Norstrom, Thor, "The Impact of Alcohol, Divorce, and Unemployment on Suicide: A Multilevel Analysis," *Social Forces* 74 (September 1995).
Osler, William, *The Principles and Practices of Medicine* (New York: Appleton, 1912).
Paterson, Dale A., *A Mad People's History of Madness* (Pittsburgh, PA: University of Pittsburgh Press, 1982).
Popper, Karl R., *The Growth of Scientific Knowledge* (Frankfurt am Main: Vittorio Klostermann, 1963).
– *Conjectures and Refutations: The Growth of Scientific Knowledge* (London: Routledge and Kegan Paul, 1963).
Porter, Roy, *A Social History of Madness: Stories of the Insane* (London: Weidenfeld and Nicolson, 1987).
– "The Patient's View: Doing Medical History from Below," *Theory and Society* 14 (1985).
Porter, Roy, and Mark S. Micale, "Introduction: Reflections on Psychiatry and Its Histories," in *Discovering the History of Psychiatry*, edited by Micale and Porter (New York: Oxford University Press, 1994).
Rawling, Bill, "Providing the Gift of Life: Canadian Medical Practitioners and the Treatment of Shock on the Battlefield," *Canadian Military History* 10 (2001).
Reaume, Geoffrey, *Remembrance of Patients Past: Patient Life for the Insane, 1870–1940* (Don Mills, ON: Oxford University Press, 2000).

Richards, Jonathan, and John Weaver, "'I may as well die as go to the gallows': Murder-Suicide in Queensland, 1890–1940," in *Histories of Suicide: International Perspectives on Self-Destruction in the Modern World*, edited by John Weaver and David Wright (Toronto: University of Toronto Press, 2009)

Roper, Michael, *The Secret Battle: Emotional Survival in the Great War* (Manchester, UK: Manchester University Press, 2009).

Roy, Alec, and Markku Linnoila, "Alcoholism and Suicide," in *Biology of Suicide*, edited by Ronald Maris (New York: Guilford Press, 1986).

Sainsbury, Peter, *Suicide in London: An Ecological Study* (London: The Institute of Psychiatry, 1955).

Shneidman, Edwin S., "The Psychological Pain Assessment Scale," *Suicide and Life-Threatening Behavior* 29 (Winter 1999).

– "The Commonalities of Suicide across the Life Span," in *Life Span Perspectives of Suicide*, edited by Antoon Leenaars (New York: Plenum Press, 1991).

– *Definition of Suicide* (New York: John Wiley & Sons, 1985).

Shorter, Edward, *A Historical Dictionary of Psychiatry* (Oxford, UK: Oxford University Press, 2005).

– *A History of Psychiatry: From the Era of the Asylum to the Age of Prozac* (New York: John Wiley & Sons, 1997).

Shorter, Edward, and David Healy, *Shock Therapy: A History of Electroconvulsive Treatment in Mental Illness* (Toronto: University of Toronto Press, 2007).

Sparr, Pamela, ed., *Mortgaging Women's Lives: Feminist Critiques of Structural Adjustment* (London: Zed Books, 1994).

Stack, Stephen, "The Effect of Divorce on Suicide in Denmark," *Sociological Quarterly* 31 (1989).

– "The Impact of Divorce on Suicide in Norway, 1951–1980," *Journal of Marriage and the Family* 51 (February 1989).

– "The Effects of Marital Dissolution on Suicide," *Journal of Marriage and the Family* 42 (February 1980).

Stearns, Peter, *Be a Man: Males in Modern Society* (New York: Holmes and Meier, 1990).

Stone, Martin, "Shell Shock and the Psychologists," in *The Anatomy of Madness: Essays in the History of Psychiatry, Vol II: Institutions and Society*, edited by W.F. Bynum, Roy Porter, and Micheal Shepherd (London: Tavistock, 1985).

Stephens, R., "Social Services," in *A Study of Economic Reform: The Case of New Zealand*, edited by B. Silverstone, R. Lattimore, and A. Bollard (Amsterdam: North-Holland, 1996).

Swazey, Judith, *Chlorpromazine in Psychiatry: A Study of Therapeutic Innovation* (Cambridge, MA: MIT Press, 1974).
Szasz, Thomas S., *The Therapeutic State: Psychiatry in the Mirror of Current Events* (Buffalo, NY: Prometheus Books, 1984).
– *The Manufacture of Madness* (London: Paladin, 1972).
– *The Myth of Mental Illness* (London: Granada, 1972).
– *Law, Liberty, and Psychiatry* (New York: Macmillan, 1963).
Tatz, Colin, "Aboriginal, Maori and Inuit Youth Suicide: Avenues to Alleviation," *Australian Aboriginal Studies* 2 (2004): 15–25.
Trovato, Frank, "A Durkheimian Analysis of Youth Suicide: Canada, 1971 and 1981," *Suicide and Life-Threatening Behavior* 22 (Winter 1992).
– "The Relationship between Marital Dissolution and Suicide: The Canadian Case," *Journal of Family and Marriage* 48 (1986).
Warsh, Cheryl Krasnick, *Moments of Unreason: The Practice of Canadian Psychiatry and the Homewood Retreat, 1883–1923* (Montreal and Kingston: McGill-Queen's University Press, 1989).
Wasserman, Ira, "The Effects of War and Alcohol Consumption on Patterns of Suicide: United States, 1910–1933," *Social Forces* 68, no. 2 (December 1989).
Weaver, John, with Douglas Munro, "Country Living, Country Dying: Suicide Inquests and Rural Hardship in New Zealand, 1900–1950," *Journal of Social History* (June 2009): 73–96.
Weaver, John, *A Sadly Troubled History: The Meanings of Suicide in the Modern Age* (Montreal: McGill-Queen's University Press, 2009).
Whitaker, Robert, *Mad in America: Bad Science, Bad Medicine, and the Enduring Mistreatment of the Mentally Ill* (New York: Basic Books, 2002).
Yang Lester, Bijou, "Learning from Durkheim and Beyond: The Economy and Suicide," *Suicide and Life-Threatening Behavior* 31 (Spring 2001).
Young, T. Kue, *The Health of Native Americans: Toward a Biocultural Epidemiology* (New York: Oxford University Press, 1994).
Zarkowski, Paul, and David Avery, "Hotel Room Suicide," *Suicide and Life-Threatening Behavior* 36 (October 2006).

Index

* *f* indicates an illustration, *g* indicates a graph, *t* indicates a table